Nursing Practice in the United States and North America

Nursing Practice in the UK and North America

Eugene Levine
Senior Advisor
Levine Associates
Maryland
USA
and
Adjunct Professor
School of Nursing
Georgetown University
Washington DC
USA

Peggy Leatt
Professor
Department of Health Administration
University of Toronto
Canada

and

Karin Poulton
Nursing Officer
Department of Health
London
UK

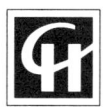

CHAPMAN & HALL
London · Glasgow · New York · Tokyo · Melbourne · Madras

Published by Chapman & Hall, 2–6 Boundary Row, London SE1 8HN

Chapman & Hall, 2–6 Boundary Row, London SE1 8HN, UK

Blackie Academic & Professional, Wester Cleddens Road, Bishopbriggs, Glasgow G64 2NZ, UK

Chapman & Hall Inc., 29 West 35th Street, New York NY10001, USA

Chapman & Hall Japan, Thomson Publishing Japan, Hirakawacho Nemoto Building, 6F, 1–7–11 Hirakawa-cho, Chiyoda-ku, Tokyo 102, Japan

Chapman & Hall Australia, Thomas Nelson Australia, 102 Dodds Street, South Melbourne, Victoria 3205, Australia

Chapman & Hall India, R. Seshadri, 32 Second Main Road, CIT East, Madras 600 035, India

Distributed in the USA and Canada by Singular Publishing Group Inc., 4284 41st Street, San Diego, California 92105

First edition 1993

© 1993 Chapman & Hall

Typeset in 10/12 pt Palatino by MFK Typesetting Ltd, Austin House, Bridge Street, Hitchin, Herts SG5 2DE

Printed in Great Britain by T. J. Press (Padstow) Ltd, Padstow, Cornwall

ISBN 0 412 33490 9, 1 56593 024 X (USA)

Apart from any fair dealing for the purposes of research or private study, or criticism or review, as permitted under the UK Copyright Designs and Patents Act, 1988, this publication may not be reproduced, stored, or transmitted, in any form or by any means, without the prior permission in writing of the publishers, or in the case of reprographic reproduction only in accordance with the terms of the licences issued by the Copyright Licensing Agency in the UK, or in accordance with the terms of licences issued by the appropriate Reproduction Rights Organization outside the UK. Enquiries concerning reproduction outside the terms stated here should be sent to the publishers at the London address printed on this page.

The publisher makes no representation, express or implied, with regard to the accuracy of the information contained in this book and cannot accept any legal responsibility or liability for any errors or omissions that may be made.

A catalogue record for this book is available from the British Library

Library of Congress Cataloging-in-Publication available

∞ Printed on permanent acid-free text paper, manufactured in accordance with the proposed ANSI/NISO Z 39.48–199X and ANSI Z 39.48–1984

Contents

Preface	vii
Biographies	ix

Part One Conceptual Background

1	Introduction	3
2	Comparative health systems	18

Part Two The United Kingdom

3	Historical evolution of the health care and nursing systems	39
4	Nursing education	56
5	The practice of nursing	72
6	The nurse at work	91
7	Nursing research	99
8	Planning for nursing	109

Part Three Canada

9	Historical evolution of the health care and nursing systems	117
10	Nursing education	129
11	The practice of nursing	146
12	The nurse at work	158
13	Nursing research	177
14	Planning for nursing	190

Part Four The United States

15	Historical evolution of the health care and nursing systems	207
16	Nursing education	225
17	The practice of nursing	237
18	The nurse at work	247
19	Nursing research	263
20	Planning for nursing	273

Part Five Conclusions

21	Conclusions	289

Index	319

The Process Archives
College of ...
Library

Accession Number: 44860

Class Number: 11A

Preface

The idea for this book originated from an article written by one of the authors (EL) entitled 'Nursing in the UK and the USA' (Levine, 1983a). It was suggested to the author by a (then) Senior Editor of the publisher, Mr Tim Hardwick, that the article be expanded into a book with, perhaps, other countries included. So began what has turned out to be a difficult undertaking.

The book has been in preparation for seven years. The length of time required to complete the book has required thoroughgoing revisions to bring materials up to date as well as to attempt to achieve some consistency of terminology, style and presentation. It was not possible to update the data to the present day because there are generally several years between the times when data are collected and when they are presented. We believe that the data contained in the book are as timely as is possible to make them. For example, in the US section, the 1988 Sample Survey of RNs was published in 1990 and the next sample, possibly in 1992, will not be published until 1994.

We believe this book is especially timely because there is considerable interest at present in comparative health systems. The US, in particular, in the face of escalating health costs and rising dissatisfaction with health care among Americans, is seeking remedies that involve an overhaul of the health system. There is keen interest in Canada's system of national health insurance, which many consider more cost-effective than the mixed, some say mixed-up, system in the US that is characterized by unevenness of distribution and access to health care. The fact that over 30 million people in the US are without any health insurance is cited as a major flaw in the system.

Also, in the area of nursing, there have been major changes recently occurring in the three countries cited. First in the US, then in Canada and now in the UK, fundamental changes are occurring in the way nurses are being educated. The trend is a movement away from apprenticeship-type training – more or less on the job – to academic preparation within the mainstream of higher education. The impact of this on the educational system for nursing, on quality of care and on the status of nursing is highlighted by the information presented.

We believe that this book is unique in several ways. It presents comparative material on various aspects of nursing in the three countries in a way that has not been done before. Moreover, it presents this material within the context of the existing health systems of the countries. Finally it has presented trends in important areas that will make it possible to project future directions in nursing education and nursing research.

We believe that 'Nursing Practice in the UK and North America' should be of interest to a wide audience, including nurse administrators, planners, educators and researchers. Students of nursing should find it useful in obtaining a quick survey of the salient features of a country's system of nursing.

In addition to the three major authors others have contributed to the production of this book. Chapter 4 was written by John M. Rogers, and Chapters 11 and 12 were written by Louise Lemieux-Charles. The chapter on nursing research in Canada was written by Marianne Lamb, Shirley M. Stinson and Marie-France Thibaudeau. Mrs Barbara Stevenson Levine worked mightily to edit the book, to attempt to achieve some degree of uniformity in word usage and layout and to enter the entire manuscript into a word processor.

The authors are grateful to the publishers, Chapman & Hall, and to their editors Rosemary Morris and Tinuke Khalidson, who patiently awaited the completion of this book over the long period of time. We hope the effort has resulted in a text that will be useful to a wide audience.

E.L.
P.L.
K.P.

Biographies

Eugene Levine PhD, MPA, BBA for nearly 30 years headed the statistical programme for the US federal government's Public Health Service, Division of Nursing. During that time he conducted many studies on various aspects of nursing manpower. With Dr Faye Abdellah he co-authored the landmark book on nursing research, 'Better Patient Care Through Nursing Research', originally published in 1965. He currently directs a project for the US federal government's Indian Health Service on health care provided by outreach personnel to Native Americans. Dr Levine is the author of Chapters 1, 2 and 15–21.

Peggy Leatt PhD, MHSA, BScN, RN, SRN is Professor and Chair of the Department of Health Administration, University of Toronto, Canada. She has conducted numerous research projects focusing on managerial and administrative issues concerning nurses and physicians. She has published extensively in the area of applying organizational theory and behaviour to the understanding of health services organizations. De Leatt is the author of Chapters 9, 10 and 13.

Karin Poulton PhD is currently Nursing Officer Department of Health, London, England. She has responsibility for nursing practice standards of care and nursing audit. Dr Poulton is the author of Chapters 3, 5, 7 and 8.

Authors of Chapter 13

Marianne Lamb RN, MN, who is currently a doctoral candidate in community health at the University of Toronto, has experience in nursing practice, teaching, research and administration. As former Director of Professional Services with the Canadian Nurses Association she worked closely with many national associations, provincial territorial associations and national committees, including the CNA nursing research committee. Her research interests include nursing ethics, nursing history, alternative health care delivery systems and health policy. She is a member of the National Council on Bioethics in Human Research.

Shirley M. Stinson RN, EdD, LLD is a generalist with experience in nursing practice, research, administration and teaching. She is Professor in the Faculty of Nursing and in the Faculty of Medicine, Department of Health Services Administration and Community Medicine, University of Alberta, and Adjunct Professor, Faculty of Nursing, University of Calgary. Author of over 70 publications and reports she is utilized widely as a consultant, nationally and internationally. Dr Stinson is a Past President of the Canadian Nurses Association, a member of several national and provincial committees, and former Chairman of the Alberta Foundation for Nursing Research.

Marie-France Thibaudeau RN, MScN is Professor and Dean of the Faculté des sciences infirmières at the Université de Montréal; has an extensive background in nursing practice, research, education and administration, and has taught graduate level research courses for some seven years. She is well known for her demonstration and evaluative research projects conducted in community health centres, focused on the primary health care of families, particularly children, and including the care of patients suffering from chronic mental illness; for her work on committees of the National Health Research Development Program, including its Advisory Committee; and as a reviewer for several research funding bodies.

Louise Lemieux-Charles PhD, MScN, BScN, RN is Assistant Professor in the Department of Health Administration and Programme Director, Hospital Management Research Unit, University of Toronto, Canada. Her research interests include impact of new organizational models in health service organizations and human resource management issues. Dr Lemieux-Charles is the author of Chapters 11 and 12.

John M. Rogers is a civil servant in the National Health Service Management Executive of the English Department of Health. Currently concerned with London's health services and the proposed radical shift from acute to primary care, he was previously Director of Personnel for the Trent Regional Health Authority. Before that he dealt with education and training issues at national level, including Project 2000, reorganizing the statutory nursing bodies and implications of the NHS reforms for education. John M. Rogers is the author of Chapter 4.

Part One

Conceptual Background

1
Introduction

The purpose of this book is to analyse and compare the nursing systems of three countries – the United Kingdom, Canada and the United States – within the context of their existing health systems. This comparison should provide insights into the present nursing systems of these countries and contribute to better understanding and closer cooperation among nursing personnel. Also the comparison may reveal how developments in one country could be beneficially applied to another. Lack of such information in the past may have prevented the dissemination of innovative programmes and techniques from one national setting to another.

However the major endeavour will be to analyse the impact of a nation's health system on its nursing system. One motivating question for this book is: does the way in which a nation's health system is organized, managed, regulated and financed make a difference to nursing recruitment, education, management and practice? The obvious answer is yes of course it does, and this book will attempt to show how and why this is so for each individual country, and why similarities and differences between nations may be important to nursing in general.

The UK, Canada and the US have strikingly different health systems. The UK has a governmentally owned and operated national health service. Canada's system, governmentally operated, provides compulsory, universal health insurance without the direct governmental control over health care providers and settings found in the UK. Finally the US has what can only be characterized as a 'mixed' system, containing within its vast and complex structure aspects of a nationalized health service for selected beneficiaries, such as veterans and Indians, national health insurance for the elderly (Medicare), a governmentally funded programme for indigents (Medicaid) administered by the states, and a multitude of voluntary health insurance programmes for other segments of the population, but with a substantial number of the population, over 30 million people, without any health insurance coverage. There are also a large number of government and private agencies offering a wide variety of health care and nursing services.

SIMILARITIES BETWEEN COUNTRIES

Despite marked differences in the health systems of the three countries, there is much in common, one reason being that the two New World countries are basically products of English law, custom and culture, although Canada also has a significant and valued French heritage.

A common background

The early history of the UK was one of numerous invasions by Saxons, Danes, Jutes and Vikings, with continuous pushing of these tribes against each other, jostling for territory and supremacy. Southern Britain was secured for Rome in the first century AD, with the governmentally sophisticated Romans staying long enough to exert a 'civilizing' effect on the native tribes. The Norman invasion of 1066 was followed by centuries of cultural adjustment and melding of Norman and Saxon until, during the strong reigns of the Tudors, the crown gained ascendency over the nobility as a distinctly English character and consciousness emerged. Succeeding centuries brought a continued development of language, literature and social customs relatively free of foreign influence, which was made possible by an isolated island situation.

From this background, in the seventeenth and eighteenth centuries, eventually came those people – the restless and adventurous, the dissenters and the dispossessed – who crossed oceans to conquer unknown lands. The accomplishment of this feat, albeit at the expense of native populations that vainly resisted encroachment, seemed to produce a type of person with the characteristic now called 'rugged individualism': independent, questioning, cantankerous and not given to 'backing down', a not entirely mythological idea held by Americans about themselves.

Language

The newcomers brought with them the common language, literature and folklore as well as the intellectual ideas and philosophies that engender a commonality of thought process and outlook. Notwithstanding the importance of French history, language and culture to Canada, the major language for all the countries is English, and language is a potent force in the communication and assimilation of ideas, customs and practices. This commonality of background aids the tendency towards philosophical and practical similarities in the delivery of health and nursing care.

The origin of modern nursing

Present day nursing education and practice in the three countries evolved from the work of Florence Nightingale. While nursing, in its particulars, has naturally moved considerably beyond Miss Nightingale's original ideas (as shown by today's emphasis on higher education, for example), the essence of the 'Nightingale system' is still in place.

Democratic traditions

In the nineteenth century Alexis de Tocqueville observed: 'The English colonies – and this was one of the main reasons for their prosperity – have always enjoyed more internal freedom and political independence than that of other nations' (de Tocqueville, 1835, 1840). This democratic attribute was hard won. Beginning with the early English kings' consultations with their councils (at which the people – at a distance – shouted approval or disapproval), through the first written statement of feudal law (the Magna Carta in 1215), the 1295 parliament of Simon de Montforte that gave representation to communities, and Edward I's agreement that the people would not be taxed without their consent, to the Restoration period when parliament gained ascendency by winning the sole right to taxation, individual rights were gradually defined. The New World colonists then incorporated these concepts of personal or individual rights into their own governments.

The characteristics of democratic societies include limits on government, particularly the executive, sovereignty of the people, respect for individual rights, freedom of press and speech, and judicial systems based on the consistent application of law. Additionally the US and Canada, were settled by individuals who, pushing across thousands of miles of dangerous wilderness, often at a distance both temporally and geographically from formal government, developed rather independent attitudes towards their political and economic systems. This individualism is often cited as the reason why the US remains the only major industrialized nation without even a minimal programme of universal national health insurance and why health care is delivered in such a heterogeneous way.

Governmental systems

The British constitution, largely unwritten, based on common law, custom and parliamentary law, and more flexible than the US federal system based on a written constitution, is the result of the continuous growth of a representative constitutional system. The central government, composed of the monarchy and the Houses of Commons and Lords, has three main elements – legislature, executive and judiciary – although the judiciary cannot rule on the validity of laws passed by the legislature, as happens in the US. Theoretically the parliament has unlimited legal power, although there are *de facto* limitations: a citizen can challenge a law through the European Court of Human Rights, and officials and citizens stand equal before the law. The system is the outcome of a centuries old struggle to gain personal liberty and a voice in government that succeeded in a way unparalleled in the rest of the world (except for its two New World offspring).

Canada's governmental structure was set by the British North America Act of 1867, which made it a federal union within the British Empire and, later, a member of the Commonwealth (Chapter 9). The US presidential system is the exemplification of John Locke's principle of separation of powers. Executive and legislature are independent of each other, and the judiciary is independent of both. All rights not granted to the federal government by the Constitution are reserved to the states. In the US the legislature has, as in parliamentary systems, primacy over other branches of government. Only the Congress may enact laws, raise taxes, appropriate money or declare war. The systems of political parties in all the countries are also somewhat similar, with two main major political parties representing so-called conservative and liberal viewpoints, although in the US there is less intraparty consistency and discipline.

Centrality of government

Both the US and Canada have federal forms of government with powers shared between the federal government and the provinces (Canada) and states (US). In Canada the provinces have played an important role in formulating and executing health policies. Until 1965 the (US) states and their local subdivisions (counties and cities) generally had a larger role in health than did the national (federal) government. The UK is more governmentally centralized than the US and Canada, with regional and local councils having responsibility for matters such as health, schools, housing and roads, with accountability to the central government in Whitehall.

Urbanization

In all three countries there has been a steady movement of the populations from rural to urban areas. In Canada and the US about three-quarters of the population live in urban areas. In the UK nine out of ten people live in urban areas.

Urbanization has significant impact on the nature of a nation's health and nursing system. Health facilities and services tend to be clustered in urban areas. These areas often have large numbers of economically disadvantaged people who may well have more severe health problems and make significantly more use of health resources than do people in rural areas.

Industrialization

Similarities exist in the degree to which the economies of the three countries are industrialized. Less than 5% of the labour force of each is engaged in farming, and manufacturing and technological industries provide the larger share of national income. An advanced state of industrialization is, in turn, related to relatively high standards of living. The *per capita* gross national products are among the highest in the world, in 1989 (World Almanac, 1991) as:

UK	$14 535
Canada	$19 020
US	$21 973

Affluence has a direct impact on a country's health system: high standards of living are associated with increased demand for health services. High income levels are also associated with improved health status, particularly with a lower incidence of infectious disease. However, high standards of living may also be associated with 'diseases of affluence', such as heart disease, stroke and cancer, the incidence of which epidemiological studies find to be associated with certain types of life-style, diet and occupation, eg lung cancer with smoking, breast cancer with diet, and mesothelioma of the lung with asbestos inhalation.

Mass education

Compulsory education to the middle-teen years is a characteristic of the three countries, which have literacy rates among the world's highest. Because high levels of education correlate with highly developed health systems, one would expect improved health status, a proposition generally true but with significant exceptions. High educational levels are also related to highly developed systems of educational preparation of health personnel as well as to a larger supply of these personnel relative to the population.

Free market economy

Although in the UK the health industry is owned by the government, the economies of all three countries can accurately be described as free market, and capitalism flourishes in all three systems. The interaction between a nation's economic system and its health system is not necessarily predictable or consistent. While totally nationalized economies like that of the former USSR do have completely nationalized health systems, there are several striking examples of countries with free market economies which have health systems largely run by the government, for example the UK and Sweden. The entrepreneurial quality of the US health care system cannot therefore be ascribed exclusively to the country's free market economic system. Other forces are the tradition of 'rugged individualism' that historically has pervaded the development of institutions in the US and the absence of a strong working class movement that might have led to a much earlier governmental involvement in health care.

Uniformity of scientific knowledge and techniques

Although there are significant differences in the ways in which health care is organized, delivered and financed in the UK, Canada and US, the scientific and technological foundations of medical and nursing care are based on intellectual activity and knowledge that have no national boundaries. The International Classification of Diseases provides a common taxonomy for discussing the signs, symptoms and pathology of disease. International exchanges of information through books, journals, conferences and other media are probably greater in health care than in any other field, so technological advances in the treatment of disease are rapidly disseminated. However, it is still necessary to understand the differences in the health care systems, for example in a government's role in planning, financing and managing care, and what these differences mean in terms of health and nursing care.

It is sufficient to say at this point that there are a number of important similarities that help to explain the particular evolution of each health system. In addition there are some important differences that will be briefly discussed as further background for comparative analysis of the three approaches.

DIFFERENCES BETWEEN COUNTRIES

Despite the number of important ways in which the UK, Canada and the US are similar, there are a few characteristics, possibly relevant to the nature of a country's health system, in which differences do occur.

Size of country

There are, of course, considerable differences in size, both geographic and of population, between the UK, Canada and the US. Geographically

Canada is the second largest country in the world (3.85 million square miles), second only to the former Union of Soviet Socialist Republics, which is over twice as large, and a little larger than the US (3.68 million square miles). By contrast the UK is quite small: a little over 94 thousand square miles.

The population of the three countries differs markedly. Recent statistics (World Almanac, 1991) show the following:

UK	57.1 million
Canada	26.6 million
US	248.7 million

Particularly significant to comparative analysis of the health and nursing systems is population density: the ratio of population to geographic area. The density varies as follows (World Almanac, 1991):

UK	606.2 persons per square mile
Canada	7.5 .. ..
US	69.0 .. ..

Canada is by far the most sparsely populated country of the three and is, in fact, the most sparsely populated major country in the world, with most of its people living along its southern border.

Population density has a direct and significant impact on a nation's health system. A widely dispersed population presents difficulties in providing adequate services. Health care providers generally prefer to live and practise in more populated, urbanized areas, in close proximity to other health care professionals and facilities as well as to more recreational and cultural opportunities. In the US considerable attention has been given to attracting health personnel to underserved rural areas, but with no great success. The Indian Health Service, with a clientele located in remote areas, is woefully understaffed. Even the UK has had problems in providing adequate services to outlying areas.

Historical evolvement

There is a substantial difference in the length of time in which the historical evolutions of the three countries have taken place. The UK has one of the longest continuous histories as a separate people among the major countries of the world, whereas the US and Canada are relatively new nations. But, because of their common heritage, the three countries have strong historical linkages, reflected in governmental philosophies, language, customs and institutions, that have survived occasional political difficulties.

Ethnic diversity

The US has been characterized as a 'melting pot', having in its early history no limits on the number or origin of immigrants and attracting people with a wide variety of economic, cultural, ethnic and religious backgrounds. In contrast, only about 2% of the UK population are classified as members of non-white ethnic groups, being mainly West Indian, Indian or Pakistani. In Canada the major non-white ethnic groups are Indians and Eskimos, making up about 2% of the population.

In the US the major non-white groups comprise nearly 20% of the population (World Almanac, 1991):

Black	12.3%
Hispanic	6.5%
Native American	0.7%

The ethnic diversity of the US population is growing rapidly. The 1980 Census of Population found over 14 million legal residents who were foreign-born. Of the most recent arrivals 1.3 million are from Latin America and 1.2 million from Asia. Ethnic diversity is often cited as a reason for deficiency in health status, of which infant mortality is the most glaring example.

Although Canada and the UK are more homogeneous ethnically as well as in other population characteristics, the current trend is towards greater diversity. Canada, in particular, is experiencing a substantial growth in the number of immigrants from Third World countries. Toronto, once described as a 'dour Scottish Presbyterian town' had as recently as 1961 eight out of ten residents who could trace their ancestry to the British Isles. Twenty years later, only one in three could make that claim (*Washington Post*, 1986). Over 6% of the UK's 55 million people are foreign-born.

Understanding the similarities and differences between the UK, Canada and US helps to set the stage for an in-depth analysis of the health and nursing systems. Also helpful is a knowledge of the major trends that have recently had an impact on the three systems.

TRENDS AFFECTING HEALTH CARE AND NURSING IN THE THREE COUNTRIES

It has been noted that the three health care systems have undergone much change in the last 30 years. This is certainly true in the US, where the year 1965 marked a turning point with the adoption of the Medicare programme, which provides governmentally administered health insurance for people 65 years of age and over. This was the first time the federal government had financed a health insurance programme, even though it was for only a small (slightly over 10%), selected portion of the population. This programme and others adopted by the federal government from 1963 to 1973 have caused major changes within the health and nursing care systems. One important result has been a huge escalation in health care expenditure. The governmental roles in health care in the UK and Canada were in place well before those in the US (and much more comprehensively), but the trends described below have also had an impact on the character of those systems of health and nursing care.

Ageing populations

A common phenomenon in developed countries is the trend towards an ageing population, which is a consequence of lowered birth rate and increased life expectancy. In contrast, developing countries have high birth rates, short life expectancies and young populations. In the US the median age is now 32.3 years and is expected to be 36 years by the year 2000. The 31 million people in the US now aged 65 years and over (about 11%) will increase to 35 million by the year 2000. In the UK the estimated figure of 10 million people – an even larger percentage (18%) being of pensionable age – also points to an ageing population.

The ageing of a country's population has major significance for its health and nursing care systems. The ageing person usually has greater need for health care services. Recent data from the US National Health Interview Survey show that one third of people aged 65 years and over rated their health as fair or poor, whereas only 6% in the age group 15–44 rated their health status as low. The length of care in short-stay hospitals per 1000 persons aged 65 years or over averaged more than 2361 days. The rate for the 15–44 age group per 1000 persons was less than 372 days.

Nursing services are in particular demand because a large proportion of the health care needs of the elderly is for those supportive and rehabilitative services best provided by nurses. The ageing of the population may well be the most important trend affecting current and future needs for nursing services.

Growth in the number of health personnel

There has been a sizeable increase in the number of all health care personnel in the past 20 years. In the US the number of active physicians has increased from fewer than 250 000 in 1963 to an estimated 600 000 in 1990 (United States Department of Health and Human Services, 1989). Active registered nurses have tripled from 560 000 to 1.7 million for the same period (United States Department of Health and Human Services, 1989). During the same time there have also been large increases in health personnel in the UK and Canada, a growth related partly to population growth in the past 20 years and partly to ageing of the population. Other factors have been filling of gaps in services and intensification of services. Government financing of health services has also grown and pushed demand for nursing services upwards.

Advances in technology

Through the centuries great technological advances have touched the lives of most of the world's people, especially those in Western countries, although it could be argued that some of the 'advances' have worked as much against man as for him. In the health field, as important knowledge has accumulated in basic scientific and social science areas as well as in clinical technology, there have also been advances in managerial techniques. Aided in part by electronic computers, the organization and delivery of health services have become more comprehensive, with greater attention paid to planning and evaluation so that services can be delivered more expeditiously and economically. Measures of performance and measures of outcome of performance, because of their continuing development and refinement, are more and more relevant in equations of health care cost/benefit ratios. The difficult task of defining and quantifying criteria for assessing the quality of health services has been recognized by researchers who have begun to focus considerable effort on solving these problems.

Clinical technology has developed more rapidly in the health field than has managerial technology, not unexpectedly since technology primarily deals with things, and managing with people. Clinical technology includes pharmaceuticals, diagnostic and therapeutic equipment, and medical and surgical procedures such as kidney dialysis and organ transplants. Medical interventions resulting in the remarkable reduction in the incidence of certain infectious and other diseases, as well as patient recovery time and the saving of lives previously lost, exist today that were unknown a few decades ago.

However the introduction of new clinical technologies has not been without cost. Although managerial technology has produced savings, clinical technology has often had the opposite effect. Clinical technology is an important factor in the recent steep rises in health care costs. On one hand it is utilized for alleviating or curing illnesses that earlier could not have been treated effectively; on the other it adds to intensity and costs of services. Moreover, by keeping people alive lnger but dependent on supportive, long-term services, the new technologies necessitate use of resources that could perhaps be more efficaciously used elsewhere. Increasingly the reality of the finite nature of economic resources forces the cost/benefit relationship of new clinical technologies to be addressed by leaders in health and government and in the religious and ethical fields.

Increase in specialization

As the health care system has grown and become more complex so has it become more compartmentalized – or fragmented – into specialties. Health care facilities have also become more specialized, with some even dedicated to a single health problem, e.g. the renal dialysis centres in the US. But nowhere is specialization more notable in the American health care industry than among health personnel. There are over 50 major specialties and subspecialties among physicians. Although specialization among nurses is not so formalized, there are approximately 50 work settings of nursing in which the structure and processes are substantively different.

The benefits of specialization in programmes and manpower are reputed to lie in the greater availability of expertise, improved productivity and cost reductions. But the negative aspects are the fragmentation of care and cost escalation because, as US data show, specialists charge more than do generalists for the same service; and, often, the outcomes of care are no different.

Greater involvement of government in health care

In the UK the National Health Service (NHS) has been in operation since 1948; in Canada universal hospital insurance has been in place nationwide since 1960, and medical care coverage since 1970. In the US only about 12% of the population, mostly the elderly, are covered by governmentally managed health insurance, while about 9% are recipients of governmental support because they are poor. These programmes have existed only in the past 25 or so years. The US federal government provides health care to a number of other groups (military personnel, veterans, American Indians and other special categories). In addition, the federal government is a major source of funds for health care research and education. Government regulation of health matters – food, drugs and the environment – is also pervasive.

Costs of health care

The most problematic trend in health care over the past 20 years is rising costs. This is as true in the UK and Canada as in the US. In 1990 health care expenditure in the US accounted for over 11% of the gross national product (GNP) – considerably more than that of the UK and Canada. The reasons for these differences in outlay will be addressed throughout the book.

Increases in a nation's health expenditure are attributable to a variety of factors, two of which – growth of population and demographic change – have already been mentioned. Table 1.1 shows the impact of major factors contributing to growth in expenditure for hospital inpatient care in the US from 1973 to 1983 (Arnett et al., 1985).

Table 1.1 Impact of various factors on the growth of hospital inpatient care in the US, 1973 to 1983

Factor	Percentage of growth attributable to factor
Overall inflation	50.9
Intensity of care provided per patient admitted	23.4
Inflation specific to hospitals above the general inflation	14.6
Population increase	6.7
Increase in admissions *per capita*	4.4

Source: R. H. Arnett *et al.* (1985) Health spending in the 1980s: adjusting to financial incentives, *Health Care Financing Review*, **6**: 1–26.

Rising costs have caused considerable concern about cost containment, a major preoccupation of health leaders in all three countries. Pervading all aspects of management and delivery of health services, it has had a notable impact on certain major health system indicators. In the US, for example, a new system for reimbursing hospitals for care provided to Medicare-insured patients, adopted in 1983 and known as Diagnosis Related Groups (DRGs), sets the payment level before treatment, resulting in a shorter average length of stay. The earlier system that had reimbursed hospitals retrospectively for all costs incurred had no inducement to reduce hospital stay. In Canada there are stronger controls on hospital and other medical care costs through the system of national health insurance.

Long-term care in extended care facilities such as nursing homes and in health centres and patients' homes is becoming increasingly important. Although on a daily basis costs of long-term care are less than those of acute care in short-stay hospitals, aggregate costs can be very high indeed.

Concern with containing the costs of health care has had a substantial impact on nursing. Tightening of health budgets and the decline in utilization of health services shifted concern from feeling that there was a shortage of nurses in the health care industry in the 1960s and 1970s to belief in the early 1980s that there was an oversupply. A recent study (Secretary's Commission on Nursing, 1988) has again found a shortage. Few nurses who want to work are unemployed and there is much advertising of job vacancies, with many inducements cited.

Quality of care

Interest in evaluating the quality of health care is at an all-time high. Numerous research projects have measured different aspects of health care quality, the questions of prestigious commissions have focused on quality of care, governmental regulations have been adopted to ensure a quality level of care, and citizen and 'watch-dog' groups monitor care practices and outcomes.

Concern with quality is a natural outgrowth of attempts to analyse the health care system in order to determine the effectiveness and efficacy of outcomes. Increasingly the following questions are being asked: What are the benefits of health care expenditures? What are the most cost-effective ways of organizing health care? How can health care be more efficiently and effectively delivered?

Developing valid measures of health care quality, especially in terms of outcomes of care, is a daunting task. Perhaps more than any other category of health care provision, nursing has tried to find measures of both performance and outcome. Much work remains, but the foundation has been laid for future developments in assessing nursing quality.

Concern with promotion of health

The health systems of the three countries are dominated by the medical model of care. Most of the money spent on health care goes to diagnosis and treatment of illness rather than to promotion of health. In the US less than 5% of health care expenditure is used for illness prevention and health promotion.

In recent years there has been rising interest in 'wellness' promotion. The former Canadian Health Minister, Marc Lalonde, has played an important role in bringing attention to bear on wellness (Lalonde, 1974). Lalonde conceptualized the health field as being composed of four elements: human biology, environment, life-style and health care organization. His thesis was that health care organization has less impact on sickness and health than do the other three elements, particularly lifestyle. Current interest in pomoting healthier life-styles through control of substance abuse, obesity, stress, accidents and other risks to good health was stimulated by Lalonde's report.

In the UK there have been some recent efforts to establish health promotion programmes although, as Levitt and Wall (1984) point out, 'too many within the NHS see health promotion as an "extra" which can be curtailed in times of financial hardship'. Two DHSS publications, in 1976 and 1981, on illness prevention and health promotion, reveal a governmental concern with wellness, but, as Levitt and Wall (1984, p. 145) indicate, this represents good intentions rather than real programmes.

In the US recent concern with promotion of health and prevention of illness stems from two sources. The first is public recognition that environmental pollutants—in air, water and food have adverse effects on people's health. This has led to the adoption of numerous programmes to remove environmental hazards, a problem of enormous dimensions, particularly in heavily industrialized areas. The second factor is the realization of the obvious fact that rising health care costs can be controlled by reducing illness. The costs of ill health and premature death were initially addressed in 1964 in a report on smoking and health by the Surgeon-General of the United States, head of the federal government's civilian health services programme (United States Department of Health and Human Services, 1964). A more sweeping report on illness prevention was issued by the Surgeon-General in 1979 (United States Department of Health and Human Services, 1979), which set goals for the year 1990 for achieving improved levels of health. Although there has been a decrease in governmental financial support of health promotion and disease prevention programmes since the reports were issued, there does appear to be greater involvement of business, industry and individuals in an effort to keep costs down.

The impact on nursing of a greater emphasis on wellness-orientated programmes can be sizeable. An important sector of nursing, the community care and public health nurses, has for many years engaged in providing preventive health services. Greater emphasis on these services would undoubtedly result in an expansion of the numbers and responsibilities of these nurses as well as of nurses practising in institutional settings who can effectively introduce techniques of health promotion and illness prevention to care of the sick.

Conclusions

The trends discussed briefly here were selected because of their acknowledged impact on the education, supply, distribution, practice and management of nursing in the three countries. They are not all the trends by any means, only the most consequential. They are also those that began in the recent past and will very likely continue into the future, where the greatest impact on nursing of some trends, for example wellness and quality assurance measures, is likely to be.

There are undoubtedly other trends common to the three countries that could be profitably discussed in the context of their impact on nursing. These include growth in education for nursing in institutions of higher learning, advanced preparation for health personnel, expansion of opportunities for women in professional roles in fields other than health care, and the movement towards the independent practice of nursing. These trends will be discussed below in chapters dealing with the specific nursing systems. Undoubtedly other trends will emerge and will be appropriately addressed in Chapter 21.

The purpose of this introductory chapter, therefore, is to provide a background for the remainder of this book. If no other point has been made by this discussion, it is clear that in analysing the health care and nursing systems of a country, we are dealing with dynamic rather than static systems. Before examining the nursing systems in detail we will present a framework for understanding the nature of the health systems in the UK, Canada and the US.

2

Comparative health systems

This chapter presents a brief general overview of the evolution of health systems, followed by a discussion of major characteristics of the health systems of the UK, Canada and the US, and their similarities and differences. The historical evolution of health and nursing systems in the three countries will be examined in more detail in later chapters. The chapter closes with a brief discussion of the interrelationship between the health and nursing systems.

EVOLUTION OF HEALTH SYSTEMS

Undoubtedly the characteristic that most distinguishes between the health systems of the UK, Canada and the US is the extent and nature of governmental involvement in financing, regulating and providing health services. In all three countries governmental involvement in health has been evolutionary. Government's earliest assumption of responsibility came in the field of public health – the control of the spread of infectious diseases. Governmental involvement in the provision of health services to individuals (except for selected beneficiaries such as indigents, armed forces members, veterans, Indians and Eskimos in the US and Canada) is a recent phenomenon. Earlier health care had been offered mainly as private enterprises. Health care was considered an item of personal consumption – like a loaf of bread – to be bought and paid for by the individual consumer on a fee-for-service basis. Health facilities were mostly privately owned. Health care providers, to the extent that they were formally trained, received their educations without government support.

The notion that provision of health care to individuals is a public responsibility is attributed to Otto von Bismarck (Roemer, 1985). An army survey had found Germany's youth to be appallingly unfit for military service, and as Germany maintained a large army, the health of the nation's youth had to be improved. In 1883 the German chancellor also promoted the adoption of compulsory health insurance for industrial workers to receive medical treatment so that they might return to productive employment sooner (thereby providing economic benefits to the whole society). From the 1920s onwards compulsory health insurance in Germany was gradually expanded to all segments of society.

Interestingly although the UK was industrially more advanced than Germany, it did not adopt a governmentally mandated health insurance system until 1911. In that year the National Health Insurance Act created a compulsory health insurance programme for low income workers that provided coverage for services of a general practitioner. In 1939 the Wartime Emergency Medical Service programme gave the Minister of Health 'responsibility for the treatment of casualites, and this enabled the central government to direct the day-to-day work of the voluntary hospitals and local authorities for the first time' (Levitt and Wall, 1984). As a result of the National Health Service Act of 1946, the National Health Service established in 1948 effected sweeping changes in the organization and delivery of health care. Financed largely by general taxation, insurance benefits were extended to the entire population to include free hospitalization (hospitals had become part of the NHS) and dental, ophthalmic, home nursing and other services.

In both Canada and the US some forms of voluntary health insurance programmes had existed since the beginning of the twentieth century, including workmen's compensation programmes and sickness funds administered by beneficial societies. In the US commercial health insurance was a rarity until the advent of the Blue Cross plan for hospital insurance (initiated in 1929). It was supplemented in the 1930s by the Blue Shield programme of coverage for medical services. These programmes grew to be major suppliers of health insurance. Today private health insurance in the US finances about a third of total personal health care expenditure (Levitt, 1985). The only national health insurance system is Medicare for people 65 years of age and over. In 1973 disabled persons, their dependents and those with end-stage renal disease were added to the scheme. Expenditure for Medicare in 1989 comprised over 20% of total US health expenditure.

The governmental role in Canada in providing health services to individuals emerged later than that in the UK, but preceded that of the US and is considerably more extensive. The Hospital Insurance and Diagnostic Services Act of 1957 initiated a programme of compulsory national health insurance administered by each province. The Medical Care Act of 1966 established a programme in which the cost of most physician services and some services rendered by other health professionals is financed by provincial medical care plans.

Thus the governmental role in the health systems of the three countries has evolved quite differently. The British NHS, financed largely by general taxation and providing essentially free care, is the system with the most government control. Intermediate is Canada with its system of

National Health Insurance operated on a decentralized basis by each province, providing universal, largely free, coverage for hospitalization and medical care, and financed in most provinces from general taxation. Finally there is in the US a health 'system' variously described as pluralistic, mixed or segmented. American health care combines the features of national health service in programmes for special beneficiaries, national health insurance for the aged and disabled through Medicare, a Federal-State programme of health care for indigents (Medicaid), voluntary health insurance through non-profit associations and commercial insurers and, sadly, 30–36 million people with no health insurance.

So far we have largely described the health systems in terms of the extent of governmental participation in *financing* health care. Health insurance is a system of financing health care costs that spreads the payment risk among all participants. Funds are collected through premiums, special (income or payroll) taxation or general taxation. The insurance programme either pay providers of insured services directly on a so-called 'service/benefit' basis or reimburse the participants on an indemnity or indirect basis. In addition there is a third type of scheme in which services are provided by the agency that collects the subscriber's funds. Here the insurance programme is a very different entity from that of the previous two situations in which the insurer acts simply as a 'third party' or fiscal intermediary. In this third type insurance is not only a financing scheme but a health care delivery programme as well. Essentially the UK's NHS is the third type of insurance scheme. In the US the Health Maintenance Organization is a non-governmental, small scale example of such a programme. In these the insured has somewhat less freedom of choice of the provider of care than in conventional schemes, a practice purported to be a shortcoming of pre-paid programmes.

SALIENT CHARACTERISTICS OF GOVERNMENT ROLE IN THE HEALTH SYSTEMS OF THE THREE COUNTRIES

Clearly the UK, Canada and the US have distinctive governmental roles in health care. In the US, despite the fact that federal government and states combined provide a substantial proportion of the funds expended on health, they do not play a very active role in the direct provision of health services to individuals. In Canada where there is universal, compulsory health insurance, administered by the provinces and jointly financed by provinces and federal government, the major role of government is as financial manager, not provider of health services. Therefore our analysis of *nursing* systems will contrast three distinctly different *health* systems. However the US and the UK are not entirely dissimilar in the matter of government involvement. Figure 2.1 shows a scale of involvement for some representative countries.

	Amount of Involvement			
Low	*Moderate*		*High*	*Total*
US	Germany Netherlands	Canada Sweden France	UK	Former USSR People's Republic of China

Figure 2.1 Scale of a nation's government involvement in health.

Today it would be difficult to find a nation with a totally private health system. Prior to this century, however, most western European countries and the US would have been placed in this category. In the category of total governmental involvement and control are countries with socialized economies such as the former USSR and the People's Republic of China, although lately there have been signs of change in even these countries. The UK does not belong in this category because a private health care system does exist, although only 2% of patients are under such care (Gray, 1985).

CHARACTERISTICS OF HEALTH SYSTEMS

The major characteristics of a health system are shown in Table 2.1.

Table 2.1 Characteristics of a health system

1. Degree of public intervention in the health delivery sphere.
2. Underlying structure and content.
3. How system is financed.
4. Scope, organization and delivery of services.
5. Providers of services and their training.
6. Facilities and technology.
7. Distribution of services.
8. Regulation and control.
9. Administration and planning.
10. Research and promotion of knowledge.
11. Quality assurance and assessment.
12. Consumer participation.

Input Characteristics	Operational Characteristics	Output Characteristics
Economic support	Organization structure	Illness services
Facilities	Procedures and processes	Wellness and prevention services
Personnel		
Commodities	Administration and planning	Regulations/monitoring
Technology		Research/knowledge
		Facilities/technology
		Health care training
	Environmental factors Governmental intervention and control Consumer participation Quality assurance	

Figure 2.2 Health system characteristics.

These characteristics are shown more graphically in Figure 2.2. It should be noted that the components interact with each other and an accurate representation would reveal a complex set of linkages and feedback loops.

Degree of governmental participation intervention

The governmental role in financing and delivering health care has already been discussed in some detail, particularly with regard to the financing and delivery of services. Other governmental activities include public control over the credentialling of health care personnel. In the US licensing of physicians and nurses is traditionally controlled by the individual states. On a national level the Pure Food and Drug Act, administered by the federal government, monitors such nationwide concerns as the quality of food and drugs and supercedes state law.

The nature of public participation in a health care system is the result of political choices. The first members of society to receive publicly supported care were the poor, who were perceived to have greatest need. Canada and the UK have adopted programmes covering all members of society, whereas the US has opted for categorical programmes – special schemes for children, the aged, veterans, the mentally handicapped, the poor and victims of certain diseases such as tuberculosis and AIDS. For most of the population health services are obtained in the marketplace. Currently the free market concept is being pursued even more vigorously by creating competition among providers. Voluntary insurance plans compete on the basis of costs and benefits, and health maintenance organizations compete against conventional insurance on the basis of costs and comprehensiveness. Hospitals and other health facilities compete for patients on the basis of services offered and other features such as schemes for alcoholics, support for cancer patients and their families, and health lectures and programmes for the general public.

Ideologically the UK and Canada stand in contrast to the US. As stated in a publication supporting the new Canada Health Act, 'the health care systems of these countries are based on the principal of health care for all regardless of their financial circumstances' (Ministry of National Health and Welfare, 1983). In the US health care is viewed as a commodity, purchasable in the marketplace. However it is not a truly free marketplace because the force of competition does not strongly influence the medical market. Physicians do not compete with each other on the basis of price, quality or any other attribute. They do not advertise freely and were in fact forbidden to do so until recently. Physicians also strongly influence the demand for health services in the ordering of tests, drugs and other therapies as well as hospital admissions and referrals. In addition they influence supply through the control of medical school admissions.

Nevertheless while the US appears to be unique among industrialized nations in its entrepreneurial approach to the organization and delivery of health care, the role of government is broadening as it attempts to cope with rapidly rising costs of health care and lack of access to care for a substantial segment of the population.

Structure and content

The structure of a health system relates to several important characteristics, one of which is the already mentioned public – private mix. Structure also relates to the degree to which the system is decentralized. The UK has the most centralized structure, although considerable decentralized authority and responsibility exists in the regions and districts. Canada's provinces have a strong role in health, while in the US the states, which earlier had the larger role, are now overshadowed, from the standpoint of funding, by the federal government.

Because of the large number and variety of governmental regulatory and private agencies that play important roles in the health system, the US structure is the most decentralized of the three. Recently however there has been a trend towards the establishment of conglomerates of profit-making health agencies – multihospital, multinursing home systems – chains such as Hospital Corporation of America and Humana, Inc.

Conglomeration results in centralized management and less 'product' diversity. Nevertheless the US system is still structurally the most complex and heterogeneous.

Content as a characteristic of a health system relates to the nature of activities performed – the procedures and processes used. In the provision of both medical and nursing services there are similarities of content in the three countries. A nurse from the US joining the staff of a hospital in the UK or Canada for the first time would quickly adapt to the work situation, finding the nursing process basically similar. Where differences do occur they are usually matters of emphasis and priority.

An important influence on the content of health care is the health problems for which people seek help. The International Classification of Diseases, used by many countries for the accounting of sickness and death, makes it possible to compare the health status of the three countries. Data show that diseases of the heart, malignant neoplasms and cerebrovascular disease account for the majority of deaths in each.

Financing health care

Broadly speaking payment for health care is derived from the following sources:

1. Direct unreimbursed payments by consumers.
2. Indirect payments by voluntary insurance.
3. Indirect payments by government-sponsored insurance.
4. Provision of prepaid services by government.
5. Provision of prepaid services by non-government agencies.

In direct payments the consumer pays without reimbursement for services received on a fee-for-service basis. Also included are direct payments for drugs, spectacles and all other health commodities.

Insurance payments are those either made directly to the consumer who, in turn, reimburses the provider for incurred expenses (indemnity), or by the insurer directly to the provider (service benefit). Finally services can be provided directly to the consumer on a prepaid basis by either governmental or non-governmental agencies. . . . The UK has the governmentally provided type. Non-governmental agencies include charitable organizations providing free services to indigents, and agencies such as health maintenance organizations in which services are prepaid, as in conventional insurance schemes.

While these are primarily the mechanisms for funding health services – direct payment for service or commodity, insurance, prepayment – actual sources of funding are varied. Direct payment comes from an individual's resources. Voluntary health insurance can be funded directly by consumer or employer, or by a combination of the two. Governmentally supported health insurance can be funded by premiums collected from individuals, special taxes earmarked for health insurance or general taxation. Services provided directly by the government can be funded, like insurance, by premiums only or by special or general taxation and may require some direct payment, usually small, from consumers of certain services or commodities. Services provided by voluntary agencies are funded by charitable contributions. Non-governmental prepaid programmes, such as American health maintenance organizations, are funded by premiums collected from individuals, from their employers or from a combination of the two.

In addition to differences in payment methods and funding sources there are large differences in the amount of money each country allocates to health. The US spends the most money in both absolute and relative terms. In 1987 nearly $2051 *per capita* was spent on health care in the US, compared to only $758 in the UK and $1483 in Canada (Schieber and Poullier, 1989).

Personal health services, by far the largest category of health expenditure, is not the only object of health care expenditure. Public health activities, a long-standing function of governments, is an important but rather small item of expenditure – less than 5% in the US. Other expenditures also within the public domain are on research, construction of facilities and education of personnel.

A generalization that can be made about the financing of health care in the three countries is the growing importance of public sources. While governmental financing predominates in the UK and Canada, the governmental portion in the US has only recently grown to the point where it is now approaching nearly half of all health care expenditure. Moreover direct payment by individuals for personal health services has declined to less than 30% from over 80% 50 years ago.

Organization and delivery of health services

Personal health services consist of a complex variety of services and delivery systems developed to address the large number of human health conditions and problems. Figure 2.3 presents a description of the major components of the US health care delivery system. A system can be described according to levels of care provided, ranging from preventive care for well persons or groups, to continuing care for those with chronic ailments or in the terminal stages of their illnesses. The types of care given at the various levels differ widely, as do the kinds of setting and provider. Nursing plays a vital role at every level of care and in every health care setting and is the major professional service most offered.

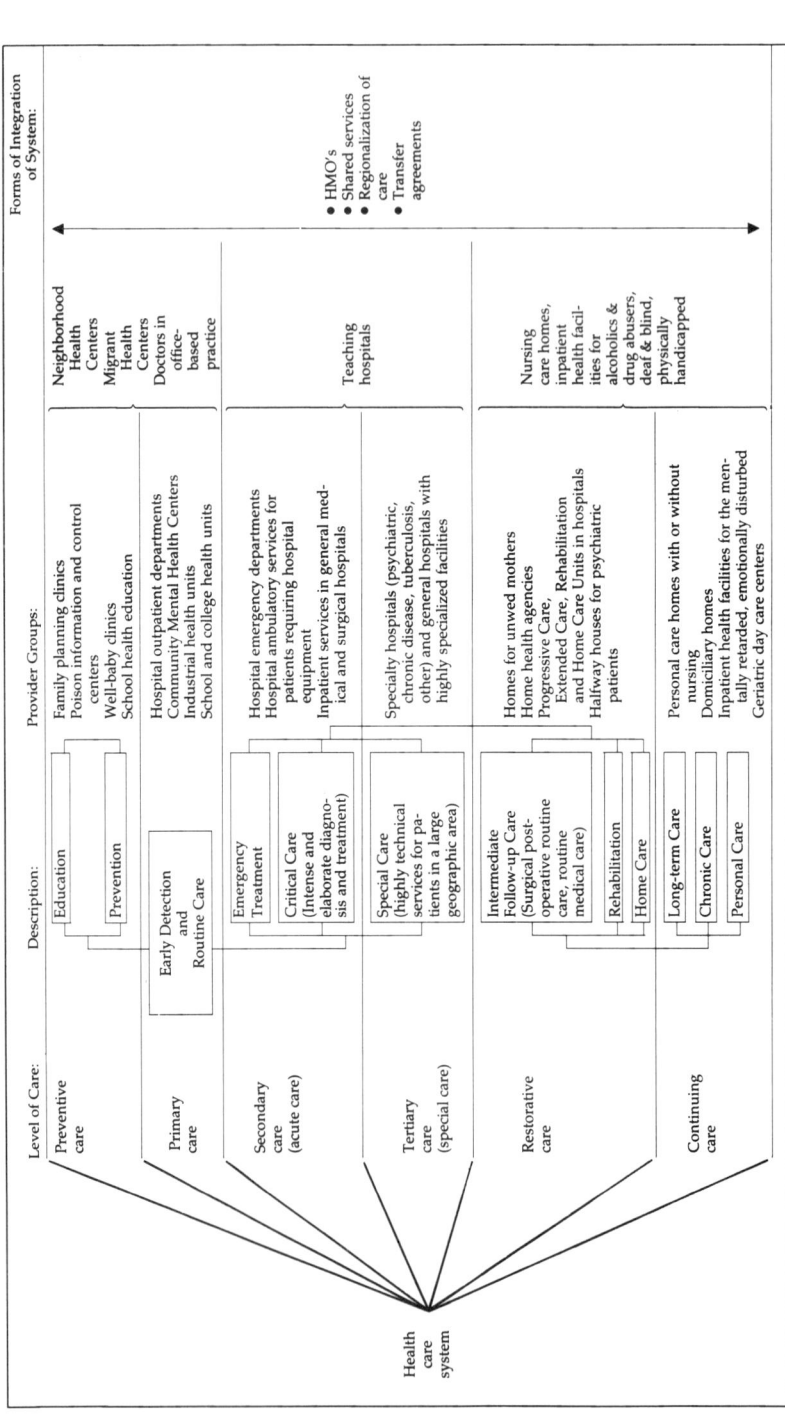

Figure 2.3 Spectrum of health care delivery. US system.

Source: Cambridge Research Institute, 1976 trends affecting the US Health Care System DHEW publication No. HRA 76-14503. Washington DC, Government Printing Office.

Distribution of services according to the various levels of care is decidedly uneven. In all three countries acute care is the single largest level of services, consuming the major share of health care expenditure. Preventive care, despite considerable recent verbal support, receives only a tiny share. Service distribution is not static. It changes with ageing of the population and a resulting increase in need for chronic and restorative care. Currently a shift away from preoccupation with acute care is discernible. However, at the same time, advances in diagnostic techniques and new therapies are increasing demands for acute care services.

New patterns of service delivery are being developed in response to technological advances as well as growth in health care expenditure. It is not too rash to predict that the health care delivery system as we know it will be significantly different in the not-too-distant future.

Providers of services

Both in number and type, health care providers have grown substantially in the recent past in the three countries. In the US, for example, the number of health personnel of all kinds actively employed has reached five million, making health the single largest employer among all industries. Similarly, the British NHS is the largest employer in Europe. In any country, the majority of health care providers are nursing personnel. Physicians, at the apex of the provider hierarchy, form only a small proportion of health manpower. Health occupations supplementary to medicine (physical therapists, laboratory technicians, X-ray technicians, etc.) are another large group of health care providers.

While the UK and Canada do not have as large a number of health personnel as does the US, they have had a similar pattern of growth. Also there are similarities in the variety of health occupations and the responsibilities of each category as well as in professional training. This training is a very large enterprise indeed. As the health personnel supply has grown so have training programmes. This is especially true for nursing personnel, whose supply has grown faster than most other occupations. Within each major occupational category are specialties, the most numerous of which are those of doctors, where educational preparation for some clinical specialties may take as long as, or longer than, the time required to become a doctor. Specialization among nurses includes both clinical and hierarchical specialization. The latter exists in large organizations such as hospitals where there is need for a chain of command extending from the director of nursing/matron to the staff nurse/ward sister.

There are important differences in the ways in which health personnel and their training are financed. In the UK most health personnel are employees of the NHS. In Canada and the US most health personnel other than doctors and dentists are not self-employed; the major employer is not government but a voluntary or, in the US, a profit-making organization.

Although physicians in the US have traditionally resisted working for others and have practised on a solo basis, the situation is changing. Some physicians have formed groups where they continue to practise on a fee-for-service basis but share expenses and facilities. They are also becoming employees of hospitals or health maintenance organizations from whom they receive salaries, a trend that Starr calls a movement towards corporate medicine (Starr, 1982). Moreover, as Starr points out, these organizations are increasingly becoming part of even larger organizations, for instance multihospital systems. Therefore the high degree of autonomy that doctors once enjoyed may be eroding. Increasingly the training of health workers is being governmentally supported. Besides the large public education systems in all countries, government loans and scholarships are provided for health professions' students.

Facilities and technology

As Figure 2.3 shows, health care is delivered in a variety of settings. The most numerous are the short-stay (acute care) and specialty hospitals. In the US 60% of all health personnel work in these hospitals, and the corresponding figure in the UK is 70%. Most hospitals in the UK are owned by the government, as are many Canadian hospitals. About one third of all US hospitals are either federally or state owned.

Hospitals consume the largest share of health care expenditure of any facility in the US – about 50%. Not included in this figure are payments to physicians for care provided to hospitalized patients. Clearly hospitals are a high cost setting. Primarily as a means of containing the high costs of hospital care, a broad array of health care settings and programmes has evolved in the US and, to some extent, in the UK and Canada. One example is of a surgical centre providing surgical services on an ambulatory basis. The number of home care programmes providing services to patients has grown rapidly in the US. This growth is especially relevant to nursing since these programmes exist to provide nursing services.

Technology

Health care facilities include not only the buildings in which services are provided but also equipment for diagnosis and treatment. With recent technological advances equipment has become an important and expensive resource in patient care settings. Technologically, acute care and specialty hospitals are the most advanced settings. The growth of free-standing ambulatory facilities has resulted in a widespread dissemination of expensive and highly sophisticated equipment.

The interaction between nursing and growth in the technology of health care is an interesting one that will be touched upon later. This interaction has had a number of influences on the education and practice of nurses as well as on the ethical issues that have arisen in the provision of health care.

The increase in health care expenditure due to new technology has caused cost-containment measures to be directed at the expensive equipment being introduced into hospitals and other health facilities.

Facilities

In the US federal financing has contributed to the large growth in the number of health care facilities. Beginning in the late 1940s the federal government provided funds on a matching basis for hospital construction in order to improve the hospital bed-to-population ratio in rural areas and to upgrade facilities and standards. Billions of dollars from public sources were provided for construction of hospitals and other health care facilities. Although the programme has now been curtailed because of an oversupply of beds, of the $3 billion spent on construction of medical facilities in 1987, nearly one third still came from public sources.

In the UK all facility construction as well as purchase of new technology in the NHS is publicly funded. In Canada investments in new health facilities are financed by all levels of government, by institutions and by private donations. Like the US the federal government in Canada which, under the National Health Grant Program, subsidized almost all hospital construction prior to 1970, terminated the programme in that year because of the perception that an adequate number of hospital beds had been provided (Soderstrom, 1978). Current Canadian federal government support is limited to educational and research facilities.

Distribution of services

The problem of equitable distribution of services that provide access to care for all citizens is widespread and is especially acute in the US with its entrepreneurial approach and multiple ways in which care is furnished. Health facilities and personnel are unevenly distributed, most notably between urban and rural areas. Within urban areas the 'inner cities' – the places of the poor – are severely underserved.

Canada, with its huge land area and concentration of population in urban centres, also has a problem of access to care in remote locations. The UK, too, is not without its problems of maldistribution. As Klein (1985) stated:

'If the North East Thames region is relatively overprovided [with health resources], taken as a whole, the picture changes dramatically when we look at the districts within it. Islington District Health Authority in inner London, is 25 per cent over target, while Southend District Health Authority, a seaside retirement area, is nearly 20 per cent below target.'

Attempts have been made in recent years to correct this maldistribution of resources. In the US a small federal programme known as the National Health Service Corps offers federally financed employment in selected 'underserved' areas to recently graduated physicians and other health personnel that 'forgives' federal loans for education. Special financial support is offered for the education of health personnel, mainly doctors from ethnic minorities, with the expectation that they will practise in places such as inner cities where populations are composed of large numbers of ethnic minorities. While some nurses have participated in these schemes, the rate of attraction to underserved areas has not been very high.

Regulation and control

In the UK and Canada there is more public control over both the organization and delivery of health services than there is in the US. While the US has very little *direct* governmental involvement in the provision of health services, there is considerable indirect involvement through regulation. State governments have had a longstanding role in licensing health personnel and facilities. The state and federal governments monitor the production, labelling, advertising and distribution of pharmaceutical products, as well as protecting the public against medical quackery and possible health hazards in consumer products. Governmental regulation also extends to health and safety standards in the workplace and to environmental protection (air, water, highways, physical structures, waste dumps, etc.).

Growth of the Medicare programme has increased federal regulatory activities. To uphold standards and control possible 'overdoctoring' the Professional Standards Review Organizations (PSROs) were established by federal law in 1972 to monitor Medicare payments. In 1983 the system of prospective reimbursement of services to Medicare patients was initiated, based on classification of patients into 467 Diagnosis Related Groups (DRGs). Instead of being reimbursed for all Medicare-incurred costs, hospitals are paid predetermined fixed fees according to the patient's DRG. In 1989 legislation was passed that imposes a uniform national fee schedule, setting the payments doctors may receive for Medicare patients. Incentives are provided to doctors who practise 'hands-on' medicine that does not rely on expensive technology. To monitor DRGs Peer Review Organizations (PROs) were created. Like PSROs, PROs consist of members from outside the government (mostly doctors).

The UK and Canadian governments have similar regulatory powers in maintaining in health and safety standards. Also, in Canada, the decentralized health system gives each province authority to regulate health insurance programmes. The review of claims, which varies from one province to another, attempts to control fraudulent billing practices (was the service provided or not? Was it provided unnecessarily?) rather than quality of service.

Direct control over quality of health services provided, both in terms of how well they were provided and their outcomes, largely falls outside the purview of government. Professional associations play an important role in this area as well as in other matters affecting health care providers. The British Medical Association and the Royal College of Nursing bargain with the government over remuneration claims. Disciplining of health professionals is also left to the Associations. Additionally professional associations have strong influence over health professions' education through standard setting and accrediting procedures.

Voluntary associations also have a regulatory impact on health facilities. An organization known as the Joint Commission for Accreditation of Hospitals (JCAH) was established in the US in 1952 by the major professional societies to review hospital performance. The National League for Nursing, one of two major nursing organizations, has an accrediting programme for home health care agencies.

Administration and planning

Of the three countries the US undoubtedly has the most complex administrative organization with its large number, layering and variety of agencies. The amount of paperwork required by this system is astounding. Studies have shown that nurses in short-stay hospitals spend a considerable amount of their time each day on paperwork, much of it related to billing patients (Levine, 1985).

While there is more homogeneity in the administration of the Canadian and UK systems, some diversity does exist. There are variations in the NHS in England, Scotland, Wales and Northern Ireland and locally among the districts. In Canada the administration of the national health insurance programme is decentralized to provincial governments.

Planning is an important component of efficient administration (Rodwin, 1984). As a governmental tool planning grew in accordance with governmental participation in health care. In both Canada and the US planning for hospital bed needs is an integral part of governmental funding of hospital construction. In the US legislation in 1974 expanded health planning considerably by dividing the nation into over 200 health system areas and by creating agencies to plan for health services and facilities on a mandatory basis. So-called 'certificates of need' gave these agencies power over construction of hospital beds and acquisition of expensive equipment. The power of planning agencies has declined with the current ideological opposition to governmental regulation and the desire to promote free-market competition.

According to Levitt and Wall it was not until 1974 and a reorganization of the NHS that serious attempts were made in the UK to systematically and comprehensively plan for health services (Levitt and Wall, 1984). As in the US, a major purpose of planning is to assist in the containment of rising health costs. In Canada the provinces are responsible for planning of hospital beds (Lalonde, 1984).

Research

An important aspect of a health system is the extent to which it engages in research. Research advances scientific knowledge and has a positive influence on both the clinical and managerial sides of health care.

Involvement of government in health care research is considerable in all three countries. This is especially true in managerial research – studies of ways to improve the efficiency and effectiveness of the organization and the delivery of health services. As an example the Department of Health and Social Security in the UK has supported several recent studies of projected nursing supply and requirements, using modelling techniques (DHSS, 1983). The federal government in Canada and individual provinces have supported numerous studies of ways to improve the efficiency of health care delivery, including some pioneering efforts to develop methodology for determining nursing workload (Giovannetti, 1973). Similarly the US federal government has been the main supporter of health services research through grants and contracts to universities and other organizations and by engaging directly in research.

In the US the support of government is predominate in health research. Of the $11.5 billion spent on non-commercial research in 1990 the federal government financed nearly 90%.

Quality of care

Rising concern with the quality of health care services is an important characteristic of our three countries. Concern with quality has grown in direct proportion to growth of public involvement in financing and delivery of health services. In the US quality assessments are federally mandated for the Medicare system. Interestingly Levitt and Wall remark that the US, despite its free-wheeling approach to health care delivery, has done more to regulate and control standards and performance than has the UK with its NHS (Levitt and Wall, 1984). In Canada the provinces have shown considerable interest in pursuing quality assurance programmes. In 1986, for example, the province of Alberta began a study to develop measures of quality of outcomes in home care programmes.

The issue of quality assurance has been an important one among the nursing profession. More than any other health occupation nursing has been concerned – perhaps even preoccupied – with measurement of quality of both performance and outcome. A not inconsiderable part of the nursing research effort is devoted to quality measurement. By contrast the medical profession is not as involved in assessing quality of performance of medical practitioners but appears more interested in improving the quality of educational preparation of doctors and evaluating the efficacy of diagnostic and treatment procedures.

A nation's interest in evaluating the performance and outcome of the components of its health care system is an indicator of the maturity of the system. It complements other techniques for rationalizing the system, such as planning and evaluating. Interest will undoubtedly grow in future as health care expenditure continues to increase and as more refined tools of measurement become available.

Consumer participation

There are a number of ways in which consumers' views and concerns influence the health care system. In democratic systems a consumer can make his views known to his elected representative. Consumers have traditionally been given representation on hospital boards, boards of public health and boards of educational institutions, and may also complain directly to medical societies and other professional associations. In addition to influencing concern over quality assurance and planning, the growth in health care expenditure has resulted in even greater participation by consumers in planning and formulating health policy and evaluating health services. In the US, for example, the health planning programme that created the planning agencies *required* lay representation of consumer participation on agency boards.

The impact on policy formulation of consumer participation on boards and other formal organizations is difficult to assess. Some critics claim that this participation is a form of 'tokenism' and that most decision making in health care is controlled by health care professionals and government bureaucrats, although there have been instances in which lay participants have had substantial impact. Outside formal settings consumer participation in health policy formulation has expanded in recent years as part of the movement labelled 'consumerism' or as part of the proliferation of voluntary organizations that promote single issues. In the US consumerism has given rise to increased governmental regulation aimed at protecting the environment and promoting safety in consumer products. Voluntary organizations on both sides of the issue of government financing of abortions have created a vigorous and sometimes combative debate and confrontation.

Another aspect of consumerism in health peculiar to the US is the incidence of lawsuits by consumers against health care providers, primarily doctors, for alleged malpractice. In the mid-1980s such lawsuits became so numerous and juries' awards so monetarily high that some medical specialists such as obstetricians left their practices because of huge increases in insurance premiums. Studies have shown that where consumer – provider relationships and communication are good, use of lawsuits to settle grievances is lessened.

IMPACT OF HEALTH SYSTEMS' CHARACTERISTICS ON NURSING

In making comparative analyses of nursing it is important to understand the essential characteristics of each nation's health systems. This chapter has presented some of them. They were selected because of their potential impact on nursing and because understanding them will enable a better grasp of differences and similarities in the nursing system. Within the context of these characteristics this chapter has given a brief description of the major ways in which the three countries are different – or similar. In later chapters descriptions of the health care and nursing systems will be more detailed. These can be viewed within the context of the characteristics outline given here.

To summarize the major points presented in this chapter, we began by saying that an important characteristic of a nation's health system is the degree of governmental involvement. Broadly speaking that involvement consists of the extent to which government finances the system and the extent to which it actually runs the system and directly provides services.

It has long been held that the US has the least governmental involvement in health. Brian Abel Smith stated in his classic *History of Medical Care* (Crichton, 1981):

'There are extraordinarily few countries in the world where there has been less public control in the medical care market than in the United States.'

The overview of health care characteristics does show that, at the various levels, governments do participate in the health care systems and influence them in a number of important ways: in planning, evaluation, regulation (including arbitrary lawsuits), training and research. These activities are less visible in the US than is direct delivery of services to patients as in the British NHS or the role of the provinces in Canada.

The important question for this book is: what does this mean for nursing? Succeeding chapters will examine, for each country, the major aspects of its nursing system. How does the fact that most nursing personnel in the UK are employees of the government affect this system as compared to Canada and, even more so, the US where most nurses are employed by the private sector? Taking another characteristic – scope, organization and delivery of services – how do the differing degrees of government participation in the health care systems affect the emphasis on ambulatory care versus institutional care or on wellness services versus care of the sick?

Finally what are the salient features of the administrative process in a unified system like the UK compared to the pluralism of the US? And paramount to all of this discussion and analysis is, what can be learned about the nursing system of one country that can be applied usefully in another country? In view of nursing's concern with improvement of the quality of its services this is indeed an important question.

Part Two

The United Kingdom

3

Historical evolution of the health care and nursing systems

The custom of human beings caring for each other stretches back into the mists of prehistory. Recent archaeological evidence shows that as long as 35 000 years ago people had cared for their elders, who were the source of wisdom and experience, and buried them with honour and respect when they died. The gradual development from then until now of a genuine social conscience has led to continuing social change, one facet of which is health care. Today's health care is the product of historical evolution of beliefs, values and attitudes spurred on by advance of medical science and lately joined by economic, technological, social, psychological and statistical principles and devices used for the betterment of the human condition.

THE EARLY DAYS

Primitive peoples coped with adversities such as sickness and death as best they could – by rituals, incantations, taboos, magic and exorcism. Many of these practices survive today in various parts of the world. However as human beings became more knowledgeable about themselves and the nature of the world in which they lived, this kind of coping was replaced by more rational practices. Evidence is found in manuscripts in India and Egypt and in the Old Testament which set forth the sanitary principles that guided the religious and hygienic practices of the Jews. The early Greek philosophers pondered the origin of disease and built temples to which people went for 'cure' of physical and mental ailments, and they established principles for physicians' treatment of patients (Hippocrates) and for biology (Aristotle). Public health measures were taken by the Romans who drained swamps and built sewers, bath houses and an extensive water supply system. All of these health principles and practices were forgotten as Europe passed through the Dark Ages.

Movement forward began again during the fourteenth century with the establishment of quarantines at European ports because of bubonic plagues that killed as much as a third of the population of Europe. In

Table 3.1 Relevant legislation health

1782	Gilbert Act
1808	County Asylum Act
1834	Poor Law Amendment Act
1845	Lunacy Act
1847	Poor Law Board Act
1848	Public Health Act
1858	Registration of Doctors Act
1861	Lunacy Act Amendment
1867	Metropolitan Poor Law Act
1871	Local Government Board Act
1872	Public Health Act
1875	Public Health Act
1890	Lunacy Act
1902	Midwives Act
1911	National Insurance Act
1913	Mental Deficiency Act
1919	Nurses Registration Act
1930	Treatment Act
1936	Mental Deficiency Act
1943	Nurses Act
1944	Education Act
1946	Mental Illness Act
1946	NHS Act
1948	National Insurance Act
1948	Family Allowance Act
1949	Nurses Act
1957	Nurses Act
1959	Mental Health Act
1962	Social Work and Health Visitor (Training) Act
1973	NHS Reorganisation Act
1979	Nursing, Midwives and Health Visitors Act

France and Germany great hospitals were established by nursing orders of both men and women. Later Protestant endeavours took the form of economic support of hospitals. Charitable care of the sick poor has always been one of the beneficent principles of great religions.

ADVANCES IN PUBLIC HEALTH

In England it was William Petty who, in 1676, introduced the idea that public health was a national concern. Nehemiah Grew produced a pamphlet for Queen Anne in 1707 that argued that a nation's prosperity rested on the good health of its population – government should be concerned with maintaining that good health (Woodward, 1974).

England had earlier built hospitals. St Bartholomew's, built in the twelfth century, is considered to be the first modern hospital. King Henry

VIII, in the sixteenth century, had chartered hospitals for the sick poor but the system fell into decay and hospitals were best avoided.

THE INDUSTRIAL REVOLUTION AND THE BEGINNINGS OF REFORM

The industrial revolution that transformed the Western world began in England because of favourable political institutions, a free trade philosophy, a favourable geographic location, an abundance of coal and a group of men who were inventors and technological innovators. It also created social and physical problems through callous exploitation and neglect of human resources. Some residues of these evils persist to this day.

Rapid urbanization, the result of industrial concentration, created hideous conditions for workers – overcrowding, long working hours, use of children and women in mines, dangerous working conditions, high accident rates and filthy living conditions that led to a general breakdown in health. Local government was incapable of dealing with problems of such magnitude. Fortunately the ideal of protecting people's health had not died. Many reformers had written treatises on various aspects of public health; a textbook had even been published.

The work of social reformers began to have an effect. Edwin Chadwick, a leading champion of reform, wrote a report on 'The Sanitary Conditions of the Labouring Population of Great Britain' (Chadwick, 1842). As a result the Public Health Act of 1848 was passed but as it lacked an enforcement clause it was ineffective. Parliament itself, before other governmental bodies, had first to be reformed before health laws would be effective. Not until the 1870s would the public benefit from the law's provisions. As conditions grew worse social reformers fought harder. Louisa Twining led the fight for workhouse and nursing care system reform. Many of the sick poor had been relegated to the workhouses and most nursing was done, or more likely not done, by 'pauper' nurses. A 'poor law' was passed.

THE POOR LAW

The 1867 Metropolitan Poor Law Act, a landmark in British health reform, established a new hospital system that had lasting effects on health care service. It bade new hospital authorities build new hospitals (infirmaries) and separate institutions for the mentally ill and infectious disease victims. However the law applied only to London so by 1871 the local boards had enacted their own laws. All the hospitals suffered from lack of trained nurses for, in spite of an increasing number of nurse training schools, demand far exceeded supply. Section 29 of the Poor Law Act allowed infirmaries to admit probationers and train their nurses, a significant step forward as nurse probationers had previously been admitted only to charity hospitals. Some remnants of these Poor Law conditions remained until the National Health Service Act was implemented in 1948.

COMMUNITY CARE

Home care for the sick, among the most ancient of health practices, became part of organized nursing service only in the mid-19th century. The idea of the health of the public, or public health, as an entity amenable to management and direction by the medical and nursing disciplines emerged with greater understanding of infectious diseases and personal and environmental hygiene, based on expanded knowledge in biology and medical science. Better maternal care, the value of vaccination and the benefits of a good diet were seen as teachable concepts and the good health of the people became a government concern for economic as well as humanitarian reasons. Edwin Chadwick, observing some unintended bad effects of the new Poor Law, continued to press for strong local government and appointment of salaried medical officers as possible remedies (Frazer, 1947). Although resisted by factory and mine owners and slumlords, and hampered by the indifference of an uninformed citizenry, the reform movement gained strength. A number of public health laws were passed; unfortunately they accomplished only conflict and confusion.

A Royal Commission (1871) recommended quick action to correct the situation. An attempt to separate public health administration from functions of the Poor Law failed. The Gladstone administration passed a Local Government Board Law Act (1871) that replaced the Poor Law Board and acquired the Register General Department and the Medical Department of the Privy Council. Another Public Health Act (1872) divided the country into sanitary authorities, each with a medical officer. The Public Health Act of 1875 consolidated many (but not all) of the sanitary authorities. The Local Government Board Act remained until the Ministry of Health came into being in 1919.

PUBLIC HEALTH WORKERS

The sanitary reformers pushed for further improvements in the living conditions of the poor. Societies of sanitary improvement and a Sanitary Association were formed. The privileged Ladies of the Sanitary Association employed women of good character to advise mothers on good health practices. The work of these women, called health visitors, was soon recognised as instrumental in improving child health and reducing infant mortality, and the association requested that the service be made statutory. Manchester City Council was one of the first to pay a portion of their salaries and bring their work under the supervision of the Medical Officer of Health.

The first education course for health visitors, classed as technical teaching and consisting of 16 lectures, was set up in North Buckinghamshire. The health visitor was considered not as a nurse but as a health educator and counsellor to the whole family. This role later changed from family visitor to one of being concerned with child and maternal death and infant mortality. This in turn led to the Midwives's Act (1902), introduced for the protection of mother and child, which required the midwife to take formal training and register with the Central Midwives Board. Health Visitors' Orders required health visitors to have either a medical or nursing qualification and a certificate from an approved society. The Royal Sanitary Association, later the Society of Health, was the certificate-granting body until 1962 when the Council of Training of Health Visitors was set up following the Social Work and Health Visitor (Training) Act (1962). Health visitors were the first nurses to be educated in higher educational institutions.

DISTRICT NURSES

Before the emergence of health visiting, nurses known as parish nurses had long cared for the sick in their homes. In the mid-nineteenth century, one, Mrs Fry, an enthusiastic social reformer, founded an Institution of Nursing (Bishopsgate) to train nurses at Guy's Hospital for home nursing. Mrs Fry had been inspired by work at Kaiserwerth (Germany) where sisters not only cared for the sick in hospital but did housekeeping, cooking and visiting patients' homes. Unfortunately the training at Guy's was unsupervised and the efforts of the institute made little impact except that the concept of providing care in the home by a trained nurse had been born (Abel Smith, 1960).

In 1859, William Rathbone of Liverpool hired a nurse from St Thomas's to work in his home. Impressed with the excellence of the service, he set up, with Florence Nightingale, an experiment whereby hospital-trained nurses were sent to care for the sick at home. From this successful beginning district nursing became firmly established on a national basis under the District Nurse Association. In 1889 the Queen Victoria Jubilee Nursing Institute, founded by the Association, received a Royal Charter. The Institute offered a six-month training course specifically for district nursing and, by the turn of the century, a strong foundation had been laid for today's community nursing service. Much legislation was passed in the early twentieth century that affected the work of the district nurse (Lamb, 1977).

Over 50% of the nursing workforce was engaged in community work at the beginning of this century (Burdett, 1905), and Abel Smith calculated from 1901 Census data that there were 69 200 full-time equivalent nursing staff in England and Wales, including those working in institutions and patients' homes. Of the total only 5700 were men and, of those, 3900 were employed in mental hospitals. It can therefore be assumed that the remaining 1800 male nurses worked in patients' homes, as voluntary hospitals did not admit men to nursing. Greater recognition of the value of skilled nursing had led to an increased demand for the services of nurses in the home. They, in turn, found work in the home less strenuous and more rewarding financially. For example in 1901 nurses in workhouses were paid £17 *per annum* and, in London, nurses' pay averaged £26.10. In contrast with room and board the nurse in the home was paid about £57 per annum (Burdett, 1901). For district nursing two guineas per week, with meal, was a common charge. How many hours district nurses worked is not known, but nurses in voluntary hospitals at that time worked about 12 hours a day.

The demand for nurses led to abuses. In London the wealthy could hire the best nurses from the voluntary hospitals, while elsewhere trained district nurses for rich or poor were scarce. The London Hospital, for example, sent out 160 nurses, including second-year probationers, unsupervised. The income from this was £4000 per annum, of which £1700 was profit (Abel Smith, 1960). Private agencies did not provide trained nurses and were considered to be a danger to an unsuspecting public. Both the British Hospital Association and the Royal British Nurses Association established cooperatives to protect nurses from exploitation (Tooley, 1906).

During the early twentieth century district nurses became more involved with public health, which was the responsibility of local authorities. Many voluntary agencies organized district nursing services, but after 1929 some county authorities also established their own services for infectious disease. In addition they provided funds to voluntary organizations but until 1939 had no power to provide badly needed comprehensive services. Under the National Insurance Act (1911) workers, but not their families, were eligible for medical care. District nurses therefore became concerned with the elderly, women and children, care being centred on the chronically sick and terminally ill and on infectious disease victims.

By the time the NHS was established in 1948, county authorities, voluntary organizations and the Queen's Institute were organizers of district nursing services. Under the NHS Act every person became eligible to register with a general practitioner and receive free care. Provisions of community nursing services included domiciliary midwives and health visitors as well as district nurses who were responsible to the local authority under the control of a Medical Officer. As more and more local authorities provided services, voluntary agencies ceased to exist.

As the work of the district nurse increased the shortage became apparent. Recruitment was difficult: nurses were unwilling to live in residential accommodation and salaries were poor. Subsequent improvements in these areas led to increased manpower. Although district nurse training was not a requirement, a six-month course, which supervised and tested candidates, was sponsored by the Queen's Institute. In areas where the Institute acted as an agent only trained personnel were employed. Where local authorities employed their own nursing staff qualifications were less emphasized.

In 1951 Ministry of Health statistics show that 8700 district nurses were employed in England and that, in Great Britain, training was provided by 55 centres, with a capacity of 913 students per annum (Ministry of Health, 1955). In 1960 the Minister of Health set up the Council of District Nursing and a panel of advisers to improve standardisation. Once local authorities provided their own training the Queen's Institute, in 1969, withdrew from training activities. Over 50% of nurses working in district nursing had no specialist training until the Nurses, Midwives and Health Visitors Act (1979) made training mandatory. A nine-month college-based programme was introduced in 1981 and is now compulsory for qualification.

MENTAL HOSPITALS

Today's large mental hospitals are the legacy of the nineteenth century. In medieval times the physically and mentally ill were usually cared for together, but by the eighteenth century the mentally ill could be found in a variety of places: prisons, houses of correction and workhouses. The wealthier were boarded privately; there were 200 such establishments (Parry-Jones, 1972). Many were cared for in the community. By the end of the 18th century attitudes towards mental illness had changed. Better understanding of psychological and emotional illnesses through expanded scientific knowledge and improvement in general medical practice gave impetus to a drive to establish mental hospitals (which also became teaching hospitals) by public subscription.

The teachings of Dr William Battle reinforced an enlightened approach that mental illness was manageable and that restraint and incarceration were counterproductive to healing. The York Retreat, founded in 1791 by William Tuke with money from the Quaker Society, was notable for compassionate treatment. The 1807 reform movement persuaded the government to set up an inquiry into the 'state of the criminal pauper lunatics in England and Wales', which led to the County Asylum Act of 1808 that laid specifications for the building and maintenance of county asylums and, eventually, a separate hospital system. The Lunacy Act of 1845, passed as a result of exploitation and abuse of patients, provided for a permanent body to inspect all asylums and private institutions. The commissioners were stringent and as staff and operating costs soared so did the dissatisfaction of the bill-paying parishioners. Only in 1861 was the Act amended and costs met from central rather than parish funds.

LACK OF NURSE TRAINING

There had been no training for personnel in this field and psychiatry had yet to become a formal discipline but the new philosophy of rehabilitation underscored the need for education and standards for care givers. Because of costs institutions had shelved training for nurses for many years. A campaign organized by the Medico-Psychological Association led by 1981 to the national examination of nurses. Improvements in this century have led to a change from mainly institutional care by poorly trained nurses to largely community-based care by highly skilled professionals.

The 1919 Registration of Nurses Act created a supplementary part of the Registry of nurses trained by the Medico-Psychological Association (RMPA), with separate sections for mental illness and mental deficiency. Under the RMPA examiners were medical superintendents and schools were not required to be directed by a trained nurse. The General Nursing Council (GNC), however, set up training courses directed by a matron and examining boards that included nurses. A compromise between the two organizations on educational and examining requirements resulted in a new training syllabus (Athlone) and in 1946 the RMPA ceased training. During its 80 years the RMPA had granted 40 000 certificates in mental nursing and 47 000 in mental deficiency nursing (White, 1985).

The 1930 Treatment Act, designed to alleviate the stigma of mental illness, raised the status of mental illness hospitals as well as attending nurses and doctors. Voluntary admission to hospital and development of advanced treatments, such as electroconvulsive and insulin therapy, and neurosurgery brought improvements to patients, and education increased public understanding and acceptance. The 1946 Act repealed the Lunacy and Treatment Acts of 1930 and 1890 and the Mental Deficiency Acts of 1913 and 1936.

Shortage of Mental Nurses

In 1948 when this service became part of the NHS recruitment of mental nurses was almost at a standstill and it was estimated that there was a shortage of 25–50% trained nurses, exacerbated by compulsory National Service for men. The General Nursing Council, which advocated attracting recruits by raising standards, encouraged general trained nurses to undertake mental care training as a second qualification. However the situation continued to deteriorate. The number of students fell by 20% in the discipline of mental illness and 25% in that of mental deficiency between 1951 and 1955 (Bendall, 1969), with about an 80% wastage rate. The patient/nurse ratio in 1953 was 6:7 patient/1 nurse in mental illness and 6:9 patient/1 nurse in mental deficiency hospitals (Ministry of Health, Annual Report, 1953).

The still-powerful medical superintendents, the highly formalized and rigid relationship between nursing, medical and administrative staffs and the isolation of mental hospitals all contributed to a perceived second class status. Because mental health laws clearly needed updating the Mental Health Act of 1959 was passed. Statutory recognition of mental health made it more important that standards and number of mental nurses, now known as psychiatric nurses, improved, although there was virtually no increase in numbers between 1949 and 1959 (Table 3.2).

Table 3.2 Mental and mental deficiency nursing staff

	Mental (hospital) nursing staff 1949	Mental (hospital) nursing staff 1959	Mental deficiency nursing staff 1949	Mental deficiency nursing staff 1959
Trained				
full time	11 056	11 415	2 613	3 343
part time	1 147	1 446	250	406
Students	5 201	6 178	1 135	1 289
Other nursing staff				
full time	2 610	7 038	1 706	3 614
part time	4 398	5 288	1 496	2 088

Source: Ministry of Health Nursing Statistics (1959).

In 1964 minimum educational standards for psychiatric nursing students were introduced, but the shortage of trained nurses persisted in spite of improved services and a change in emphasis from custodial and treatment care in hospitals to community care. The most recent effort to improve quality of care as well as nurses' education has been the 1982 syllabus of education based on principles of sociopsychological pathology.

NURSING AS A PROFESSION: 1850–1900

The introduction of nurse training in the latter part of the 19th century played a vital role in the making of the profession. St John's House began training nurses in 1848 and King's College in 1856. Florence Nightingale, the most influential of the reformists, founded a nurse training school at St Thomas's Hospital in 1860, based on the teachings and philosophy of Pastor Fliedner's Institute at Kaiserwerth. However her most lasting contribution to nursing may have been the installing of a spirit of dedicated service (Smith, 1982) like that she had observed in the deaconesses at Kaiserwerth.

A person of great determination and influence, Miss Nightingale was able to use circumstances to achieve her goals. Not only were trained nurses badly needed to cope with advances in medical technology stemming, for example, from the work of Joseph Lister, Louis Pasteur and James Simpson, but also respectability for the new profession would fill a social need by providing an outlet for the social consciences and frustrated energies of single Victorian women (Abel Smith, 1960).

The St Thomas's Hospital school attracted young ladies of the highest social class and it was not long before the potential of nursing as suitable for the upper class women was realized. By 1903 the school had issued 1907 certificates (House of Commons Select Committee, 1905). These women became Miss Nightingale's missionaries in nursing reform as training schools proliferated. Because infirmaries and workhouses attracted only lower social class girls it became apparent to some that the only way to secure status was to standardize examinations and centralize registration in order to guarantee quality of care. A battle for power to control nursing labour and education developed but, by the end of the century, it was accepted in voluntary hospitals that the matron was the head of the independent department.

Mrs Bedford Fenwick, a nurse and feminist, was one of the originators of State Registration, which Miss Nightingale firmly opposed. The argument about registration was not just a battle of principles: the real issue (one writer called it a 30-year war) was a battle of status conducted in an atmosphere of rampant snobbery and militant feminism. Further conflict arose when the Hospital Association set up its register, prompting others to form the Association of British Nurses (ABN) in 1893. The ABN started its register, requiring three years training of its students, a decision that had far reaching effects on future length of study. The group wanted registration *and* national standards and urged all hospitals to set up boards of education. To gain more support they also founded the Matrons' Council of Great Britain and Ireland in 1894, which was instrumental in promoting an International Council of Nurses (ICN). The National Council of Nurses of the United Kingdom came into being in 1904 to represent British nurses on the ICN.

An important precedent for nurses was the Midwives' Act 1902, which required registration with the Central Midwives' Board. Each year between 1901 and 1904 a nurse registration bill was laid before parliament without success. The war years brought great upheaval as nurses were needed in unprecedented numbers. Demand was met by recruiting untrained personnel, known as the Voluntary Aids Detachment (VAD), to work in hospitals, while trained nurses cared for the wounded. VADs, however, found their way to the wounded and worked alongside trained nurses and Red Cross volunteers. Lack of coordinated organization among nurses led to the suggestion of a College of Nursing to promote nursing and the advancement of nursing as a profession. The College was registered in 1916 and its business controlled by Council (Baly, 1980).

There was considerable friction between the Royal British Nursing Association an the College of Nursing (CN), each organization presenting its bill on registration to parliament. The CN presented its bill to the House of Lords, the Royal British Nursing Association its bill to the House of Commons, and the government brought in its own bill under which the Minister of Health appointed the Council. In December 1919 the Minister's bill received Royal Assent. The Nurses Registration Act 1919 contained four parts: distinctions between general, mental illness and children's nurses and a separate register for men. There were separate councils for England and Wales, Scotland and Northern Ireland.

NATURE OF THE REGISTRATION ACT

Official recognition of nursing by the Registration Act did not create greater unity among the professional organizations. Undisputedly the College of Nursing, which in 1928 received its Royal Charter (thus becoming the RCN), became the major voice of the profession. Its main purpose became (RCN, 1984) and still is to:

1. promote the science of nursing and better education and efficiency of nurses;
2. promote the advance of nursing as a profession in all branches;
3. promote the professional standing and interests of members of the nursing profession;
4. promote, through international agencies and otherwise, the foregoing purposes in other countries;
5. assist nurses who by reason of adversity, ill health or otherwise are in need of assistance of any nature;
6. institute and conduct examinations and grant certificates and diplomas to those who satisfy the requirements of the Council of the College.

As hospitals and local authorities clamoured to employ registered nurses, the shortage of well trained nurses became acute. Recruitment became somewhat easier between the two World Wars but, according to a survey by the General Nursing Council, the proportion of untrained staff in hospital rose steadily.

Pressure from a profession concerned about shortage, wastage and education led the government to set up a Committee of Nursing Services in 1938 under the chairmanship of Lord Athlone. The survey showed that in 1937 there were 113 700 hospital nursing staff in England and Wales, an increase of 13% since 1933. Of nurses 86% were female, 30% were trained nurses and midwives, 38% were students and 25% were untrained. The proportion of untrained nursing staff had risen by 3% in four years but the number of trained staff had also increased by almost 1% (Athlone, 1939).

THE SECOND WORLD WAR

During the Second World War it was anticipated that 67 000 nurses would be needed. The Emergency Nursing Committee was set up to organize a Civil Nursing Reserve that, in 1939, attracted 7000 trained nurses, 3000 assistant nurses and 20 000 auxiliaries. These people were divided into three grades, with little definition of standard. The Ministry of Health thus became the largest employer of nurses and so created a Division of Nursing at government level.

To plan for the post-war period, a Committee of Reconstruction was set up under the chairmanship of William Beveridge, which reported on Social Insurance and Allied Services (1942). The proposals, designed for a pluralistic society, resulted in interrelated legislation in four crucial social services areas: Education Act (1944), National Health Act (1946), Family Allowance Act (1946) and National Insurance Act (1948).

In 1943 the Nurses' Salary Committee, under the chairmanship of Rushcliff (England and Wales) and Taylor (Scotland) prompted the Nurses' Act 1943 and provided a starting point for the first Nurses and Midwives Whitley Council, 1948. Under this Act the enrolled assistant nurse became subject to a professional code of conduct and to the discipline of the General Nursing Council. The Ministry of Health was empowered to restrict the title 'nurse' to those with recognized training. Following the war there was an acute shortage of nurses and midwives and 30 000 beds were closed for lack of staff. The Armed Services in contrast, had no shortage of applicants.

THE NATIONAL HEALTH SERVICE

The NHS was established in 1948 under the 1946 NHS Act. The entirely new principle of universal coverage provided for free medical care, available equally to poor and rich and free at the point of delivery. There were already 19.5 million people covered by national health insurance and, by the end of 1948, 21.5 million additional people had registered with a general practitioner. Doctors reported a marked increase in demand for services and many more patients were referred to hospital outpatient departments. Dentists and opticians were flooded with demands for service.

The introduction of the NHS was a major administrative undertaking, particularly in the establishment of planned and coordinated hospital services. It also involved major changes in relationships, especially for the medical profession, and adjustments by the various segments did not come easily (Abel Smith, 1978). The NHS consisted of three parts: hospital services, family practitioner services and local authority services that included health visiting, midwifery and district nursing. In 1949, in England and Wales, there were about 130 000 nursing and 12 000 midwifery staff working in hospitals and 12 000 health visitors and district nurses in the community (Ministry of Health statistics). Health services were administered by Regional Hospital Boards and day-to-day business left to Group Hospital Management Committees, including a nursing committee. In the UK the cost of the NHS in 1949 was 3.9% of the gross national product; by mid-1980s this had almost doubled.

Nursing and midwifery services in hospitals remained under the control of the matron or chief male nurse, and in the local authorities under the chief medical officer of health. The NHS Reorganisation Act 1973 brought all health services, except family practitioner committees, under the health authorities. Changes most affecting nurses during that period were the increasing acceptance of male nurses, married nurses and, by implication, part-time staff. This period also saw educational changes responding to modern needs. The 1949 and 1957 Nurses' Acts were passed and specialization of post-basic education became an important element. A number of committees concerned with nursing practice and education also had their influence, such as:

Committee	*Chairman*
Nursing Reconstruction Committee	Lord Horder (1943–9)
Recruitment and Training of Nursing	Sir R. Wood (1946–7)
Work of the Nurse in Hospital Wards	H. A. Goddard (1948–53)
A Reform of Nursing Education	Sir H. Platt (1961–4)
Report of the Committee of Senior Nursing Structure	B. Salmon (1963–5)
Report of the Committee of Nursing	A Briggs (1970–7)
Committee of Inquiry into the Pay and Related Conditions of Service of Nurses and Midwives 1974	Rt Hon the Earl of Halsbury

There is no doubt that the last 20 years have been the most eventful for the nursing professions. Science has made tremendous advances, medical technology and psychology have provided tools undreamed of before and nursing research has established itself. Changes in nursing practice, education and management were therefore inevitable. The Salmon Report of 1965 had far-reaching effects on the organizational structure of the nursing service. Based on an industrial model, it created a three-tier structure of reasonable span of control, first line, middle and top management. Emphasis was being placed on management skills and roles had to be redefined.

When the NHS was reorganized in 1974 creating health authorities, areas and districts were formed and top management nurses became members of the management team. One of the problems of the structure was the number of tiers of command and in 1979 a Royal Commission on the NHS recommended the abolition of area health authorities, which was effected in 1982.

As with the introduction of the senior nursing staff structure, the unification of the NHS and its subsequent fine tuning, the nursing service had experienced radical change. The most recent change, in organizational terms, saw the introduction of general managers to head the management of health authorities, the result of recommendations by a working party on management arrangements (Griffiths, 1983). One of the provisions affecting nursing in this arrangement was the new advisory role on professional matters given to general managers and health authorities.

One of the major changes in education, and indeed the profession, was the introduction of the Nurses, Health Visitors and Midwives Act 1979, which brought the three entities under one control on a UK basis. The United Kingdom Central Councils for Nursing, Midwifery and Health Visiting (UKCC) took over the function of the General Nursing Councils, the Council of Training of Health Visitors and the Central Midwives' Boards, previously responsible for registration, and is responsible for education within UKCC legislation. It also took on the Joint Board of Clinical Nursing Studies, England, Wales and Scotland and the panel of District Nursing for post registration education and qualifications.

During almost 40 years of the NHS nursing manpower has increased not only in total volume, to over half a million whole-time equivalents in the UK in 1991, but also in the proportion of qualified nurses, which has increased to 61.5% compared to less than 50% at its inception. In addition some 40–50 thousand nursing staff are employed in the independent sector. The private sector is relatively small compared to the size of the NHS but over the past few years activities of private hospitals have greatly increased. This will have implications not only for the total supply of qualified nurses and midwives but also for nurse education, which will need to take this into consideration in future years.

Budget

The NHS is mainly financed by central government funds through taxation and, to a much lesser extent, by NHS contributions and patient charges (Figure 3.1).

Figure 3.1 National Health Service funding in England

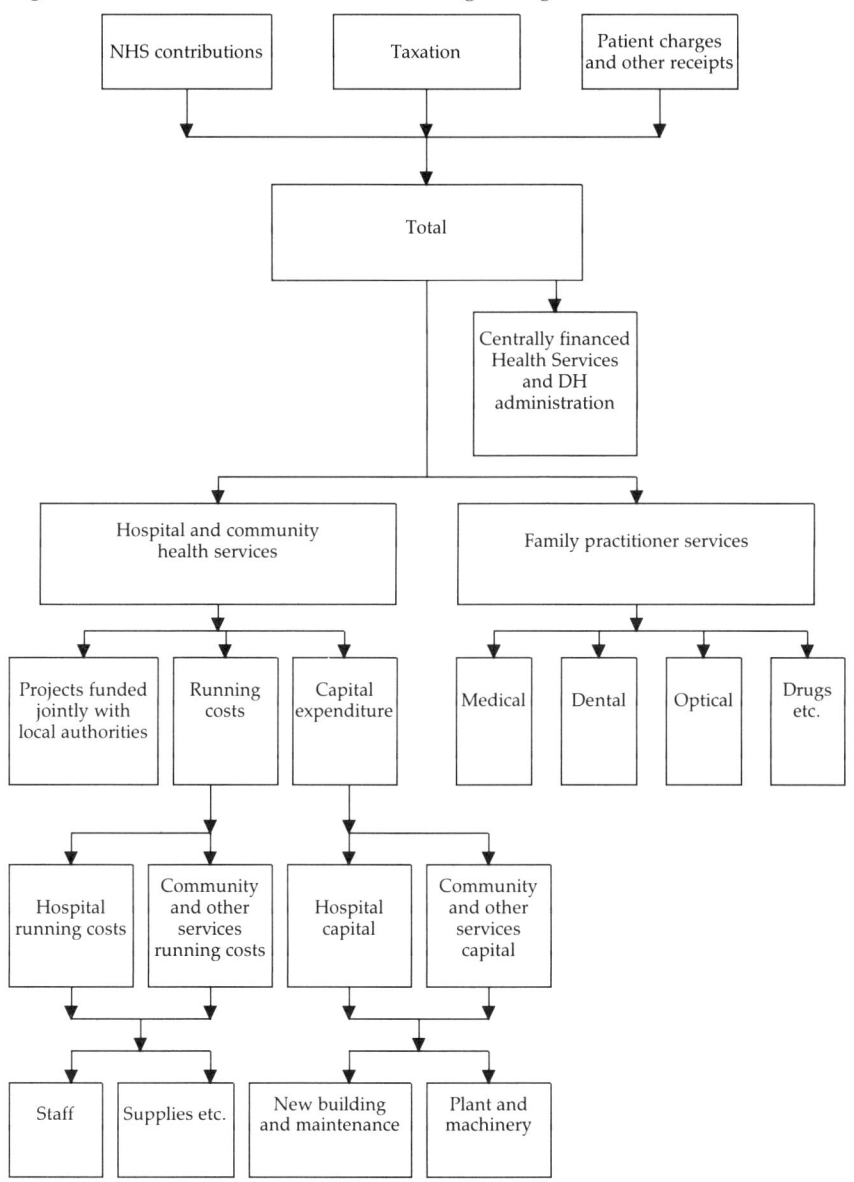

Expenditure on health services in the UK amounted to over 6% of the GNP. Since the 1978/9 financial year spending on the NHS has more than trebled. Hospital and Community Services consumed 72% of this and Family Practitioner Services the remaining 38%. Table 3.3 gives some demographic data.

Table 3.3 Some demographic statistics for the UK:

Area (sq. miles)	94 226
Population (in 1990)	57 121 000
Population density (per sq. mile)	
urban (in 1985)	601
rural	7.5
GNP (in 1989)	$843 billion
per capita	$14 535
Life expectancy (in 1989)	
male	72
female	78

Government allocates resources to regions, responsible for distribution in line with government policy. The aim has been towards achieving equity of access to the population and a service to the point of delivery. For more than ten years this policy was underpinned by allocation of funds according to a complex formula partly based on mortality indicators (Resource Allocation Working Party RAWP). Despite considerable progress towards equalization large variations in the levels of service and the cost persisted at sub-regional level. Medical consultants, who are largely responsible for determining spending levels, had so far had little incentive to count the cost.

The recent review of the National Health Service, 'Working for Patients' was the most radical yet and resulted in the NHS and Community Care Act 1990. The Act received Royal assent on the 29th June 1990 and proposed a programme for action which came into effect on April 1st 1991 with two main objectives:

1. To give patients a better quality of health care and greater choice of service available;
2. To provide greater satisfaction and reward to those working in the NHS who successfully respond to local needs and preferences.

The overall effect of the measure is expected to make the health service more responsive to patients. Accountability for resources will be improved and medical consultants, in particular, will be encouraged to play a greater part in the management of hospitals.

The most radical part of the NHS reform is changes in the funding arrangements. Funding of the health care is separated from its provision.

Budget holders – general practitioners and health authority managers – will buy services by competitive tender from competing public and private suppliers of care (hospitals and community units). Now and in the future the cost and, more importantly, the outcome of treatment will need to be known so that best use can be made of resources. Funding allocation will therefore be determined by a managed marketplace for decades to come.

The NHS and Community Care Act 1990 brings with it many changes that require the development of a new organisational culture, which spells not only new freedoms but also new responsibilities. For those who buy health services through the contractual process it means identifying the population's health needs and obtaining and monitoring value for money. Health authorities are required to establish a public health function whose actions in the health field can be better directed towards needs, that is to prevent disease, prolong life and promote health by understanding the determinants of disease in a given population – the epidemiology of health and service, the establishment of mechanisms to institute effective action.

This change will affect the objectives and priorities of health services, which will no longer be directed by historically determined patterns of service provision. For those providing care it means planning and managing health care that is responsive to the direction and priorities defined by the contractual process. The organizational developments will have a profound influence on human resource planning and education. The planning process is being decentralized and most health manpower supply and demand needs are expected to be determined at operational level. As part of the implementation process of the NHS reform the government issued a number of working papers on, for example, the establishment of National Health Service Trusts, the role of new district health authorities, information requirements and resource management, medical audit and education and training.

4

Nursing education

John M. Rogers

Chapter 3 traced the history of nursing in the UK and some of the major legislation and developments affecting the education and training of nurses. This chapter describes the current system of education and training and some possible future developments.

THE STATUTORY FRAMEWORK OF NURSE EDUCATION

The 1972 Report of the Committee on Nursing (The Briggs Report; DHSS, 1972) made recommendations concerning both statutory framework and content for nurse education. The legislative result of the Report was the 1979 Nurses, Midwives and Health Visitors Act, which joined a number of separate bodies for each of the professions into one statutory framework by establishing the United Kingdom Central Council for Nursing, Midwifery and Health Visiting (UKCC) and a National Board for each of the four UK countries.

The UKCC has the following principal functions:

1. To establish and improve standards of training for nurses, midwives and health visitors ('training' is the terminology of the Act) and to set qualifications for entry and kinds and standards of training;
2. To maintain a Register of those who qualify after training;
3. To establish and improve standards of and provide advice on the conduct of nurses, midwives and health visitors.

The National Boards have the following principal functions:

1. To provide or arrange for others to provide at Board approved institutions:
    (a) courses of training leading to qualifications and registration or recording of additional qualifications in the Register;
    (b) courses of additional training for those already registered;
2. To ensure that courses meet UKCC requirements on content and standard;
3. To hold or arrange for others to hold examinations;
4. To collaborate with the UKCC in improving training methods;
5. To investigate cases of alleged misconduct, referring those where a

prima facie case is established to the UKCC for disciplinary proceedings.

In educational terms, then, the UKCC sets the broad framework of qualifications for entry to training, the general method of training and the competencies to be achieved, while detailed syllabuses and approval of institutions that carry out nurse training are the responsibility of the national boards.

CONSTITUTION OF THE UKCC AND NATIONAL BOARDS

The UKCC consists of 28 members nominated by each National Board and 17 members appointed by the government. It elects its own Chairman. The Boards consist of members elected by the professions and those appointed by the government. The National Board elects and appoint some of their members. The Boards also elect their own Chairmen [1].

WHAT HAPPENS IN PRACTICE?

The preceding brief outline of the statutory framework omits to mention a third major influence on nurse education, that is the health authorities and boards that manage the NHS. The following section concentrates, for clarity, on the position in England, although there are some differences in the organization of both the NHS and nurse education in the other UK countries, and on the position prior to Project 2000, the reform of nurse education partially introduced in 1989.

The UKCC established standards of training through the Nurses, Midwives and Health Visitors Rule Approval Order 1983. The UKCC shall produce its own rules, which have statutory force but which must be approved by government ministers. This Order sets minimum qualifications for entry to nurse training. The 'first level' nursing (that is training for qualification of Registered General Nurse, Registered Sick Children's Nurse, Registered Mental Nurse and Registered Nurse for the Mentally Handicapped) qualification was, from 1st January 1986, 5 'O' (Ordinary) levels in the General Certification of Education in England and Wales or the Scottish or Northern Irish equivalents. Examinations for 'O' levels were usually taken at age 16; by contrast, university or other higher education entry usually requires two or more 'A' (Advanced) levels, taken at age 18. Entry to 'second level' training (the Enrolled Nurse) requires no formal academic qualifications. The Order sets the minimum statutory age for entry to training as 17½ years.

The Order also sets general content and standards of nurse training. For first level nurses training must enable the student to accept responsibility for personal development and acquire competency to:

1. Advise on promotion of health and prevention of illness;
2. Recognize situations detrimental to the health and well-being of an individual;
3. Carry out activities involved in conducting a comprehensive assessment of a patient's nursing requirements;
4. Recognize the significance of observations and use them to develop an initial nursing assessment;
5. Devise a nursing plan based on the assessment, with the cooperation of the patient to the maximum extent possible, taking into account the medical prescription;
6. Implement planned programmes of nursing care and, where appropriate, teach and coordinate other members of the nursing team; also to be responsible for implementing specific aspects of the nursing care;
7. Review the effectiveness of nursing care provided and, where appropriate, initiate any required action;
8. Work in a team with other nurses, medical and paramedical staff and social workers;
9. Manage the care of a group of patients over a period of time and organize appropriate support services.

Competencies are all to be related to the care of the kind of patient the student will encounter once registered.

Competencies required of a second level nurse are:

1. To assist in carrying out comprehensive observations of patients and help in assessing care requirements;
2. To develop skills to assist in the implementation of nursing care under the direction of a first level nurse;
3. To accept delegated nursing tasks;
4. To assist in reviewing the effectiveness of care provided;
5. To work in a team with other nurses, medical and paramedical staff and social workers.

The rules also fix the minimum length of training: three years for first level nurses (three years and ten weeks in England) and 18 months for second level nurses (in practice two years in England). Entry and other requirements for midwifery are similar but health visitor training is taken as post-basic training after registration in another part of the register. (Although it is possible to undertake a three-year midwifery education along the same broad lines as nurse education, few such courses are available in practice and most midwives undertake an 18-month training following qualification as a nurse.) District nursing is not part of the register but is a recordable post-basic qualification.

Within this general framework the National Boards prepare syllabuses to meet UKCC criteria. They also provide, or arrange for others to provide, training courses. The English National Board (ENB) conducts no courses directly. These are provided by NHS nursing or midwifery schools (administered by health authorities) or institutions of higher education (universities or polytechnics).

Health authorities influence training in three ways: first, with most learners being on their payrolls they effectively determine the numbers in training; second, they arrange for the practical element of training; and, third, they influence the number of courses offered. 'Learners' is the generic term for both students (those training for first level nursing) and pupils (those training for second level nursing). The ENB has established Educational Advisory Groups in each English health region, which advise on the distribution of Board funds to schools of nursing within the region and, in theory, act as a forum for resolving the sometimes conflicting demands of the service and education requirements. In practice health authorities can, at short notice and usually for financial reasons, cancel intakes to nursing and midwifery schools.

In addition to preparing syllabuses and arranging for courses the ENB approves institutions providing training. In practice this duty is exercised primarily for NHS schools of nursing and midwifery; the Board does not 'approve' in the same way whole institutions of higher education or universities that provide nurse education as a minor part of their overall activities. The Board employs professional headquarters staff to inspect institutions, report to the Board and advise the institutions. Criteria considered during inspections include the number and quality of tutorial staff, the physical environment and the proportion of qualified staff in clinical areas where learners receive practical experience. The Board generally approves an institution for a period of time, usually five years, although in some instances a shorter period of approval is given and sometimes (usually by agreement with the authority concerned) approval is withheld and training ceases while improvements are made.

FINANCING OF NURSE EDUCATION

There is a wide range of funding sources for nurse education. Almost all funding is from taxation, the private health sector contributing little. The main sources are given below.

Health authorities

Health authorities, with funds almost all provided from taxes, pay the training allowances (salaries) of most learners. That learners are paid a salary, rather than a grant or bursary, is in part recognition that they make significant regular contributions to patient care. In addition learners are eligible for special duty payments (nights or weekends) and overtime, although they work fewer unsocial or extended hours than qualified staff. Learners are included in health authority staff for manpower planning and control purposes. Also health authorities pay the salaries of most qualified staff taking additional basic training in a different specialty. Exceptions to these general rules are undergraduate nursing students who generally receive grants from local authorities and whose tuition costs are covered by the higher education (HE) funding bodies. Those taking health visitor, district nurse, community psychiatric nurse and community mental handicap nurse training do so within higher education (polytechnics, etc.). Health authorities pay salaries and part of tuition fees for all but a small number who pay their own expenses; the balance of tuition fees is met by the HE funding bodies. Health authorities also finance 'on-the-ward' teaching costs of learners, that is loss of time to patient care due to the purely educational contribution of ward staff as well as any extra time taken over normal ward duties because of the presence of learners. In addition health authorities maintain NHS schools of nursing and midwifery and pay heating and lighting costs and local taxes.

The UKCC and National Board

The UKCC is primarily financed from registration fees, paid on a basis of periodic three-yearly fees. The National Boards, on the other hand, are almost entirely dependent on direct government funding, although a small proportion of their income derives from examination fees paid by the health authorities. From this the ENB pays salaries and other costs of its headquarters administrative and professional staff, and the salaries of most teaching staff in NHS schools of nursing midwifery. It also pays the salaries of administrative, clerical and support staff in schools, although there are minor variations throughout the country in cost apportionment between the ENB and health authorities. The Board also pays the cost of preparing teachers of nursing, midwifery and health visiting in the HE sector.

For England the Board makes arrangements for controlling and monitoring expenditure. In each region the Regional Treasurer, or an officer nominated by him, is designated as the Board's local financial agent. He is also a member of a non-statutory regional Educational Advisory Group (EAG) established by the Board (there is provision in the 1979 Act for statutory local training committees but these have never been established). The Board submits estimates of expenditure to the Department of Health and, after approval of a national cash limit by the Department, notifies each financial agent of the region's cash limit for the year. The agent, in consultation with the EAG, then apportions the cash limit among schools and advises each Director of Nurse Education (DNE), as budget holder for the school, of the budget. The DNE may incur expenditure against the budget within the Board's guidelines and on advice of the EAG. Adjustments to the borderline between Board and health authority expenditure may not be made without agreement of the Board. (There are minor variations among regions.) Support for the DNE is provided by District Treasurers (e.g. with regard to payroll services, financial information and budget monitoring). Expenditure is not incurred directly by regions for nurse training but regions charge the EAGs for support and accommodation services.

Higher education

All district nurse, health visitor, community psychiatric nurse and community mental handicap nurse education occurs in HE institutions and requires basic nursing qualification. In addition some schemes of basic nurse training occur in HE institutions and a small number of nurses obtain registrable professional qualifications in conjunction with a university degree. Tuition fees for most health visitor and district nurse courses are subsidised from the HE funding pool, distributed by the Polytechnics and Colleges Funding Council (PCFC). The pool constitutes the direct taxpayer subsidy to HE. HE tuition for undergraduate courses is paid by local education authorities but is subsidized by the general taxpayer's contribution to HE costs, via the Universities Funding Council (UFC) and the PCFC.

The overall cost of nurse education

From the previous discussion it follows that, given the complexity of funding arrangements, estimating the true costs of nurse education is difficult. The only recent reasonably comprehensive study is a 1984 Discussion Paper from the Centre for Health Economics, University of York (Hartley and Goodwin, 1985). This study concentrated on the training of Registered General Nurses (RGNs) and Enrolled Nurses (General) (ENGs) and concluded that the main components of the training costs of the groups were:

1. ENB expenditure;
2. District health authorities, i.e. costs of running and maintaining the 168 schools of nursing in England;

3. 'On-the-ward' teaching costs, i.e. costs of the teaching contribution of ward staff, in particular the ward sister/charge nurse;
4. Net salary costs, i.e. gross salary costs of learners minus costs of replacement staff that health authorities would have to employ in the absence of learners, in recognition that learners contribute to service during training.

While stressing that calculation of net cost is sensitive to assumptions about the service contribution of learners, the authors concluded that the gross cost of training general nurses in 1982–3 was £330 million and the net cost, after allowing for the service contribution, £126 million. The main reason for the real terms increase in costs of training between 1963 and 1983 (271% for RGNs; 516% for ENGs) was the significant rise in salaries of learners relative to qualified staff and unqualified nursing auxiliaries. Net costs in real terms probably will have declined since 1982–3 with the significant decrease in the number of pupil enrolled nurses in training.

THE PROJECT 2000 REFORMS OF NURSE EDUCATION

The picture described in the preceding section has undergone radical change since 1989. In the Spring of 1986 the UKCC published its initial Project 2000 proposals for the reform of nurse education. After consultation with the nursing, midwifery and health visiting professions and detailed work on the cost and manpower implications of the proposals, revised proposals were formally presented to the government in February 1987. These were agreed with some modification. In their final form the proposals have emerged as follows:

1. There should be a new, single level of registered practitioner, competent to assess the need for care, provide care, monitor and evaluate care in both institutional and non-institutional settings. Second level training would be discontinued. The new practitioner would be capable of working in both hospital and community settings rather than, as in the past, requiring further specialist training for community work.
2. All branches of nursing should share a common foundation programme of education in the first 18 months of training, followed by specialization in the second half of the course. Branches would consist of mental illness, mental handicap, adult and child nursing. The separate branches would continue to be separately recorded in the Register.
3. Nursing qualifications would have academic currency at higher education, AG Diploma level. This implies that NHS schools of nursing

would have to seek academic validation of their courses from a local AG institution or become part of AG.
4. Students should be supernumerary to NHS staffing establishments through most of their course. Previously general students, for example, made a major contribution to services to patients, being on rostered duty for some 50–60% of the training period; under Project 2000 this rostered service contribution reduces to 15%.
5. Instead of salaries, students should be paid bursaries, which would remain NHS-controlled but be derived from a separately identified education budget. Bursaries have been set at a level only slightly below that of the net income of the average salaried student nurse.
6. The UKCC proposed that all teachers of nursing, midwifery and health visiting should have teaching or other qualifications at degree level. This proposal was not specifically endorsed by the government but, in practice, an all-degree teaching workforce is emerging rapidly.
7. There should be a new grade of helper, with formal training, directly supervised and monitored by the registered practitioner.
8. Midwifery education was excluded from the Project 2000 proposals. In practice, in some locations, nursing and midwifery students were to undertake a substantial amount of shared learning with nursing students even if they were not a formal part of the Project 2000 common foundation programme.

These proposals had profound implications, in terms of delivery of service and of finance, for the NHS. To explain these fully it is necessary to provide some background data about the nature of the NHS nursing and midwifery workforce. The total number of nursing and midwifery staff in Great Britain rose from 240 000 whole-time equivalents in 1962 to just over 480 000 in 1984. This total includes professionally qualified staff, learners and unqualified auxiliary staff. The proportion of registered (first level) nurses stayed relatively constant at around 35% throughout this period but, at the same time, the proportion of enrolled (second level) nurses rose from 7% to 18%. The proportion of students (first level), however, declined sharply from 27% to 15%. The proportion of pupils (second level) started at 3–4% in the early 1960s, rose to around 7% in the early 1970s but dropped back to 3–4% in the mid-1980s.

Over the 20 years leading up to the preparation of the Project 2000 proposals there was a gradual decline in the service contribution made by learners during training – particularly marked in mental illness and mental handicap training – following the introduction of new syllabuses in 1982. In times past intakes to training were dictated as much by the need

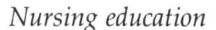

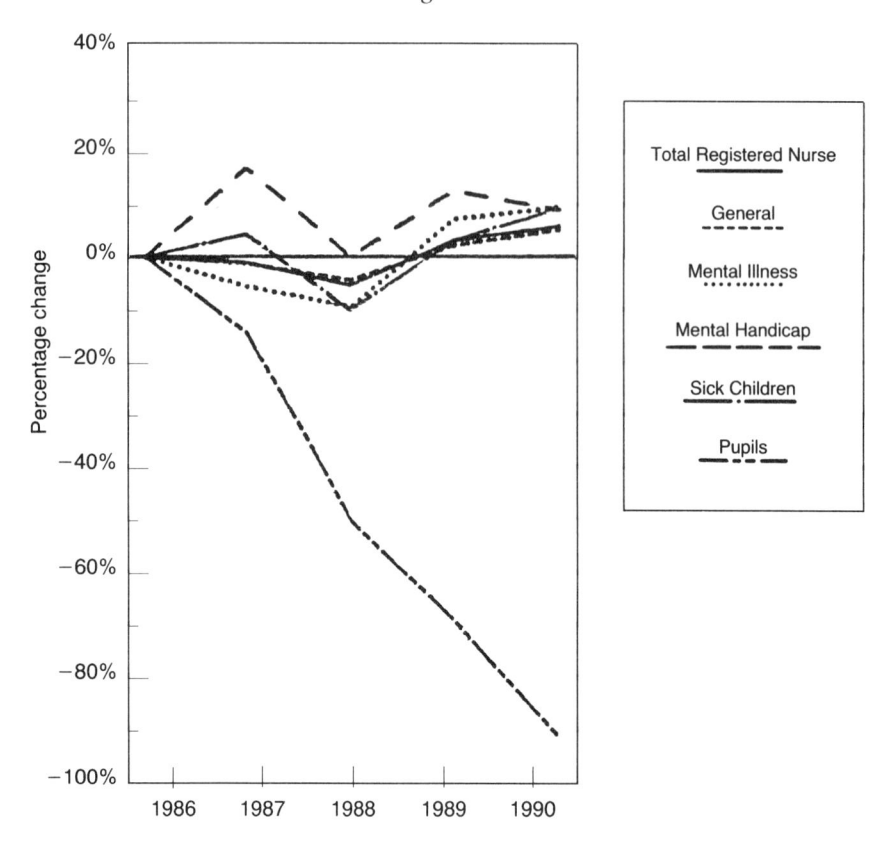

Figure 4.1 Intakes to pre-registration nurse training in England, Percentage change March 1986–90. Source: English National Board for Nurses, Midwives and Health Visitors, 1991.

for the service contribution learners made as by the need to provide newly qualified staff. During the 1980s the need for replacement qualified staff was generally estimated at around 10% a year. Two-thirds of this was met from learners qualifying and one third by qualified staff returning after a break in service. However wastage during training and failure to practise on qualification meant that the number of learners needed to be around 10% of the current stock to make sure of meeting replacement needs. On that basis the mid-1980s England intake of students and pupils, of around 25 000 a year, was adequate for a stock of 240 000 whole-time equivalent qualified staff. However, at the same time, there was evidence that the participation rates of qualified nurses (that is their propensity to remain active in the workforce) was growing in line with the behaviour patterns of the female workforce generally. Although conclusive evidence will not be to hand until the detailed results of the 1991 Census are available, there is little doubt that replacement needs were declining through the decade.

The other major factor affecting numbers in training is demography. In the mid-1980s it was estimated that nursing was taking between 20% and 25% of all female school leavers with between 5 'O' level and 2 'A' level passes. This group was projected to decline sharply from 73 000 in 1982–3 to 53 000 in 1991–3 as the result of the declining birthrate in the 1970s. If recruitment continued to be mainly from this age group and if second level training were to be phased out with the number of pupils replaced by students, nursing could be trying to recruit over 40% of the cohort. This was inherently unlikely.

The relevance of these and other factors to the acceptance of the Project 2000 proposals is complex. The reduction in the service contribution of traditional nurse learners, and the change in participation rates leading to a reduction in the numbers of replacement staff needed, made the proposals cheaper to implement than they would have been in previous decades. (It is worth noting that, in broad outline, the Project 2000 proposals were not dissimilar from proposals that had been made at various times over the preceding 40 years.) At the same time the decline in the number of school leavers meant that nurse education needed to be made more attractive to intending students, as well as efforts being made to widen the recruitment base, particularly by recruiting older entrants to training. Government plans to expand significantly the number of students in HE suggested to many that nursing qualifications needed to have academic currency if nursing was to compete effectively with other forms of education as far as school leavers were concerned. A further contributory factor may well have been the way in which nursing issues, vigorously promoted by professional organizations and trade unions, were placed higher on the political and managerial agendas than hitherto.

Nevertheless the cost and organizational implications of implementing Project 2000 were considerable. Organizationally the need to replace the lost service contribution of students, the requirement to link nurse education to AG and the need to give additional training to a substantial proportion of the existing workforce in order that they could supervise Project 2000 students effectively all required a major managerial effort. Consequently the government agreed to phase in Project 2000 over a number of years. A start was made in England in 1989 when 13 schools of nursing were approved by the ENB to introduce Project 2000, with funding provided by the Department of Health. A further 16 sites followed in 1990. By 1991 49 colleges had introduced Project 2000 and 50% were directed on the new training schemes (Table 4.1).

Table 4.1 Intakes to training by course of study – England: years ended 31 March 1986 to 1990

Specialty and trainee class	1986	1987	1988	1989	1990	change 1989/90
A. Pre-registration nurse training (1)						
Registered nurse training: total	18 597	18 422	17 642	19 183	19 688	2.6%
Traditional training: total	18 597	18 422	17 642	19 183	18 618	−2.9%
General	14 208	14 002	13 581	14 473	14 094	−2.6%
Mental	2 707	2 559	2 458	2 896	2 794	−3.5%
Mental handicap	894	1 040	893	1 003	926	−7.7%
Sick children	788	821	710	811	804	−0.9%
Project 2000: Total	–	–	–	–	1 070	–
Adult	–	–	–	–	806	–
Mental illness	–	–	–	–	164	–
Mental handicap	–	–	–	–	45	–
Child	–	–	–	–	55	–
Pupils: total	5 105	4 391	2 625	1 694	591	−65.1%
General	4 204	3 665	2 303	1 517	484	−68.1%
Mental	704	524	205	106	54	−49.1%
Mental handicap	197	202	117	71	53	−25.4%
B. Post-registration training						
Midwifery students (2)	2 961	2 759	2 720	2 707	2 595	−4.1%
Health visitor students (3)	872	856	847	823	847	2.9%
District nurse students:	1 221	1 216	1 131	1 211	1 241	2.5%
Registered general nurse	946	927	935	898	845	−5.9%
Enrolled nurse (G)	275	289	196	313	396	26.5%
C. Other post-registration training (4)						
General intensive care	436	502	394	462	555	20.1%
Coronary care	60	61	70	70	74	5.7%
Paediatric intensive care (5)	–	–	23	61	75	23.0%
Neonatal intensive care	278	393	291	309	395	27.8%
Renal	132	140	143	160	182	13.8%
Operating department nursing	272	249	192	227	233	2.6%
Community psychiatric nursing	243	212	273	274	306	11.7%
Community mental handicap nursing	84	48	90	81	97	19.8%

Source: English National Board for Nursing, Midwifery and Health Visiting.

Notes:
1. These figures relate to all nurse learners entering nurse training, including those undertaking training for a further pre-registration nurse qualification.
2. Includes direct entry midwifery students.
3. These figures relate to entrants in the previous September.
4. These figures relate to registered nurses and midwives.
5. The first intakes to this training occurred during 1988.

Other developments

In July 1986 the government published a White Paper 'Working Together – Education and Training' which announced the creation of a new National Council for Vocational Qualifications. The task of the Council is to establish, on a voluntary basis, a national framework for vocational qualifications designed to extend coverage of formal qualifications, establish links and ladders between non-professional and professional qualifications and create links and equivalencies with academic qualifications. The Council's initial remit is to concentrate on non-professional vocational qualifications but the professions, including the health care professions, will be involved in due course. The Council has established a framework for vocational qualifications at four levels, with degree level professional qualifications to be brought into the framework at level V and above in due course. This framework leaves nursing qualifications, predominantly diploma rather than degree level, in an uncertain position. They are clearly not part of the existing levels up to level IV but there is lively debate about their position in the new framework. However an early priority for the Council was the creation of a qualification for the non-professional helpers of a number of health care professions, and a Health Care Assistant qualification at levels I and II was agreed in 1990. Work is proceeding on qualifications in this field at level III, which may provide an alternative entry gate into professional education in due course.

In 1990 the UKCC published a consultation document on a new framework for continued education for staff already qualified. This argued that nurses should demonstrate a minimum commitment to continued education as a condition of registration (midwives have had statutory, compulsory refresher training for a number of years). The UKCC also proposed rationalization of the current multiplicity of National Board-approved post-qualification courses and 'credit-rating' for academic purposes of continuing education. At the time of writing the outcome of these proposals is not certain. Mandatory refresher training will have a cost and it is not clear in what proportion this will be borne by employers or individual professionals. Meanwhile developments in continuing education are rapid and sometimes confusing. Traditionally advanced clinical education has been delivered by NHS schools of nursing and others in conjunction with clinical centres of excellence. Increasingly, however, there is a move to deliver specialist training in participants' own workplaces, with substantial use of distance modes of learning as far as the theoretical component is concerned. Among employers, and some educationalists, there is considerable emphasis upon multidisciplinary training and development programmes and a blurring of the distinction between what are conventionally regarded as 'management' and 'professional' development.

POST-REGISTRATION EDUCATION

District nurses and health visitors

Training for these professions is different but they are considered together for a number of reasons. Health visiting may only be undertaken as a post-registration qualification following initial training as an RGN. Courses have for some time been located in higher education and similarly require an initial RGN qualification. District nurse training is now mandatory for first level nurses working in the community. Unlike in health visiting, a registrable qualification in its own right, district nurses receive only the National Certificate in District Nursing. Most district nurses and health visitors are seconded on courses by their health authority and receive a full qualified nurses' salary in training, although a minority undertake training independently.

Midwifery

The large majority of midwives take an 18-month post-registration course in an NHS School of Midwifery. Direct entry midwifery course of three years duration to those without previous nursing qualification is now being offered by a number of schools throughout the UK.

NURSING DEGREES AND DIPLOMAS AND OTHER COURSES IN HIGHER EDUCATION

There are 14 courses in England combining acquisition of a degree with registered nursing qualification. Some 250 or more students enter each year. (There are seven courses elsewhere in the UK.) Most courses are a little over four years in length and most involve practical work during holidays. In addition there are three full-time and six part-time degree courses in England for those who already have nursing qualifications and three courses for nurses and professions supplementary to medicine. An unknown number of nurses are pursuing degrees elsewhere (e.g. the Open University).

However the proportion of the nursing workforce with degrees of any kind is small (about 5%), although it is higher among certain groups (e.g. almost 50% of nurse educationalists have degrees).

The Diploma in Nursing is an advanced qualification providing evidence of a high standard of knowledge and skill in nursing practice. The syllabus, prepared by the University of London, is offered in a number of centres around the country of the basis of three years' part-time study in a technical college, polytechnic or college of education.

Continuing education

In addition to various forms of post-registration training mentioned above there is a wide range of post-registration clinical nursing courses. Two kinds of course are controlled by the ENB:

1. Certificate courses prepare nurses for practice in a particular area and develop professional expertise to a high level, for example in intensive care, community psychiatry or oncology.
2. Statement (or attendance) courses are shorter courses for experienced nurses, designed to keep them up to date with current trends and practices; these are, for example, in family planning, care of the dying and stoma care.

The length of courses is from two to 18 months for a certificate course, or up to 30 days (usually on day release) for a statement course. Additional training is also available in ophthalmic nursing (Ophthalmic Nursing Diploma) and occupational health (Occupational Health Nursing Diploma). Health authorities also run local in-service training courses. A wide variety of management training courses is available for staff from ward to senior management level.

An initiative by the Department of Education and Science and the NHS Training Directorate seeks to improve continuing education for nurses and other health care professionals. Health Pickup (the health care part of a national initiative for professional updating and development) is designed to be the major contribution for continuing education and training of nurses, midwives, health visitors and professions supplementary to medicine. The programme embraces clinical updating, management and skills (e.g. quality assurance and client relations) common to all the professions. It will be modular and designed to accumulate credits so that individuals may progress to degree level or other nationally recognized qualifications. The programme is designed to rationalize the current plethora of opportunities for continuing education, to improve it in terms of personal and professional development and to provide links with other qualifications. In the last respect and in its multiprofessional nature Health Pickup is a major departure from most types of previous continuing education.

OTHER UK COUNTRIES

The above description has concentrated on England. The major differences in other countries are summarized briefly below.

Wales

The pattern is broadly the same as in England, but because there is no intermediate regional tier between the Welsh Office and Welsh Health Authorities there is a simpler network of relationships and communications. The Welsh National Board for Nursing, Midwifery and Health Visiting has not replaced previous Welsh statutory bodies (education has been controlled on a joint England and Wales or UK basis, depending on specialty); hence, Welsh courses and syllabuses are broadly similar to those in England. Two points may be noted: general nursing courses are largely modular and cooperation with the Central Council for Education and Training in Social Work in terms of joint training has gone further than in England.

Scotland

Similarly in Scotland there is no intermediate regional tier between the Scottish Home and Health Department and health boards (not authorities as in England and Wales). The National Board for Scotland (NBS) relates directly to health boards that act as NBS agents for disbursement of funds for basic nursing and midwifery education. The NBS controls funds for the same purposes as the ENB and it also may allocate funds for all continuing education. Programmes of training for first level nurses were reorganized in 1982. They are now modular and in two stages: Stage 1 is semi-comprehensive, containing modules relating to at least two parts of the Register; Stage 2 is directed to a specific specialty. Choice of specialty is normally made at the beginning of training but there is limited scope for decision in the latter part of Stage 1. There is also a 16-week bridging course for second level nurses wishing to convert to first level by taking Stage 2. Midwifery training is also modular. Scotland is nearer than any of the UK countries to a common foundation approach to nurse training for all specialties.

Northern Ireland

The health service in Northern Ireland is organized very differently from that in the rest of the UK in that health and social services are administered jointly by four Health and Social Services Boards under the Department of Health and Social Security (Northern Ireland). Responsibilities of this Board are also different in that it administers directly to colleges (rather than schools) of nursing, mental health nursing and midwifery. The Health and Social Services Boards, however, continue to determine the numbers in training and to pay their salaries. Actual course content is broadly similar to that of the rest of the UK, although there is one educational institution that provides a common foundation for general and mental illness nursing followed by specialization before registration.

Note [1]After 8 years the Constitution of the UKCC and National Boards is changing. The government has accepted that there should be a change of emphasis on the respective roles of the bodies. This will result in elections to the UKCC and smaller government-appointed National Boards.

5

The practice of nursing

The previous chapters have dealt with the history leading up to recent reforms of the health service and education. The reform of the health service has wide-reaching consequences on the need, shape and mix of the nursing workforce, nursing practice and the arrangements governing nurse education.

People in the UK increasingly expect the NHS to deliver a good quality service when and where they need it. They are beginning to play a more active part in voicing their consumer views and raise complaints as they see fit.

There is no doubt that the general public is increasingly better informed about health, care and illness and their rights as well as their responsibilities, although they are more likely to be more concerned with rights than responsibilities. The government recently published a Citizen's Charter, of which the Patient's Charter forms a part. The rights and standards set out in the Patient's Charter are an essential part of the programme to improve and modernize the delivery of a national health service to the public while continuing to reaffirm its fundamental principles. The Patient's Charter is about delivering a quality health service and puts the government's Citizen's Charter initiative into practice.

One of the standards in the Patient's Charter is that every patient should have a named qualified nurse, midwife or health visitor responsible for nursing or midwifery care. This is a big achievement by the nursing professions and a long standing objective of the Chief Nursing Officer at government level.

To put this into context the Strategy for Nursing was published by the Department of Health in 1989, a culmination of three years' work of leaders of the nursing professions, aimed at preparing nursing to meet health care challenges reaching into the next century. It sets out a framework for achievement through targets over the next decade for nursing practice, the workforce, education, leadership and management. The strategy's core is nursing practice. The workforce, education, leadership and management provide the infrastructure to enable and enhance practice. The strategy highlights the importance of partnership with patients and other disciplines and emphasizes the need for flexibility to be responsive to health care changes and to new developments, including specialties, practitioner roles and nurse-led roles.

THE NURSING WORKFORCE

The NHS is a labour intensive industry and its most precious and costly commodity is its staff. It employs over one million people and is the biggest single employer in Europe. The nursing and midwifery workforce in the UK in 1990 totalled just over half a million whole-time equivalents with a further 50 000 being employed in the independent health care sector. The term 'nursing workforce' is a collective term that denotes the level and category of nursing personnel; the discipline of nursing is extremely complex. In the UK nursing in this context includes registered first and second level nurses, midwives, health visitors and district nurses holding a qualification on part of the United Kingdom Central Council (UKCC) Register. It also includes students and pupils undertaking pre-registration nurse education, qualified nurses studying for a second qualification or attending post-registration courses and unqualified auxiliaries and health care assistants.

The distribution between countries of whole-time equivalent nursing staff in 1990 was as follows: England 79%, Scotland 12%, Wales 5.3% and Northern Ireland 3.7%. In comparison the general population of 57 million has a somewhat different distribution: England 83%, Scotland 9%, Wales 5% and Northern Ireland 3%. The variation of ratios of nursing staff to population, therefore, ranges from 0.95 in England to 1.33 in Scotland.

In Great Britain the NHS in 1990 employed some 494 000 whole-time equivalent nursing staff, which in terms of individual nursing personnel is considerably higher as some 38% work part time (Table 5.1). This makes the NHS the major employer of nursing staff. Of these 494 000 61.5% were qualified nurses, health visitors and midwives (ILO level 1). The remaining 38.5% were learners (14.5%) and auxiliary nursing staff (24%). Nursing staff comprise the largest single group of NHS employees and form half the workforce, cost 45% of the salary bill and account for 34% of NHS revenue expenditure.

Nursing and midwifery staff are an essential part of the NHS, not only because they are in the majority but also because most are in direct contact with the public. As key ambassadors of the service, and because of the nature and philosophy of nursing, they are one of the patients' or clients' main advocates. The nursing workforce therefore, by implication, has tremendous influence on determining standards and quality of care delivered, especially of nursing care. Also the NHS provides the training resources and environment for nurse education. This is important not only in defining standards of care but also because of implications of future supply of adequate numbers and suitably qualified nurses and midwives.

Table 5.1 Health service directly employed staff by main staff group including other statutory authorities; Great Britain (1) – at 30th September each year; whole time equivalents, 1986–1990

	\multicolumn{5}{c	}{Whole-time equivalents}	\multicolumn{2}{c	}{Change Sept 1986–90}	\multicolumn{2}{c}{Change Sept 1989–90}
	Sept 1986	Sept 1987	Sept 1988	Sept 1989	Sept 1990	WTE	%	WTE	%
Nursing and midwifery (2)	492 900	495 400	495 900	498 000	494 000	1 200	0.2	−3 900	−0.8
Professions allied to medicine	39 200	40 500	41 600	42 800	43 300	4 100	10.5	500	1.2
Scientific and professional	12 300	13 000	14 000	14 500	15 200	2 900	23.4	700	4.9
Other professional and technical	39 400	40 800	39 900	39 800	41 700	2 300	5.9	1 900	4.7
Medical and dental (3)	52 400	52 500	54 200	55 800	56 800	4 300	8.3	900	1.6
Total direct-care staff (4)	636 200	642 100	645 600	650 900	651 000	14 800	2.3	100	0.0
Ancillary	159 200	148 500	138 800	129 600	120 100	−39 100	−24.6	−9 500	−7.4
Administrative and clerical	132 600	136 200	137 900	144 000	153 500	21 000	15.8	9 500	6.6
Maintenance	23 800	23 100	21 800	20 800	20 000	−3 800	−15.8	−800	−3.7
Works	7 200	7 100	6 600	5 900	5 000	−2 200	−30.4	−900	−14.6
Ambulance (including officers)	22 500	22 500	22 300	22 400	21 700	−800	−3.4	−700	−3.3
Total directly employed staff	981 400	979 500	972 900	973 700	971 300	−10 100	−1.0	−2 400	−0.2

Sources: Department of Health (SM13) Annual Censuses of NHS Medical and Non-Medical Manpower; Welsh Office; Scottish Health Service Common Services Agency

Notes:
1. Includes staff at the Dental Estimates Board, Prescription Pricing Authority, London Post-Graduate Special Health Authorities and Family Practitioner Committees (and equivalent bodies in Scotland and Wales). Figures rounded to the nearest 100 whole-time equivalents. All changes calculated on unrounded figures. From 1987 other statutory authorities are included, for example Public Health Laboratory Service, NHS Training Authority and Health Education Authority.
2. Includes agency staff.
3. Includes all permanent paid, honorary and locum staff in hospitals and primary health care services, hospital practitioners and part-tme medical/dental officers. From 1987 includes agency locums.
4. Direct-care staff consists of nursing and midwifery, medical and dental and professional and technical staff.

It is not anticipated that the number of nursing staff will increase at the same rate as it has done over the past decade but supply will need to be planned carefully to meet future needs. Because the practice of nursing has changed considerably over the past decade the structure and composition as well as the number of the nursing staff will be an even more important factor in planning for the future.

Historically the nursing workforce has grown in response to the demands of social and political pressures. Nursing as a vital part of the health care system must contend with rapidly changing roles in order to meet modern requirements within equally rapidly changing social expectations, technological advances and health care needs of the increasing proportion of the elderly.

Demographics

A major factor influencing the practice, size, skill mix and work setting is a change in demographic structure. Between 1983 and 1993 the UK population is expected to grow by over one million (Figure 5.1). The proportion of those aged 65 and over is 15% and is expected to increase at a faster rate than that of total growth. The largest proportion of growth will occur in the 75 year old and over group. People in this age group make significantly greater demands on both health and social services, which by implication affects the level of nursing staff required.

The number of young children has been increasing since 1976 after falling for 13 years. This has significant effects not only on midwifery services but also on services for children such as child development, health education and prevention programmes, with considerable workload implications for nursing and midwifery.

Management of nursing services

Nursing and midwifery personnel are employed in every specialty and involved with every client group. The profession and its various organizations are committed to improving standards of care and quality of service. During the past few years the level of qualified nursing staff has increased and the distribution of specialties has changed in line with policy; therefore nursing staff needs demands and an adequate supply of suitably qualified nursing staff must be considered within the total health care system (Chapter 8).

Nursing workforce by distribution of staff category

In England between 1979 and 1989 the largest proportion of increase was

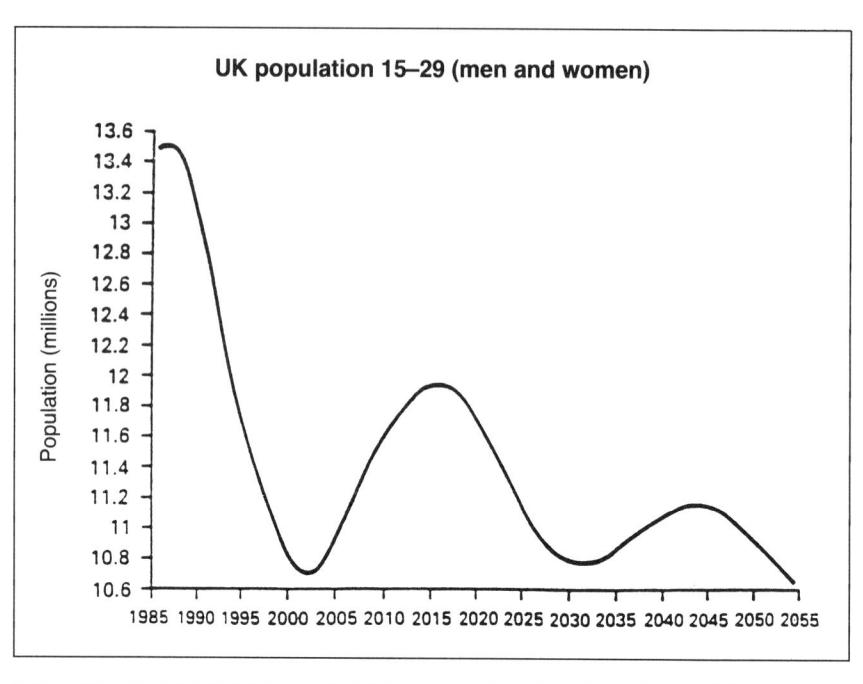

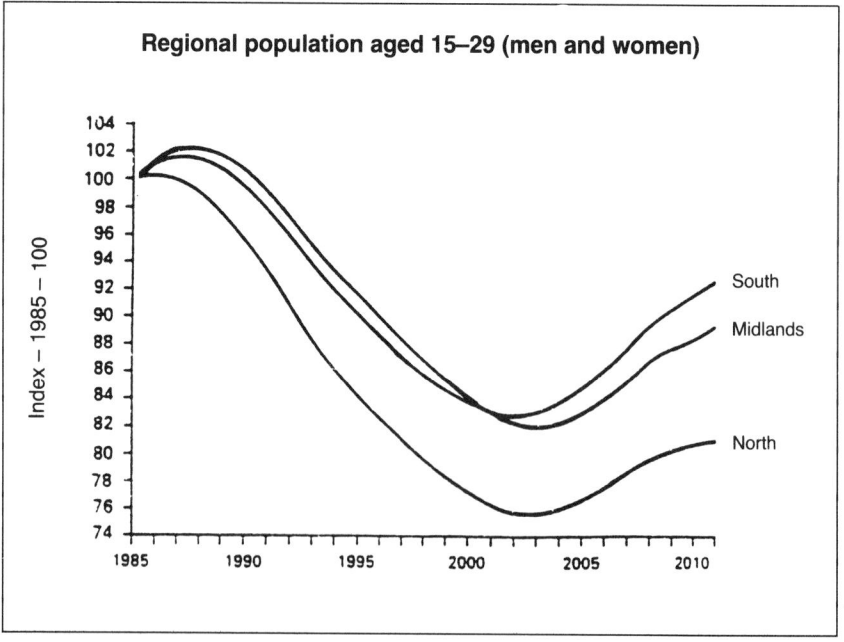

Figure 5.1 Estimated changes in UK population. Source: Institute of Manpower Studies, University of Sussex, UK. Report No. 52, *Employees' response to the decline of school leavers into the 1990s*.

among qualified staff, from under 200 000 to 244 000 whole-time equivalents (a rise of 27%) respectively. Some increases also occurred in midwifery and unqualified staff and there was a small drop in the number of health visitors, student health visitors and student midwives. The biggest reduction was in pre-registration students, from 24.6% to 14.5%.

There are some concerns about the effect on the availability of qualified staff in future in relation to the number of people entering training and issues of recruitment retention and redeployment are being addressed by NHS managers.

Nursing workforce by specialty and area of work

There are two distinct aspects of work concerning nursing staff distribution. First, a distinction is made in terms of specialty. The main historical groupings are general, mental illness, mental handicap, paediatric, midwifery, health visiting and district nursing. General, mental illness and mental handicap nursing qualifications are obtained through pre-registration courses. The paediatric qualification is either taken as a post-registration course or in combination with general nursing. Midwifery can be taken by a direct entry route, although many schools provide a post-registration course only. District nursing and health visiting can only be taken as post-basic qualifications. Project 2000 (Chapter 4) now has a pre-registration level for paediatrics. The second distinction is made by location: all nursing and midwifery staff work either in hospitals or the community, and some work in both.

For a number of years health authorities have pursued a policy of directing more resources towards community-based services and groups such as the elderly, mentally ill and mentally handicapped. Patients' stays in hospital are shorter with the practice of early discharge, and an increasing amount of nursing care is now provided in patients' homes. One of our main aims is to provide the best possible service in the most efficient way when and where it is needed.

Table 5.2 shows the distribution and trend in numbers of all nursing and midwifery staff by specialty in Great Britain between 1986 and 1990. During the earlier years between 1986 and 1990 the nursing workforce increased but it is now at the same level as in 1989 (Figure 5.2). Over the same period general nursing numbers decreased by about 6% and distribution among specialties changed. There was little increase in the number of mental illness and mental handicap personnel. The numerical balance between midwifery and other maternity work shifted towards midwives, and there were considerable increases in the care of the elderly and paediatric nursing personnel. The proportion of acutely ill patients needing nursing care and the increased number of complicated technical

Table 5.2a Nursing and midwifery staff by broad area of work – staff in post 1986–90, Great Britain – at 30th September each year; whole-time equivalents (Excluding agency staff)

Area of work	Total staff						Qualified				
	1986	1987	1988	1989	1990	1986	1987	1988	1989	1990
Total staff:	487 270	489 040	489 570	490 540	487 010	287 720	291 390	294 830	299 530	299 070
Hospital	430 370	432 090	432 300	434 450	430 310	239 470	243 150	246 360	252 460	251 660
Primary health care	49 640	49 500	49 710	49 500	50 510	42 510	42 340	42 480	42 270	43 130
Centrally-based services	3 100	3 200	3 190	3 470	3 570	1 580	1 690	1 670	1 710	1 720
Administration	4 170	4 250	4 380	3 120	2 610	4 150	4 220	4 330	3 100	2 560
Within hospital services:										
General nursing	212 890	210 180	208 260	200 430	198 930	115 170	115 370	115 980	113 870	114 760
Care of the elderly	46 500	45 600	44 320	51 300	51 070	25 260	24 820	24 370	28 440	28 470
Paediatrics	10 160	10 450	10 570	11 810	12 290	6 860	7 300	7 650	8 880	9 310
Mental illness	73 420	72 390	72 840	73 810	74 010	41 170	40 510	40 660	41 920	42 660
Mental handicap	37 980	37 830	37 770	38 480	38 420	15 340	15 060	14 820	15 430	15 550
Maternity/midwifery:										
Midwifery staff	23 010	23 360	23 440	23 370	23 160	17 680	18 260	18 330	19 000	18 860
Nursing staff	11 040	10 670	10 300	9 830	9 490	3 990	3 810	3 900	3 990	3 860
Education	7 620	7 810	7 880	8 270	8 720	7 620	7 810	7 880	8 270	8 720
Other/unspecified	7 750	13 880	16 920	17 160	14 220	6 380	10 210	12 770	12 670	9 470
Within primary health care:										
Health visitors	14 000	13 930	13 950	13 040	13 500	13 030	12 990	13 000	12 030	12 570
Other health visiting	820	1 030	1 070	820	780	600	770	830	610	570
District nurses	13 090	12 590	12 460	12 860	13 560	12 290	11 790	11 710	12 160	12 840
Other district nursing	9 540	10 010	9 970	8 900	9 390	6 140	6 510	6 510	5 470	5 770
Midwifery	4 370	4 350	4 330	4 540	4 610	4 370	4 350	4 330	4 530	4 610
Other	7 740	7 500	7 850	9 270	8 580	6 010	5 840	6 000	7 380	6 680
Education	80	90	90	80	80	80	90	90	80	80

Sources: Department of Health (SM13) Annual Census of NHS Non-Medical Manpower; Welsh Office; Scottish Health Service Common Services Agency.

Area of work	Unqualified 1986	1987	1988	1989	1990	Learners 1986	1987	1988	1989	1990
Total staff:	116 410	118 570	117 450	116 090	117 420	83 150	79 080	77 280	74 930	70 510
Hospital	109 530	111 590	110 350	108 770	109 790	81 370	77 340	75 590	73 220	68 860
Primary health care	5 350	5 430	5 540	5 530	5 730	1 780	1 740	1 690	1 710	1 650
Centrally-based services	1 520	1 510	1 520	1 770	1 850	–	–	–	–	–
Administration	10	30	50	30	50	–	–	–	–	–
Within hospital services:										
General nursing	35 870	35 860	34 490	30 410	31 630	61 840	58 950	57 790	56 150	52 540
Care of the elderly	21 240	20 790	19 950	22 860	22 600	–	–	–	–	–
Paediatrics	2 340	2 340	2 260	2 330	2 330	950	810	660	610	650
Mental illness	22 530	22 640	23 400	23 030	22 960	9 720	9 230	8 780	8 860	8 390
Mental handicap	19 120	19 440	19 700	19 820	19 880	3 510	3 340	3 250	3 240	2 990
Maternity/midwifery:										
Midwifery staff	–	–	–	–	–	5 330	5 100	5 110	4 370	4 300
Nursing staff	7 050	6 860	6 390	5 830	5 640	–	–	–	–	–
Education	–	–	–	–	–	–	–	–	–	–
Other/unspecified	1 370	3 670	4 150	4 490	4 750	–	–	–	–	–
Within primary health care:										
Health visitors	220	260	240	210	210	970	940	950	1 010	930
Other health visiting	–	–	–	–	–	–	–	–	–	–
District nurses	3 400	3 500	3 460	3 430	3 620	810	800	750	700	720
Other district nursing	–	–	–	–	–	–	–	–	–	–
Midwifery	1 730	1 670	1 840	1 890	1 900	–	–	–	–	–
Other	–	–	–	–	–	–	–	–	–	–
Education	–	–	–	–	–	–	–	–	–	–

Sources: Department of Health (SM13) Annual Census of NHS Non-Medical Manpower; Welsh Office; Scottish Health Service Common Services Agency.

Table 5.2b Nursing and midwifery staff by broad area of work – changes in staff in post 1986–90, Great Britain – at 30th September each year; Change 1986–90 (Excluding agency staff)

Area of work	Total WTE	Total %	Qualified WTE	Qualified %	Unqualified WTE	Unqualified %	Learners WTE	Learners %
Total staff:	−270	−0.1	11 360	3.9	1 010	0.9	−12 640	−15.2
Hospital	−60	−0.0	12 190	5.1	260	0.2	−12 500	−15.4
Primary health care	860	1.7	620	1.5	380	7.0	−130	−7.3
Centrally-based services	480	15.4	140	9.1	330	22.0	—	—
Administration	−1 550	−37.2	−1 590	−38.3	40	337.7	—	—
Within hospital services:								
General nursing	−13 960	−6.6	−410	−0.4	−4 240	−11.8	−9 310	−15.0
Care of the elderly	4 570	9.8	3 210	12.7	1 360	6.4	—	—
Paediatrics	2 130	21.0	2 440	35.6	−10	−0.4	−300	−31.6
Mental illness	590	0.8	1 500	3.6	430	1.9	−1 340	−13.7
Mental handicap	440	1.2	210	1.4	750	3.9	−530	−15.0
Maternity/midwifery:								
Midwifery staff	150	0.6	1 180	6.7	—	—	−1 030	−19.4
Nursing staff	−1 540	−14.0	−130	−3.3	−1 410	−20.0	—	—
Education	1 090	14.4	1 090	14.4	—	—	—	—
Other/unspecified	6 470	83.4	3 090	48.4	3 380	246.7	—	—
Within primary health care:								
Health visitors	−500	−3.6	−460	−3.5	—	—	—	—
Other health visiting	−40	−5.0	−30	−4.8	−10	−5.5	—	−4.3
District nurses	470	3.6	560	4.5	—	—	—	—
Other district nursing	−150	−1.5	−370	−5.9	—	—	−90	−11.1
Midwifery	240	5.4	240	5.4	220	6.4	—	—
Other	850	10.9	680	11.3	170	10.1	—	—
Education	0	−4.0	0	−4.0	—	—	—	—

Sources: Department of Health (SMI3) Annual Census of NHS Non-Medical Manpower; Welsh Office; Scottish Health Service, Common Services Agency.

Table 5.3 Nursing and midwifery staff by broad area of work – skill mix distributions 1986 and 1990, Great Britain – at 30th September each year.
(Excluding agency staff)

Area of work	1986 Qualified %	1986 Unqualified %	1986 Learners %	1990 Qualified %	1990 Unqualified %	1990 Learners %
Total staff:	59.0	23.9	17.1	61.4	24.1	14.5
Hospital	55.6	25.4	18.9	58.5	25.5	16.0
Primary health care	85.6	10.8	3.6	85.4	11.3	3.3
Centrally-based services	51.0	49.0	–	48.2	51.8	–
Administration	99.7	0.8	–	98.0	2.0	–
Within hospital						
General nursing	54.1	16.8	29.1	57.7	15.9	26.4
Geriatrics	54.3	45.7	–	55.7	44.3	–
Paediatrics	67.5	23.1	9.4	75.7	19.0	5.3
Mental illness	56.1	30.7	13.2	57.6	31.0	11.3
Mental handicap	40.4	50.4	9.3	40.5	51.7	7.8
Maternity/midwifery:						
Midwifery staff	76.8	–	23.2	81.4	–	18.6
Nursing staff	36.1	63.9	–	40.6	59.4	–
Education	100.0	–	–	100.0	–	–
Other	82.3	17.7	–	66.6	33.4	–
Within primary health care:						
Health visitors	93.1	–	6.9	93.1	–	6.9
Other health visiting	72.7	27.3	–	72.8	27.2	–
District nurses	93.8	–	6.2	94.7	–	5.3
Other district nursing	64.4	35.6	–	61.5	38.5	–
Midwifery	100.0	–	–	100.0	–	–
Other	77.7	22.3	–	77.9	22.2	–
Education	100.0	–	–	100.0	–	–

Sources: Department of Health (SM13) Annual Census of NHS Non-Medical Manpower; Welsh Office; Scottish Health Service, Common Service Agency.

procedures that nurses perform have had major effects on the nursing workload in hospital and community, and demands are escalating for the supply and deployment of nursing manpower to meet the new needs.

General nursing – hospital services

The largest number of nursing staff are employed in general nursing in general acute hospitals. This includes all general specialties such as high-intensity technical nursing, orthopaedics, neurology, general medicine

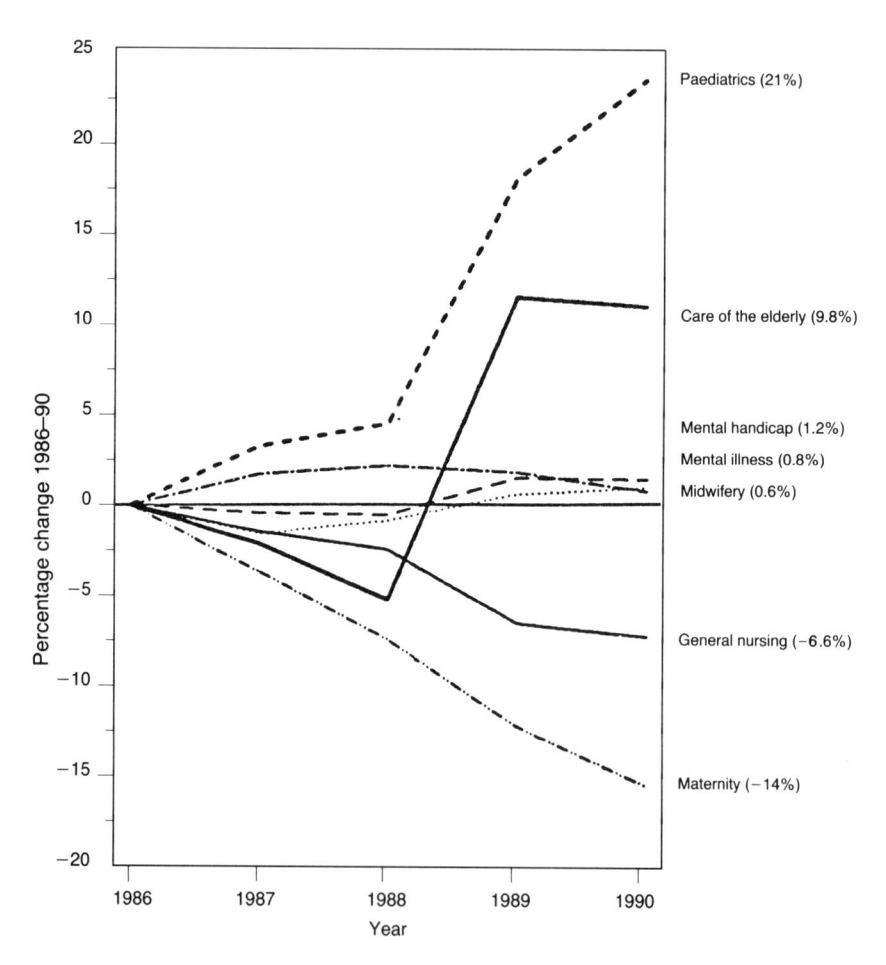

Figure 5.2 NHS hospital nursing and midwifery staff by broad area of work at 30th September. Percentage change 1986–90 – Great Britain.

Source: Department of Health (SM13) Annual Census of NHS Non-Medical Manpower.

and surgery. The overall number of whole-time equivalents decreased from 213 000 in 1986 to 199 000 in 1990, a drop of about 6.6%. In 1986 the proportion of qualified nursing staff was 54%, that of learner nurses 29% and that of nursing auxiliaries 17%. The rising turnover of patients per bed and increasing activities in out-patients and accident and emergency departments, new technology, medical and nursing advances and the rising average age of the patient have all had workload consequences for nursing staff as well as support services.

Care of the elderly hospital services

This is a growing area and in terms of rehabilitation and remedial care is especially time consuming. Although many elderly receive care at home hospital services are an important resource.

Hospital services deal mainly with acute episodes where care is focused on assessment, treatment and rehabilitation. The average length of stay in hospital is decreasing. The number of nursing staff in this area increased from 46 500 to 51 000 between 1986 and 1990, an increase of 10%. In 1990 the proportions of qualified and unqualified nursing staff were 55.7% and 44.3% respectively.

Overall the numbers have improved considerably but the proportion of qualified nursing staff is somewhat lower than in acute services. Greater emphasis on specialization, advanced education programmes and increasing numbers of post-registration courses now provide greater opportunity to improve overall depth of knowledge in this specialty.

Paediatric nurses – hospital services

In paediatric nursing emphasis is on keeping a sick child within the family setting. If a child is to be admitted to hospital, stay is kept to a minimum. This intensifies the workload per patient and means a heavier commitment for community services.

It is policy in England that children in hospital should, whenever possible, be nursed in paediatric wards supervised by a qualified paediatric nurse (Memorandum, 1971). The proportion of staff in this field is relatively small compared to most other specialties and the supply of qualified paediatric nurses does not meet present demand. Project 2000 paediatric branch programmes should also help to close the gap. It is nevertheless encouraging that the overall number increased by 21% between 1986 and 1990.

Maternity services

Maternity services are provided on a joint hospital-community basis; sometimes midwives are involved in both community and hospital care but most work either in hospital or the community. Most women have their babies in hospital but antenatal and postnatal care also occurs in out-patient departments or in general practitioners' surgeries and clinics. Midwives are independent practitioners accountable for supervision, care and advice before and after childbirth, and for delivery and care of the newborn child and its family. Although expectant mothers are normally under the overall supervision of an obstetrician, the midwife is the senior person present for 75% of deliveries. Obstetricians are called only if complications are anticipated (Royal Commission NHS, 1979).

Over the years midwifery personnel numbers have increased. Although the number of maternity staff between 1986 and 1990 did not change significantly, the trend of increasing numbers of qualified midwives continued up to 1989. In 1986 23 010 whole-time equivalents were qualified midwives, compared to 23 160 in 1990. The number of student midwives has decreased from 5300 to 4300 (by almost 20%). For purposes of replenishing the profession student numbers have always been relatively high. Historically midwifery training additional to a nursing qualification also opened many career opportunities, for example entry to a health visiting course. This is no longer the case but even now, only just over half of newly qualified midwives continue to practise for any significant length of time. There are now increasing numbers of courses offering direct entry to midwifery training (Chapter 4).

Mental illness and mental handicap services – hospital and community

These two specialties are usually managed separately, with different education programmes for mental illness or mental handicap nursing. Hospital and community nursing services are normally provided by a joint administrative service under the control of a director of nursing service or service manager. Hospital services are contracting and the emphasis is more on community care. Many alternative care options, such as smaller community units or sheltered housing with some nursing care support, are being provided. Much of the care is also provided in day hospitals or patients' homes. Admission to hospital is less frequent and stay is kept to a minimum. The move from institutional to community care has required not only redeployment and relocation of nursing staff but also new nursing skills and knowledge.

Community psychiatric nursing courses were introduced in the early

1970s but, with a changing scene requiring new skills, it became apparent that a new training programme was needed for psychiatric nurses. In 1982 a training syllabus for both parts of the Register – mental illness and mental handicap nursing – was introduced, which contained the social skills and community care components.

There is a long-term problem of adequate supply of qualified psychiatric nurses and nurses for the mentally handicapped. Psychiatric nursing staff form the second largest group in terms of specialty and in 1990 comprised 73 420 whole-time equivalents. Of those 57.6% were qualified, 11% were in training and the remaining 31% were unqualified auxiliaries.

Nursing staff levels in psychiatric services have increased considerably over a number of years. Since 1986 levels have risen slightly, due mainly to an increase in the number of qualified nursing staff and to a lesser extent in the level of auxiliaries. Numbers leaving have decreased by nearly 14%. That the number of learners entering training has fallen over the past few years is of considerable concern as it affects the overall supply of newly qualified nursing staff. One important factor in supply and demand in the field of psychiatry is the ratio of men to women. Men comprise 32% compared to a national proportion of 10% of nursing workforce overall and present a potential untapped pool of recruits.

Mental handicap services

The number of nursing staff concerned with care of the mentally handicapped was 38 420 in 1990. The increase over the past years has been minimal and is mainly due to the increase in the level of qualified nurses. Provisions for the mentally handicapped are changing, the emphasis now being on health and socialization rather than illness and custodial care. Nurses in this area are dealing with entirely new concepts and the question of nurse as social worker or 'carer' is much debated. A recent seminar on training and education discussed the way forward and a number of joint education schemes between the NHS and the Department of Social Services are being set up in an attempt to explore the benefits.

Because of changing requirements and social attitudes it is difficult to attract a sufficient number of people to undertake training. As in psychiatry the proportion of men is high and recruitment for training is directed towards this potential market.

Community nursing services

Community nursing services are part of primary health service and, by tradition, are provided by district nursing and health visiting staff. In recent years school nursing, which in the past formed part of the health visitor's responsibility, has developed as an associated specialty and is now carried out in many areas by school nurses. Apart from these main groups there are a number of other nursing staff working in treatment rooms and in general practitioners' surgeries. The role of nurses in primary health care services was described in a health circular as follows:

> The health visitor is a family visitor and an expert in child health care. She is trained to understand relationships within the family and the effects upon these relationships of the normal process of growth and aging and events such as marriage, birth and death. She is concerned with the promotion of health and the prevention of ill health through education, advice and support, and by referrals to the general practitioner and others where help is needed. She is leader of a team that may include registered and enrolled nurses, and on some occasions, nursing auxiliaries working in schools and clinics. The scope for the employment and supporting staff, and the nature of the task that health visitors delegate to them, vary according to the needs of the population.
> The school nurse is involved in health surveillance and education of school children. In some areas school nurses work directly with health visitors and much benefit is derived from close integration of the school nurse into the primary health care team.
> The District nurse is an integral part of the community nursing team. The qualified District nurse is responsible for giving skilled nursing care where required to all persons living in the community. She is the leader of the District nursing team within primary health care services, working with a team of qualified nurses, enrolled nurses and nursing auxiliaries. The District nurse is professionally accountable for assessing the needs of patient and family, and for monitoring quality of care. It is her responsibility to ensure that help, including financial and social, is made available as appropriate, and to delegate tasks as appropriate to her team members.

Although these roles are distinct, they can on occasion be combined. Some nurses in rural areas undertake all the functions. In 1990 in Great Britain community nursing staff totalled 50 510 and constituted over 10% of the nursing workforce. Professional community nursing staff, although small in number, are among the most highly qualified nurses. District nurses and health visitors require a mandatory statutory qualification that can only be gained after pre-registration nurse education. Community nurses work either from a health centre or clinic or a general practitioner's surgery, within a primary health care team.

The ratio of health visitors to population has not changed significantly and the number of health visitors in 1990 was 12 570 whole-time equivalents – a ratio of one health visitor to 5000 population. In addition there are 1000 unqualified nursing staff. Compared to other nursing services this is a relatively small proportion of unqualified staff.

The nature of the work of district nurses also requires a different skill mix. Of about 23 000 whole-time equivalent district nursing staff about 50% are qualified district nurses, 30% qualified nurses, 5% student district nurses and the remaining 15% unqualified nursing staff.

Community nursing services have been under increasing pressure and although resources are being directed towards priority services such as care of the elderly, changes in health and social services with which they are intrinsically bound have had their effects. A government review of community services (DHSS, 1986) suggested the establishment of neighbourhood nursing services to make better use of nursing skills and qualified district nurses and health visitors. It also recommended that primary health care teams be strengthened by clear objectives and, significantly, that the concept of nurse practitioners be adopted. The review, taken in conjunction with a document on primary health care, has had its effects. With the publication of *Health of the Nation* (1991) the process is likely to accelerate.

An expanding professional role

Within nursing, many levels of skill and different roles are needed to give the necessary care in the most efficient and effective way. Basic preparation leads to registered nurses (Chapter 4) with a number of different branches of nursing, that is general adult, paediatric, mental illness and mental handicap. There is also a small number of courses that combine nurse training with an undergraduate degree programme.

The expansion of knowledge in medical science and the legitimacy of nursing research have affected the way in which nurses respond to new challenges. Goal-oriented nursing care plans are now widely used and total patient care is becoming a reality. More services are developing primary nursing and the concept of patient partnerships. The Patients Charter standard on a named nurse, midwife or health visitor responsible for nursing or midwifery care of individual patients will focus on possible models to take this forward. Nurses do not work in isolation, and with each gain in knowledge there is a need to integrate the work of various health care professionals in order to achieve the best service for the patient. Nurses' and doctors' roles are on the whole complementary but may on occasion be interchangeable, as indeed they may be with those of other health care professionals such as physiotherapists and occupational therapists.

The nurse's role is expanding in some areas and extending in function. For example there is increased recognition that nursing care is a major health need of groups such as the chronically sick and elderly. Nursing staff in this case take the key role in management of these patients, which enables them to prescribe nursing care and mobilize other services such as occupational and physiotherapy. The Royal College of Nursing Report on the extended clinical role of the nurse (1979) supported this move.

In 1974 an interdisciplinary working party, looking at the range of nursing duties, identified an increasing number of activities that were clearly extensions of usual functions. As a result of specialization extended roles such as renal dialysis, intensive care in the neonatal area and cardiology have developed. Advances in health science and technology require doctors and nurses to pioneer new roles, often, by implication, leading to special expertise and advanced roles in nursing, a process that seems a natural evolution of professional maturity.

One resulting concern is that the extension of the nurse's role will not be at the expense of the caring function and that technical procedures will not detract from essential nursing care. One initiative to encourage nurses to remain clinically involved was the negotiation of a flexible clinical grading structure that would enable nurses to widen their scope of work and make careers in the clinical field (Clinical Grading Review). This provides the opportunity to combine a high level of clinical expertise with responsibility to promote quality of care, research and advanced education in nursing practice.

Above all ward sisters and charge nurses are the key managers of clinical areas such as the ward or department or, in the case of the community, a caseload of patients. They normally work with a team of staff nurses, enrolled nurses, auxiliaries and, if it is a teaching area, learners. Much effort has been invested in research to establish the role and function of the ward sister, her influence on the ward and the skills and abilities required for efficient management of a clinical area. As role models develop there is little doubt that the ward sister holds the key to determining standards of care and the quality of service delivery, and the clinical team's interface with patients is the pivot of the health services. To clarify the scope and responsibility the UKCC published guidance – *The Scope of Professional Practice* – which provides the framework for action for an accountable registered practitioner.

NURSING DEVELOPMENTS

As already mentioned, in 1989 the Department of Health published a Strategy for Nursing, which addresses areas with the aim of delivering a health service of the highest standard while taking into consideration available resources. The four areas were practice – the core of nursing – manpower, education and management and leadership. The strategy pulled together many of the initiatives hitherto taken forward without a framework. The strategy included targets for action and in response to practice, targets of nursing care and teaching material were developed by the Department of Health (Measuring the Quality, 1990). Two other relevant publications concerned with practice, resource management and the NHS Reform were 'A Framework of Audit for the Nursing Services' (1991) and 'Using Information in Managing the Nursing Resources' (1991).

With the introduction of the NHS Reform in April 1991 and the new arrangements concerning purchaser, provider roles and the establishments of Trusts, many combinations of responsibilities and job titles have emerged.

The scope and development opportunities for nurses, midwives and health visitors are extensive. For example nurses are members of the executive boards of provider NHS Trusts with wide-reaching responsibility, and the development of clinical roles allows them to become expert practitioners and clinical lecturers.

NURSING DEVELOPMENT UNITS

Throughout the UK centres of nursing excellence are demonstrating how to recruit, motivate and develop staff and how this in turn provides high quality cost-effective patient care. Some of the earlier examples of this are the Oxford experiment and the Tameside Care of the Elderly Unit.

Since then there have been a number of developments of centres of excellence which are now known as nursing (or midwifery or health visiting) development units (NDUs). These are wards and clinics with an explicit commitment to improving clinical practice. In a climate where nursing creativity is encouraged and each person's contribution is acknowledged and valued, staff are producing a rich variety of initiatives concerned with good practice, resource management, recruitment retention and return to nursing and nursing leadership. These are all nursing challenges embodied in the Strategy for Nursing. Nurses are also beginning to evaluate the initiatives in order to modify them in a ceaseless search for improvement.

Each NDU selects its own priorities within the framework of its organization, in which the organization plays an important part in providing the climate and framework for the NDU to grow and develop.

Oxford and Tameside Health Authorities NDUs have been in existence for several years and the example was followed by Brighton, Camberwell, Southport and West Dorset. These units have received a grant from the

King's Fund Centre and the Department of Health is funding an evaluation of those four units in addition to Tameside. Recently a further 20 units have received a small grant from the King's Fund and the Department of Health has made over £3 million available to establish a further 30 units.

All units are based in ordinary NHS wards or units, ranging from long-term elderly care to intensive care areas. They are not privileged, elitist or different in any way except for the small amount of extra resources that some are receiving to accelerate their development. Experience suggests that many more NDUs could be established with a little support. The emergence of an NDU usually arouses competitiveness amongst neighbouring wards, which raises standards throughout the unit.

Evaluation of NDUs

Internal auditing goes on within each NDU, and a few have secured resources for evaluation by external researchers. Key conclusions are:

1. Better use is being made of nursing skills through adjusting skill mix, improving team work and staff developments;
2. Staff motivation and morale have improved;
3. Recruitment and retention rates are improving, partly because people are more satisfied with their jobs and partly because NDUs act as 'magnets' for staff;
4. Care is more patient focused;
5. Local strategic planning and goal setting is going on, often for the first time.

NDUs are not a panacea but they provide persuasive evidence that nurses at the grass roots are able and willing to come up with long-term solutions if the climate is right and their potential is developed.

6

The nurse at work

'It is probable that with the exception of motherhood, no occupation has ever been so richly remunerated in terms of lip service and so poorly regarded in terms of practical consideration. But at any rate it enjoyed the lip service. The public became nurse-conscious' (DHSS Working Party on Midwives, 1949). Those words were written in 1949, yet the ideas they draw together – an occupational group held in some esteem, but with a confused public profile and, up to recently, a history of relatively low pay – retain some validity when considering the nurse in the 1990s. The National Health Service (NHS) in the UK employs more than 500 000 people in nursing roles (i.e. professionally qualified, unqualified auxiliaries and learners). Other arms of the public sector, as well as the private sector, also employ qualified nurses. Nurses comprise about 2% of the total UK workforce. They are distinguished as a group possibly only by an ability to seek internal conflict at the cost of public misperception of specific nursing care while experiencing a history of relatively moderate pay.

The bases of nurse employment practices in their widest sense in the NHS are considered in this chapter, which first reviews historical influences and then examines the way nursing fits into the broad NHS, both in a structural and a mechanistic sense. This latter consideration of negotiating machinery leads into the social demographic structure of the nursing profession. The final section reviews the political issues in and for the profession.

In the following sections the phrase 'nursing', will unless the text indicates otherwise, cover both qualified and unqualified staff employed on NHS nursing grades, whereas the phrase 'the nursing profession' refers to the qualified cadre only. The discussion will concentrate on the NHS as it is the principal source of nursing employment and has been the principal determinant, directly or indirectly, of nursing developments since its inception of 1948.

HISTORICAL INFLUENCES

To the public, to paraphrase Gertrude Stein, 'a nurse is a nurse is a nurse', and even to many inside the health field, the distinctions between general nurses, nurses for the mentally ill or mentally handicapped, midwives, health visitors and district nurses are less than clear. Indeed to those inside the professions the distinctions remain central and battles are fought to preserve them. The causes of this continuing conflict are twofold: first, a perpetual crisis of identity for the nursing profession as a whole, the resolution of which is seen by some to require an emphasis on diversity; and, second, a range of social and philosophical bases espoused by particular people on the nursing scene to which, is some ways, they remain loyal.

Taking first the crisis of identity, a good definition is Etzioni's concept of a semi-profession (Etzioni, 1969), which describes a group with less autonomy than a fully fledged profession but which encompasses more than traditional white – or blue – collar work. Autonomy can be claimed by a group but can only be granted by society where the group can clearly be seen by society to be necessary and unavoidable for the course of normal activity. Even where that autonomy is fully granted it will always be under challenge. In the health field such examples are the challenges to medicine, both from those alleging malpractice by individual practitioners and from those attacking the rationale for the profession itself. In a wider context law is a classic 'profession', yet do-it-yourselfers are always fighting to open up areas of work to the public. It is arguable that the hallmark of a recognized profession is its ability to set the rules of debate about its roles and boundaries and to redefine them as necessary to protect its own – an analysis of all professions as essentially imperialistic.

Sense of identity

In this paradigm of professionalism the nursing occupational group suffers the considerable disadvantage in that its core expertise is perceived not to be unique to its members: everyone can claim to be a 'nurse' at some time, in a way in which they would not claim to be a doctor or lawyer or pharmacist. Similar difficulties beset the professions of teaching and social work. Responding to this challenge to the nursing profession's self-perceptions has generally thrown each group back not on a common core concept but on its particular expertise (with the underlying and perhaps unconscious suggestion that only it of all the nursing groups really is a profession). At a time when what is needed is unity in the cause of professionalism, energy is dissipated in internal rivalry and strife.

Two examples from widely different areas at widely different times may serve to make the point that pay has been an issue in NHS nursing since 1948 and was a negotiating issue until 1983. During the 1950s mental nurses as a group had characteristics that potentially offered considerable negotiating benefits to nursing as a whole: there was a large population of male nurses (hence pressure for wages that could support families) who were paid for overtime when general nurses were not. However the staff interests in the Whitley Council were split between trade unions that largely represented mental nurses and professional bodies that did not admit mental nurses to membership. In spite of the possible immediate benefits of using mental nurses as a pay vanguard, debates about union versus profession and quality of mental nursing took such precedence that mental nurses pressed for separate negotiating machinery (White, 1985). It was not until the late 1950s that mental nurses' characteristics were in fact 'exploited' to the financial benefit of all nurses (White, 1985).

The second example relates to the debate resulting from publication by the United Kingdom Central Council for Nursing, Midwifery and Health Visiting (UKCC) of its report 'Project 2000' (UKCC, 1986). At one level of analysis this report, with its emphasis on a common core of supernumerary training for all qualified nurse professionals, offers an opportunity to build what could clearly be seen as the basis of a peculiarly professional expertise, thus moving professionals towards full rather than semi-professional status in the public's perception. Yet for reasons which, in their own terms, are undeniably important; a substantial volume of midwifery opinion is arguing that midwifery needs to be based on a health rather than sickness model and cannot therefore be conjoined to the Project 2000 proposal (Flint, 1986).

Profession and trade union

Turning from the issue of crisis of identity to the question of bases from which particular 'actors/actresses' on the nursing scene come, one difference already touched upon is the trade union male culture in mental nursing as opposed to the professional body female culture in general nursing. Tensions between the two cultures remain visible in the staff side of the negotiating body. However there are discussions within each culture that also remain influential, at least in terms of impact at crucial points in the past.

Again, two examples will serve. The first is the existence not of a single but three professional bodies, each of which operates in a professional and a trade union role. The Royal College of Nursing (founded in 1916 and chartered in 1928) is in essence a professional body coming late to a leading trade union role. The Royal College of Midwives draws its strength from the professional role of the midwife as specified originally in the Midwives Act. The Health Visitors Association, established in 1929 though avowedly professional, is unlike the two Royal Colleges in that it also holds TUC membership. That any profession or would-be profession contains various specialties within its broad church is a statement of the obvious; it seems a waste of valuable energy to maintain separated organizations to fight for certain specialties. 'United it stands, divided ...'.

The second example is equally rooted in the past but still survives, in its effects if not in its reality. This is the way in which, as is perhaps inevitable with professional bodies, high counsels of the profession have been dominated by its more senior members – the former General Nursing Council, for example, with its heavy representation of matrons and tutors. The result is development of professional policy by those for whom managerial concerns are as immediate an issue as long-term professional changes. To note that is not to argue for pure professional policy, an essentially meaningless phrase since policy can neither exist nor be implemented in a vacuum, but simply to point out that short-term managerial solutions may militate against long-term professional development. This stress has to be acknowledged, and the profession needs to seize opportunities and to react positively to opportunities for change.

In 1948 the NHS acquired the pre-existing structures of the hospitals it took over. In structural terms that meant staffing by matrons, deputy and assistant matrons, ward sisters, staff nurses and nursing auxiliaries (plus state enrolled assistant nurses, later to become state enrolled nurses). Two points are clear about this structure. First, while within wards there was a clear and manageable hierarchy, above that the situation changed: one matron, to whom sisters tended to see themselves as responsible, with 'administrative' deputies or assistants. Second, a structure did not extend beyond one hospital. Links between hospitals were largely informal. There were some teaching links, but they were not central to the profession's development (DHSS, 1972). In essence, therefore, the structure was designed to service wards with horizons limited largely to wards and hospitals, and a Hospital Management Committee responsible for several hospitals might receive different nursing advice from the matrons of each.

The Salmon Report

The influential Salmon report (Ministry of Health and SHHD, 1966) led to changes. A coherent managerial structure was created, retaining the grades up to ward sister, then adding – in increasing rank – nursing officer, senior nursing officer, principal nursing officer and chief nursing officer. Matrons were replaced by one of these grades. A small hospital might have in charge a senior nursing officer or even a nursing officer, whereas a large one would have a principal nursing officer. Equally important was the move to hierarchical principles, each level of officer reporting to an officer one level, or sometimes more, higher. These changes unified nursing within each group, or unit of management, and fitted nursing for the managerial changes brought about in the NHS upon its 1974 reorganization.

A structure similar to that recommended by Salmon was instituted in community services by Mayston (Ministry of Health, 1969) and it greatly eased the amalgamation of ex-local authority community nursing services with the hospital service in 1974.

The next stage was an additional refinement – the move to new grades consisting of senior nurse (levels 1+ down to 8) and director of nursing services (levels 1+ down to VI). In essence grading factors were determined that allowed each local unit of management to have as its head of nursing an appropriate director of nursing services (DNS) level, supported by adequate numbers of and properly graded senior nurses.

The above brief sketch, deliberately over-compressed, is designed to make the point that the successive reorganizations were managerial, not professional, in nature. Nursing was moving to establish a recognized professional hierarchy paralleling the administrative hierarchy, a classic example of the dominance of managerial over professional approach.

Clinical grading

After many years of discussion, negotiation and job evaluation, all of which proved fruitless, a major step forward was taken with the introduction of the clinical grading structure. The essence of this structure is that staff previously graded between nursing auxiliary and senior nurse have had their posts re-examined and regraded according to duties and, although it led to a significant rise in nurses' salaries, it is also fair to say that it caused significant dissension within the profession, because individuals who had previously shared the same job title, e.g. enrolled nurse or staff nurse, and had received the same salary now found that they were paid differently.

A stated aim for the introduction of the new structure was to obviate the necessity for well-motivated nurses to move into management or teaching in order to secure a higher salary. The extent to which this aim will be met will be decided in future years. The key question for them to answer will be whether clinical grading has improved patient care by maintaining the pressure of a cadre of well-qualified, well-motivated nurses in 'hands-on' patient care.

These organizational changes required negotiation with the profession, which formed, for this purpose, the Staff Side of the Nurses and Midwifery Whitley Council (now the Nursing and Midwifery Negotiating Council). Established in 1948 as part of a Whitley structure encompassing all NHS employers (from which the medical profession rapidly decamped in all but name), Staff Side consists primarily of the three professional bodies (RCN, RCM, and HVA) and the four trade unions (COHSE, NUPE, NALGO, and GMBATU), although a number of other bodies (e.g. the Association of Supervisors of Midwives and its Scottish equivalent, and the Scottish Health Visitors Association) have or have had seats. It is a coalition of interest groups, the position of which at any time reflects inevitable internal compromise, just as any individual Staff Side constituency will in itself reflect internal compromise.

Nursing and the NHS

The history of NHS negotiations with the nursing professions is a long one, too long to be set out here, but it is worth sketching the broad outline of NHS nurse employment patterns to demonstrate that, in general terms, employment as a nurse in the NHS is on reasonable terms and conditions. Briefly nurses are conditioned to a 37.5 hour week, with four or five weeks' annual holiday (depending on grade) plus public holidays. Work at night and weekends attracts premium payments. Extra hours worked qualify for time off *in lieu* of payment; if this cannot be taken paid overtime can be given. There is a contributory, inflation-linked NHS pension scheme run by the government, and female nurses may retire at 55 years of age.

Nursing pay, however, is a more complex story. It was originally a Whitley Council subject and very early a cause of contention. In 1949 the government's policy stressed the need to restrict personal incomes. As a result the Management Side of the Nurses and Midwives Whitley Council was asked to delay a settlement due for public health nurses. Dissatisfaction with pay, overtime compensation and the way in which the Whitley system operated grew and led to three independent reports – the National Board of Prices and Incomes report in 1968 (National Board of Prices and Incomes, 1968), the Halsbury Committee report in 1974 (DHSS, 1974), and the Clegg Report in 1980 (DHSS, 1980). In 1982 there were serious industrial disruptions and the removal, with Staff Side consent, of pay from the negotiating arena. Instead the government established an independent Review Body, which paralleled one already established for the medical profession, and stated that it would implement the Review Body's recommendations except where there were 'clear and compelling reasons to the contrary'. The Review Body has so far reported from 1984/5–1991/2. Its recommendations, although sometimes staged, have been implemented and, as a result, nurses' salaries measured against retail prices have returned to and broadly exceeded the levels set by Halsbury in 1974.

Certainly for a professional group in the UK as large as nursing to have done comparatively as well over the years 1984–9 is a considerable achievement. But it must be noted there was considerable debate when the Review Body was being established about the inclusion – or otherwise – of unqualified auxiliaries in its terms of reference. Perhaps inclusion of unqualified auxiliaries in the review seemed threatening to the profession.

Who are the nurses?

It may reflect the confusion in both the public's and the profession's minds, but hard data on nurses are largely lacking. In 1947 a Working Party on Nurse Recruitment and Training (Wood, 1947) referred to:

> the almost complete lack of reliable statistical data necessary to provide essential background information showing the composition and structure of the existing nursing profession. Such statistics as were available were at best inconclusive and at worst actually misleading.

Little changed between 1947 and 1985, and the Public Accounts Committee reported to the House of Commons in monotonously similar terms.

However some data are available. As of September 1990 the NHS in England, Wales and Scotland employed some 494 000 whole-time equivalent staff, including auxiliaries and learners, some 1 in 50 of the working population of the UK. They are predominantly (90%) female, although the proportion of men rises significantly the higher the position in the hierarchy. Although the evidence here is scant many come from the professional, managerial, non-manual and skilled manual groups rather than from the semi-skilled or unskilled groups (HMSO, 1972).

Now, however, there is a great deal of interest in the area of nurse manpower and it seems likely that in a few years there will be better 'defined' nurse profiles.

POLITICAL ISSUES IN AND FOR NURSES

Work on nurse manpower has gained momentum for a variety of reasons, including the NHS's need to make as cost-effective a use of possible of all resources available to it. But there are two major developments that together have forced the pace and raised issue central to the future of nursing: demographic changes and a review of nurse education and training.

In brief the decline in the birth rate in the early 1970s compromises the ability of the NHS to maintain current intakes and training patterns. NHS nursing would need not 22% of the available school leaving cohort but 39% – scarcely a realisable number in a publicly financed system. In addition the UKCC's Project 2000, now being implemented, prescribed a new training pattern resulting in the loss of a very large part of the learner's service contribution and the phasing-out of the second level qualification, the enrolled nurse. NHS nursing looks unlikely to remain as it is.

The question is, how will nursing be shaped? The move is towards a more classically professional model: higher standards of training for fewer people, leading to higher status practitioners. This ties in with pressure for rewarding clinical expertise other than by promotion out of the clinical area.

Other interest groups in the area of health – managers, doctors, paramedical professions – will all have views on nursing's direction. These views might not be coherent or convergent but they do exist, and it is proper that they be expressed in order to strengthen the debate.

Enoch Powell in 'Medicine and Politics' (Powell, 1976) described the NHS's 'vested interest in designation'; to improve the NHS more money is necessary, and no matter how successful an Exchequer funded service, 'complaint and dissatisfaction are essential to extracting more money'. The nursing professions, coming as they do from different bases and different agendas, may well have found it easy to pursue the good of the NHS by coalescing around the chorus of complaint and dissatisfaction designed to yield Exchequer funds. That tactic succeeds when the outcome is unlikely to be threatening. Something more may be needed if a perceived threat is to become an opportunity.

7

Nursing research

Among the bequests of Florence Nightingale to the nursing profession was one of a role model for scientific research, one that nursing was slow to take up. Through the years, however, there has been a growing awareness by health and social professions of the need for research. Nightingale was one of the first in the UK to collect and use social statistical information to support arguments for improvement in hospital facilities. Following her experiences in the Crimea Nightingale's main concern was to improve conditions for the care and treatment of war casualties, in particular for members of the armed services.

BACKGROUND

Nightingale's participation on the Commission of the Sanitary Conditions of the British Army in India and her work on planning military hospitals in Britain provided a unique environment for her to develop her interests in medical architecture and scientific forms of enquiry with regard to health status (Woodham Smith, 1950). Her work in the Army Medical Service had considerable influence on public interests of the late 19th century in the provision of hospital accommodation and estimates of health status. Her initiative in this field formed the basis for the collection of modern health statistics. Although Nightingale directed her analytical skills to questions of public health, she did not use those skills to address the questions of nursing services, choosing rather to focus on the need to develop a structured programme of training for nurses (Prince, 1982).

Nursing research did not appear as a serious issue in nursing literature until Briggs, in his report on nursing, stated: 'Nursing should be a research based profession' (DHSS, 1972). That report gave considerable impetus to a growing awareness of research in the profession and encouragement to those who had been attempting to establish research as a legitimate function. As with any emerging field of knowledge, nursing research has passed through various developmental stages, beginning with descriptive studies and progressing to experimentation and evaluative types of research. Nursing research has not developed uniformly across the whole field. While evaluative studies have been possible in some areas of nursing, research is only beginning in others.

Development of nursing research

One of the first nursing research studies done in England was a description of nursing in hospital wards. This work was prompted by the recommendations of the Working Party on the Recruitment and Training of Nurses (Ministry of Health, Wood, 1947). Although the group attempted a type of job analysis of nurses' work, they were only able to demonstrate the inherent difficulties of this type of study in nursing and show the considerable need for reliable information on the range and type of work that nurses do in hospitals. In 1953 Nuffield Provincial Hospitals Trust published a report entitled 'The Work of Nurses in Hospital Wards' (Nuffield Provincial Hospitals Trust, 1953) based on work by Goddard and others who had attempted a job analysis of nursing in general hospital wards. The report was given wide publicity and received much criticism because of methods employed and conclusions drawn. Despite the unfavourable reception the report was a milestone in British nursing research. It remains a classic study that has yet to be duplicated. A major finding of Goddard and colleagues was the wide diversity and complexity of tasks and skills required in nursing. Subsequent descriptive studies have not attempted such a wide undertaking. More recent descriptive studies have attempted to delineate the roles of various specialist groups of nurses, e.g. the midwife (Robinson, 1980), community nurse (Dunnell and Dobbs, 1982) and ward sister (Pembury, 1980). It can be argued that Goddard's work will only be superceded when all the main groups of nurses have been studied. It should then be possible to conduct a theoretical piece of research to synthesize the essential points of these studies and extract common themes and issues. At that stage it may be possible to answer the question posed at the beginning of the Wood Report, 'What is the proper task/role of the nurse?'

The scale and variety in nursing is such that research is invariably at an uneven stage of development. While descriptive studies remain necessary in some areas, others have moved on to experimental-type research aspects of nursing practice and nurse education. Hayward (1975), in his study of post-operative pain, examined the effects of pre-operative information on levels of pain that patients experienced. Bendall (1975) and Alexander (1980) have both studied ward learning environments. These separate studies have been used as the basis for further research that has helped to build up the field of nursing research. Current experimental nursing research includes controlled laboratory studies of the development of pressure sores and the aetiology of infections among patients on urinary catheter drainage. This type of scientific as opposed to social scientific research has a small but important relevance to nursing. However, as the nature of nursing is concerned with the delivery of a service of care to individuals, the social sciences provide the most recently used methods in the study of nursing.

Types of study

Nursing research studies with an evaluative approach are much less well developed and much more recent. The types of study carried out include the evaluation of a ward sister training programme (Lathlean, 1988 and research on the provision of nursing care services to elderly people in nursing homes (Bond, 1984). Evaluative research includes, among other methodologies, action research. This method builds on information from descriptive and experimental research. It is a complete integration of research into the professional discipline of nursing and achieves change through research-based information.

A BASIS FOR FUNDING NURSING RESEARCH

Within the UK nursing research has developed in a way not dissimilar to that in other advanced industrialized societies. The crucial factor is always availability of funds for nursing research and nurses' ability to argue for funding in the research marketplace. In the UK the main source of funding for scientific research is one of the five Research Councils. Two of these Research Councils (the Medical Research Council and the Economic and Social Research Council) have direct interests in the health services while a third (the Medical Sub-Committee of the Science and Engineering Research Council) has a partial interest.

In the absence of a Nursing or Health Services Research Council nursing research has no natural or central location. The professional nursing organizations involve the full range of staff associations, from wage bargaining to professional education. Nursing research has been accorded low priority within the various organizations. Given the lack of both a focus and a professional impetus the main responsibility for nursing research has been assumed by central government through the Department of Health.

In 1974 Lord Rothschild carried out a study of the British government's support of research and development and recommended that, in general, government departments should only be involved in supporting research relevant to the policies of that department. He also argued that policy-related research should be commissioned using the industrial model of a customer/contractor relationship. The DHSS adopted Rothschild's recommendations and in 1983 Kogan and Henkel evaluated them. In practice the principle requires the various policy groups in the department to act as customer and formulate a shopping list of research requirements. Once these are converted into the department's; priorities and funding is secured, a research contractor is then found to do the research. The whole programme of research is coordinated by a medical, nursing and social service team involved in liaison on health and personal social services research and directed by a chief scientist.

Apart from government-sponsored research concerning nursing there are several other ways to obtain funds, such as the already mentioned Medical Research Council, as well as locally organized research funds held by regions and trust funds. Skills to obtain these funds must be developed and one of the functions of research nurses at regional and district level is to help nurses with the design of protocols.

ORGANIZATION OF NURSING RESEARCH

Research in the UK is organized into four settings: designated research units, academic departments of nursing, health authorities and independent commercial clinical research centres. All research undertaken in these settings is supporting endeavours to assist in the formation of policies that result in improved quality of care provided by the health care profession. Within that four general objectives for nursing research are:

1. To support development of a research expertise in nursing;
2. To extend the corpus of research-based knowledge and information available to nurses;
3. To disseminate findings of nursing research to the professions and other interested researchers;
4. To promote implementation of research findings in order to bring about change and improvement in the practice of nursing.

These objectives are common to the four nursing research settings, although each may have different emphasis within the four aims.

Research units

Within the UK there are five research units designated for the study of nursing. Each unit has a permanent staff of full-time researchers commissioned by the funding agency to undertake specific pieces of research. Three of these units are funded by government departments; the unit in Scotland is funded by the Scottish Home and Health Department and the English and Welsh units are funded by the Department of Health. With central support these units have rolling contracts that allow them to undertake longer-term research projects than is possible in units with less secure financial bases. One of the other two nursing research units is funded by the Royal College of Nursing and the other by a charitable organization. The emphasis of the research programmes in each unit is expansion of the body of nursing knowledge. Each unit does, however, have a commitment to develop the research expertise available in nursing and to disseminate its findings to the profession. Each is, to a lesser extent, involved in the implementation of findings. The research units function as centres of excellence where methods for nursing research can be refined and advice on project work obtained.

Departments of nursing

Academic departments of nursing have a commitment to the development of research in nursing through postgraduate courses and doctoral students. In this situation the research undertaken is invariably in areas of the student's interest rather than on policy-relevant topics. Departments of nursing in the UK by and large, have not developed interest in specific areas of nursing. Consequently topics selected for doctoral theses vary considerably with any given department. The emphasis of research undertaken in these departments is development of a research expertise. Through the postgraduate courses they also contribute to dissemination and implementation of research findings.

Health authorities

Within the NHS health authorities a number of senior nurses' posts have as part of their work responsibility to coordinate and advise nursing staff on carrying out or participating in research projects. The purpose of such responsibilities is not so much to carry out research as to heighten practising nurses awareness and knowledge of research findings, and to point out the problems of practising nurses utilizing research findings, and the problems and pitfalls of embarking on research projects without appropriate support and advice. The broad objectives emphasized in this situation are, therefore, the dissemination and implementation of research findings.

Clinical research centres

Centres such as these tend to be associated with equipment evaluation or clinical trials conducted by the pharmaceutical industry. Many studies employ nurses to conduct a part of or a whole study without being the main grant holder. The emphasis of this activity is on doing the actual research. There is not much involvement by participants in this work in any of the other objectives, namely developing the research expertise of those involved in the studies or ensuring that findings are disseminated to or utilized by nurses.

Although research in nursing within the UK has established its own organizational structure, with a number of broad objectives for overall development of nursing research, there are gaps in the structure that need to be considered in future development. Reference has been made to research units that focus on research in nursing. There are a number of multidisciplinary research units involved in studies of the health care service. Because there is a discrete area of nursing research nurses make an important contribution to health care research, although this opportunity has been developed in only a limited way.

It can be argued that benefits from research conducted in academic departments by postgraduate nursing students could be greatly increased if they, like the research units, were developed as centres of expertise in a specific area. It is well recognized that the field of activity has been identified, as nursing is widely diverse. Consequently it may be more effective to have one department focusing on one aspect rather than all departments trying to address the whole field.

The links between nursing research and charitable trust funds or commercial enterprises remain rather tenuous. Nurses in the UK are not well acquainted with the research funding marketplace. In this nursing is particularly unfortunate as it means that nursing has only a limited number of sources from which it can obtain funds. The government departments that currently support approximately 85% of nursing research invariably commission policy-related studies, which may not be in accord with the pressing research needs of the profession.

NURSING EDUCATION AND NURSING RESEARCH

Nursing education in the UK is regulated by Acts of Parliament – currently the Nurses, Midwives and Health Visitors Act of 1979. This Act established the UKCC and the four National Boards (Chapter 4). The broad aim of the UKCC is to establish and improve standards of training and professional conduct and to protect the public from unsafe members of the profession. The broad aim of the National Boards is to arrange courses of basic and post-basic training, including examinations, and to conduct investigations of alleged misconduct.

The need for nursing to place greater emphasis on research was identified in two separate but significant developments in British nursing during the early 1970s. The Report of the Committee on Nursing (DHSS,

1972) made several references to the need for nursing to become research based. Prior to the publication of that report, in 1970, the Joint Board of Clinical Nursing Studies was set up to 'co-ordinate and supervise' post-basic clinical nurse education. This body existed for 13 years and, in that time, became the focus of innovation and experimentation in the content and conduct of educational courses for nurses. The Joint Board drew up curricula and monitored a wide range of clinical nursing courses. The curricula identified the educational objectives to be achieved, which were categorized in terms of skills, knowledge and attributes. All courses included a research objective. As these were examined courses the objectives had to be achieved, and those taking the courses had to achieve a research objective. Lord Briggs' Committee supported a general philosophical stance and the Joint Board then changed the pattern of nurse education to ensure implementation of that stance. The General Nursing Council for England and Wales (GNC E&W) followed the example of the Joint Board and, in 1977, an appreciation of nursing research was included in the syllabus of training for the General Nursing Register. It was not until 1983 that the GNC published a policy document outlining the need for the nursing curriculum to reflect changes in the structure of society and to prepare nurses 'for the resolution of ethical dilemmas based on research evidence'. The organizations that have replaced the GNC and the Joint Board have continued to foster an appreciation of the need for nurses to use research findings and to develop an expertise in research methodology.

While the Joint Board included a research objective within the post-basic clinical courses, it also organized a number of research appreciation courses to assist in heightening nurses' general awareness of research findings and research issues. These courses remain popular and have the objective of promulgating research-mindedness through development of an enquiring attitude of mind, a logical approach to problems relating to nursing, an awareness of the existence of research reports and the ability to read, evaluate, select and make use of relevant findings.

Simpson (1981) has argued that research appreciation courses should disappear as research understanding is built into education for nurses; we are none the less still a long way from that goal. She went on to claim that the use of research in policy making is in its infancy and, as indicated above with respect to manpower planning, part of the problem is the dearth of research evidence to support decision making.

A major difficulty when promoting research awareness in basic and post-basic programmes of nurse education and training is the ability of nurse teachers to use research in their teaching sessions. Courses of preparation for nurse teachers have not responded as quickly as have organizers of clinical courses to this developing situation. If research is to become an integral part of all nurse education, as it should be, teaching sessions should encourage students to utilize research findings through problem solving, decision making and self-awareness.

In the UK, at present, fewer than 10% of all newly qualified nurses are graduates who have completed their nurse education on a university or polytechnic course. Those who do are exposed to more vigorous research-based educational programmes; they are, however, the minority and investment has to be directed towards the basic nurse education system. Addressing this problem is the diploma programme in nursing (University of London). A part-time course run in several centres throughout the country, it is organized in six modular sections, one of which is research.

In 1967 the then DHSS provided funds to support a nursing research studentship/fellowship scheme. Awards have been made annually since then and, to date, 122 nurses have used the scheme as a means of achieving a higher degree and education and training in the methodology of research. Over the years of its existence the type of support provided has changed to meet the changing demand for research education. Whereas the majority of awards were at one time given to nurses who taught research courses, they are now only given to graduate nurses who are pursuing doctoral studies on a part-time basis. One of the main aims of this scheme has been to develop a research expertise in nursing and this is being slowly achieved. Those who held an award under the scheme in the early years have gone on to take up posts in academic nurse education. More recently a number of former students have gone on to take posts in health authorities with responsibility for disseminating research to practising nurses. A secondary outcome of the DH scheme has been that it has been used as a model for other funding agencies such as charities or health authorities.

In 1987 the first post-doctoral research fellowship, established by the DH, provided an opportunity for nurse researchers to work above the level of PhD study. A specific objective of this award is to encourage nurse researchers to become involved in multidisciplinary health service research. While there is a specific area of work that can be identified as nursing research, the much larger sphere of the work of health services research requires multidisciplinary participation, with nursing as an integral and important part. In terms of personnel development it is participation in multidisciplinary research that must be a major focus for nursing research in the future.

DISSEMINATION AND IMPLEMENTATION OF RESEARCH

The dissemination and implementation of findings to improve quality and standards of nursing care is a major aim of nursing research, whether this is through improving personnel policy issues, such as raising morale among staff, or better knowledge about specific aspects of direct care. Dissemination and implementation of research findings takes much effort and tends to be slow in showing a return on investment. Dissemination has mainly been in the form of top down activity, for example in the setting up of the 'Index of Nursing Research', funded by the Department of Health and published at quarterly intervals.

In 1958 in London the first research discussion group was set up, which in 1974 became the Royal College of Nursing Research Society. This has led to a network of small research interest groups throughout the UK that meet regularly to discuss developments in research and provide local peer support. Other means of disseminating research are through nursing journals, conferences and seminars. The Chief Nursing Officer of England and the government health departments focus attention on major nursing research reports by issuing a research letter. The RCN publishes research work through a research series and has also established the Steinberg Collection, which houses PhD and MPhil nursing research theses.

In 1972 a number of research nurses were appointed at regional level to promote nursing research in the NHS. Their role was broadly two-fold: they were expected, first, to promote awareness of systematic enquiry and, second, to translate this into practice. Doreen Norton and Arnold Lancaster were two of the pioneers in this field who promoted 'the need for research at the patient level'. They attempted to set up a network of nurse researchers at district level, some of whom were more successful than others. But throughout the UK the practice of bringing about change through decisions made as a result of knowledge based on research grew. These nurses brought research closer to patient care and began to demonstrate the value of solving problems through systematic enquiry. The range of enquiry included clinical practice, such as research into incontinence and healing of pressure sores (Norton, 1970), patient management with specific groups (Redfern, 1991), roles of the ward nursing team (Pembury, 1980), care in the community (Kratz, 1978; Poulton, 1981) and research into nursing education, both basic and post-basic (Bendall, 1975; Fretwell, 1985; Stapleton, 1986).

At that time nurses were also trying to obtain research funds from various funding bodies, such as the Medical Research Council, locally organized research funds and trust funds. Salter (1981) suggests that nurses were not very successful in this. Another function of research nurses at the regional and district level has been to help nurses with research design and protocols.

KEY AREAS IN NURSING RESEARCH AND FUTURE PRIORITIES

Much of the research to date has been descriptive rather than experimental in nature. Testing long-term effects of certain nursing actions is uncommon and the question of 'What difference does it make if, for example, the composition of the health care team is changed?' has been slow to be addressed. Identification of research priorities is an important area. There is a need to distinguish between those problems that need management action and those that need scientific investigation. The influence of nurses in the community is one area of importance, given the commitment to the World Health Organisation Alma Ata declaration that aims to achieve health for all by the year 2000.

The efficient and effective utilization of scarce professional health care manpower is high on the agenda. The question of providing the most cost-effective education pattern for the 'future' health carer, including nurses, and, in particular, the possible effects of proposed education strategies (Chapter 4) will no doubt be seen as important areas for research. Supply of the necessary numbers of suitably qualified nurses to meet future needs is of crucial importance and demands attention.

In terms of addressing client satisfaction issues, quality of care and productivity are bound to form a focus for nursing research. Not unlike other Western countries, it seems that the primary need is to develop appropriate new methodologies for nursing research. Development of sensitive indicators to measure outcomes and, with confidence, relate them to identified processes is essential.

The research index shows that these areas are being looked at and, as this research develops, questions such as 'What difference does it make if certain changes are made in nursing practice and how much does it cost?' can only then be adequately addressed.

8

Planning for nursing

THE PLANNING PROCESS

The role of the Department of Health is essentially strategic, with responsibility for the level of funding of the National Health Service (NHS), and with ministers giving strategic guidance on national policies and priorities, broadly indicating ways in which they look for development in the service and where economies should be sought.

In pursuit of providing the best possible health care service within available resources in response to national and international goals, such as better health for all by the year 2000 (World Health Organisation, 1976), the Department of Health published in 1991 'The Health of the Nation'. It set out what will need to be achieved by way of further improvements to the nation's health.

A number of areas for further development have been identified as either priority client groups or priority services for elderly people, especially the most vulnerable and frail, the mentally ill, mentally handicapped, and physically and sensory handicapped; also highlighted are maternity and neonatal services, primary health care, services for young children at risk and care and treatment of young offenders.

The limited growth of financial resources, coupled with large priority groups, requires health authorities to assess carefully the utilization of resources through the contracting framework. They often face conflicting pressures from different groups and categories and, at the same time, must deal with rapidly rising costs in some service sectors, especially hospital services. The last few years have seen higher levels of activity in acute and maternity services, coupled with a reduction in the number of available hospital beds, increased use of high technology, equipment and procedures, increasing rates of early discharge from hospital and the development of community care for the main client groups – the elderly, mentally ill, mentally handicapped and disabled and children.

Planning nursing services and the workforce to achieve stated goals is an integral part of planning total NHS services. Over the past decade regions in England prepared their strategic ten-year plan, agreed with the Department of Health, and produced annual operational plans. Underpinning this process is a system of monitoring and review on an annual basis.

Since the reform of the health service and the introduction of the provider/purchaser functions, roles and responsibilities have changed to take on board new market force concepts.

The Department of Health Performance Management Directorate is the main arm of the NHS Management Executive responsible for the monitoring process. Activities are changing as relationships between purchasing regions or districts and provider units change. This is particularly prominent in the dialogue with NHS Trusts who relate directly to Department of Health and therefore 'bypass' regions.

Planning and managing nursing resources, however, remains high on the agenda. The supply/deployment and demand for nursing services involves all levels of the service. Regions mainly hold the nurse education budget for pre-registration training and are therefore responsible for contracting pre-registration nursing and midwifery education to colleges and other education establishments.

Units are responsible for ensuring that they are able to obtain sufficient numbers of nursing staff according to their needs. Manpower planning at unit level is becoming more important and will help to establish their need for new qualifiers to inform about the regions' purchasing (of education) intentions.

Districts are responsible for ensuring that their contracts for services with units include quality indicators to ensure a high quality service for their population. Such indicators may, for example, be a stipulation of ratios of qualified to unqualified staff, specialist experts or service outcome indicators.

In this new era of delivering health services, and the operating market forces, cost containment, efficiency and value for money, the focus is sharply on nursing practice and the efficient use of nursing resources.

The question of how many nurses, midwives or health visitors we need is not new. The National Audit Office undertook a study on manpower issues from a value for money and efficiency viewpoint. It published a report in December 1985 that was critical of the Department of Health and health authorities for not being systematic enough in determining future demand for manpower. The report also made a number of detailed recommendations concerning nurse rostering, shift overlaps and skills utilization (National Audit Office, 1985).

Development of nursing services is part of the overall planning for such services but there are no nationally prescribed methodologies for planning either supply or demand for nursing manpower. Since the development of resource management, however, there are excellent examples of successful methods employed at local level.

To turn first to supply it is Department of Health policy that, in broad terms, each region in England should be self-sufficient in recruiting and training of its skilled nursing workforce. The position in Northern Ireland is somewhat different in that nurse emigration from this country has always been a factor, and it is therefore necessary to include some degree of over-training in order to ensure an adequate supply of staff. For much of NHS history planning the supply of nurse recruits has not been a significant issue. That is to say health authorities have been able to rely, with occasional exceptions in specific localities or for specific nursing specialties, on a ready supply of qualified recruits. There have been occasional periods of recruitment difficulty and the demographic prospect for the UK is of a prolonged period of difficulty in the years ahead.

The NHS is the biggest single recruiter of academically qualified female school leavers in the UK. The supply of such school leavers has declined by 25% over the 1982–92 period, at a time when, over approximately the same period, demand for such staff grew. During the mid-1980s much higher demand for qualified staff was predicted, which led to a renewal of interest in supply modelling, both in terms of modelling future demand in the labour market and modelling the output from the existing training capacity. However it must be said that the 1984 round of strategic plans showed little evidence of extensive use of supply modelling. Indeed the Department of Health, which had in the early 1980s modelled the supply emerging from the training system on a national basis discontinued this use of modelling. This decision resulted not from lack of interest in the findings of such modelling but from the fact that NHS manpower statistics were notoriously out of date. This caused results from the national model to emerge up to two years after the year to which they related, making them of little use for practical planning purposes.

The work of the United Kingdom Central Council for Nursing, Midwifery and Health Visiting (UKCC) in examining the future of nurse education and training (Chapter 4) has also stimulated interest in supply issues on a national basis. In particular the UKCC undertook a major study on future manpower prospects for nursing, which concluded that a combination of future demography and a decision to phase out second level (enrolled) nurse training (thus increasing demand for recruits qualified to enter first level training) could, on certain assumptions, produce a 20% shortfall compared to planned demand for qualified nurses by the end of the century. Over the last several years health authorities have increasingly conducted their own local supply studies, ranging from demographic and educational surveys of their traditional recruiting areas to local labour market surveys to identify the pool of qualified nurses currently not in nursing who are being encouraged to return and, in some cases, use models of training capacity to attempt to identify the effect of action to decrease the rate of wastage during training.

There has also been a considerable interest in stimulating direct entry midwifery training. The vast majority of midwives in the UK undertake midwifery training as a second registration, having already trained as a nurse (Chapter 5). Not only is this considered to be expensive but it is also arguable that, in a period of recruitment difficulty, it is wasteful of scarce human resources, hence the interest in recruiting and training midwives specifically for the profession.

Information needs for planning

A further consequence of the growing awareness of potential difficulties with supply has been the Department of Health decision to collect, as part of the latest round of short-term programmes, more detailed information about the training intentions of health authorities than has hitherto been collected. This information is being set alongside prediction of stock of qualified staff at various stages through the strategic planning cycle.

Supply modelling presents very different problems from demand modelling. That is to say the overall dimensions of a future supply problem are readily identifiable without use of sophisticated modelling techniques. What is more difficult is the modelling of the effect of different kinds of management action to overcome future supply problems and estimating their chances of success. Some of the most difficult decisions facing the nursing profession in the UK today concern the efficacy and feasibility of alternative methods of reducing wastage in training, reducing wastage from stock, encouraging the return of qualified nurses not currently working in nursing and, perhaps most crucial of all, devising ways of widening the entry gate to nurse training without sacrificing quality.

Much more effort has been put into demand modelling. There are a number of widely used methods as well as a series of comparative studies of methods. Most of these comparative studies, carried out by operational researchers, have frequently been criticized because they lack adequate professional input. Furthermore, in general, nurse workforce demand models have concentrated on the demand for acute hospital nurses and relatively little attention has been paid to demand modelling for mental illness, mental handicap or community nursing.

Essentially methods in general use can be divided into 'bottom up' and 'top down' methods. Bottom up methods define operational requirements at ward or hospital level to meet the nursing workload and convert them to required establishments of nursing staff. In some cases the methods are used to adjust day-to-day allocations, for which purpose they were often designed in the first instance. Top down methods relate aggregate key factors as a proxy workload to nursing staff numbers, generating expected staff levels that can be compared with existing levels. Application of this method lends itself primarily to determining strategic demands and planning new services.

Most bottom up methods seek to establish a statistical or arithmetical relationship between nursing workload and number of staff required. This can be done in two ways: first, by adding up standard times (by dependency) for patients on the ward and then adding in (according to method) times that take account of type of ward and the way it is operated; and, second, by giving patients in each dependency group a weight which is multiplied by the number of patients in a group to give a workload for a ward of patients, summing these workloads and deriving a nurse-time equivalent from a regression relationship that has previously been established. A frequent criticism of such methods is that, although they all make extensive use of statistical and arithmetical relationships or formulae, all contain significant elements of subjective judgement that the models do not make explicit.

In contrast a completely different form of bottom up method is provided by the Telford model, which seeks to collect, in a structured fashion, professional judgements of experienced ward sisters about the staffing required for their patients on the basis of simple dependency classification. In some variants of this method results are subjected to regression analysis and judgements that prove to be outliers subjected to further questioning and scrutiny. The various methods have been subjected to a degree of comparative analysis, which suggests that results from application of the Telford method are not significantly different from those produced by more sophisticated methodologies.

Top down methods all use multiple linear regression analysis to examine the relationship between various proxies for nursing workload and current establishments. The results may be used either to monitor existing establishments, and to seek to change those that are significantly out of line, or to predict establishments in new developments for strategic planning purposes. Use of such approaches is sometimes resisted on two grounds:

1. Variables that are not statistically significant are often 'felt' to be so locally and their exclusion from the formula damages the chances of its acceptability.
2. The methodology is rooted in current practice and cannot take account of future changes in nursing practice or other developments that may affect nursing workloads.

There is thus considerable diversity upon which little attempt has been made to impose any central conformity. Some steps in this direction have been taken in Scotland and Wales but in England the Department of

Health has confined itself to publishing descriptions and analyses of the different methodologies. This state of affairs has been criticized by the National Audit Office and the Parliamentary Accounts Committee but the Department of Health position is that all methodologies currently in use have limitations or flaws and that uniformity is not possible, given the diversity of conditions in England. A comprehensive information pack provides the NHS with considerable guidance on managing nursing resources and covers workload, skills and management, human resources management, quality and finance (DOH, 1991). This and other recently published material referred to in these chapters forms the essential armour for all nurses in the new world and will equip them well to enter the new millennium.

Part Three

Canada

9
Historical evolution of the health care and nursing systems

The history of nursing in Canada must be seen in relation to the history of the country itself as well as the unique fabric of Canadian society, social conditions and economic development. Canada is a relatively young country; only in 1534 did the Frenchman Jacques Cartier arrive in the area of what is now Canada. The vastness of a country that spans 4000 miles, with its inherent geographic and environmental contrasts within that area, has presented special challenges to Canadian nurses.

THE EARLY SETTLERS

In the early 1600s the first nurses in Canada, from French nursing sisterhoods, settled along the St Lawrence River. The sisters, highly vocational and having intense missionary zeal, often found their dedication and courage tested in the primitive conditions then existing. Deadly epidemics occurred frequently in the first 150 years of Canadian history and had it not been for the brave French sisters, many Huron and Algonquin Indians and white people would have died who in fact survived (Gibbon and Mathewson, 1947). The major health problems in the early years were epidemics (smallpox, typhus and cholera) and nutritional deficiencies (scurvy and rickets) (Hastings and Mosley, 1966). Much is known about these conditions because of local (parochial) registration of deaths as well as births and marriages, required as early as 1608.

Hospitals and growth of the country

In 1629 a French garrison hospital was built at Port Royal in Acadia (Nova Scotia). This hospital did have trained male attendants but, in the early days of Canadian nursing, French nuns carried the burden. The first *Canadian* nurse was not a sister. She was Marie Hubou, widow of a French surgeon who had come to Canada, who devoted much of her time to caring for the sick sent to her by the Jesuit fathers (Mussallem, 1968).

The first civilian hospital, established on the shores of the St Lawrence River, was the Hotel Dieu of Quebec (1639), originally staffed by nursing sisters from Dieppe. Life at this time was harsh and brutal and the sisters needed much courage to live in such primitive and dangerous conditions. Montreal's first hospital, the Montreal Hotel Dieu, was built in 1645, largely by the efforts of Jeanne Mance. That determined woman made frequent trips to France often bringing back women to serve as nursing assistants. The original hospital measured only 60 ft by 24 ft plus an adjoining chapel. As often happened with wooden structures it burnt down completely (in 1721) but was rebuilt, with subsequent additions to accommodate a growing population. At the time of the original hospital Montreal had a population of just 65, difficult to imagine in these days of over two million inhabitants. The first Canadian-born women began to join the nursing sisterhood by the late 1600s. The first Canadian midwife, Catherine Guertin, was apparently elected by the women of Ville Marie (Montreal) in 1713.

One of the most important groups to contribute to nursing in the pioneer days were the Grey Nuns (Soeurs Grise), part of a medieval order dating from the 13th century. The Grey Nuns were known as the 'tippling sisters' because they sold liquor to the Indians. They wore grey-brown habits and were founded in Canada by Madame d'Youville, who in the mid-1700s started what is now called district nursing and home visiting.

Immigrants and epidemics

In the late 1700s and early 1800s a wave of immigration, first of Americans and later a steady influx of English, Irish, Scots, Dutch and Germans, increased the urgency to build new hospitals. These new immigrants were often in poor health from nutritional deficiencies and diseases, often acquired in transit. One especially difficult problem was cholera, which had no known effective treatment except for 'herbal cures' learned from the Indians, and nurses died along with their patients. This and other infectious diseases spread very rapidly from seaports despite attempts to control them by quarantine of passengers.

Montreal General Hospital, built in 1819, was the first to have a lay (non-sister) nurse as matron. (In 1829 this hospital became the Medical Faculty of McGill University.) Conditions in hospitals in general were appallingly unhealthy and wiser people endeavoured to stay out of them. Dr I. J. Shephard, in a history published by the Montreal General Hospital nursing school alumni, said (Mussallem, 1986):

> In my day (the late [18] sixties and after), age and drowsiness seemed the chief attributes of the nurse, who was ill-educated and was often made more unattractive by the vinous odor of her breath. Cleanliness was not a feature, either of the nurse, the ward or the patient; each one

The early settlers

did as best pleased her, and the 'langwridge' was frequently painful and free. Armies of rats frequently disported themselves about the wards, and picked up stray scraps left by the patients, and sometimes attacked the patients themselves.

In the mid-1800s a movement westwards began by homesteaders (mostly Metis, the offspring of French Canadians and Indians) to the vast fertile lands of the prairies, but Scottish settlers also went west via the Hudson Bay, along with Americans, Germans and Swiss. The Grey Nuns bravely followed. Settling in St Boniface (Manitoba) they expanded their services to the Northwest Territories and Bytown (Ottawa), nursing mostly in the homes of the settlers (Gibbon and Mathewson, 1947). In the prairies, a Father Lacombe, who travelled and nursed across the vast lands, is especially remembered for his work among the Indians.

In 1848 anaesthetics were introduced by Dr James Young Simpson from Scotland and procedures were set up following Florence Nightingale's 'Notes for the British Army'. Because many Canadians had served in the Crimean War two hospitals were built in Canada by the British government, in Halifax and Esquimalt, Vancouver Island.

Further movement westward to the Pacific coast was spurred by the lure of gold as well as flourishing fur and timber trades. The British Columbian coast was settled by Indians, Orientals, Scandinavians and Britons. The first hospital there was the Royal Columbian, founded in New Westminster in 1862 and financed by the city council and private donations from gold miners. As towns grew (the trans-Canada railroad being a major factor) building of hospitals could be justified, although they mainly served the poorer classes and were regarded as places of last resort because of high mortality rates (Hastings, 1985).

The health problems of the continuing influx of immigrants were serious. There was also a major public health problem in trying to control the filth and garbage that accumulated in larger towns from the hygienically uneducated. Repeated epidemics snuffed out many lives because of lack of adequate care in spite of the dedicated work by the few nurses available.

Confederation

The federation of Canada was formally enacted in 1867 when the British North American Act, passed by the British parliament, united several of the Canadian colonies, which were then given the status of Dominion. The Act formed the constitutional framework for the governance of Canada. Following the confederation the land monopoly of the Hudson Bay Company was bought by the British government and a new province of Manitoba was formed, the rest of the prairies still being designated the

Northwest Territories. Winnipeg was the first city in Canada to organize a public general hospital (1872).

HEALTH AND THE FEDERAL GOVERNMENT

The terms of the North American Act with respect to health were quite meagre since, at that time, government was seen as having a limited role in health matters. The federal government had responsibility for quarantine regulations, marine hospitals, veterans, Indians, prisoners, sailors and arrivals from abroad. The provinces had responsibility for the management of hospitals, asylums and other institutions (Soderstrom, 1978).

In the late 1880s each Canadian province, starting with Ontario in 1884, passed a public health act that required each municipality to appoint a local board of health, a medical officer of health and a sanitary inspector.

Nurse training schools

The first training school for nurses in Canada was established in 1874 by Dr Theophilus Mack, in conjunction with the General and Marine Hospital at St Catherines, Ontario. Canadian schools of nursing were patterned on the Florence Nightingale model and were typically a part of the hospital rather than an independent entity. Montreal General Hospital sought advice from Florence Nightingale, who sent Maria Machin, a Canadian-born student at St Thomas' school, to assist in developing a school in Canada. The training programme extended over two years and included practical instruction on the wards as well as lectures. In 1881 the Toronto General Hospital established its training school and there began a growth of specialized hospitals, including the Hospital for Sick Children and Women's College Hospital in Toronto as well as provincial psychiatric hospitals in Ontario.

The Victorian Order of Nurses (VON) was established by Lady Aberdeen in 1898. Initially centred in Ottawa the services of the VON quickly spread across the country. The Grey Nuns and the Sisters of Providence had done home nursing; the VON was to supply trained nurses to hospitals and districts, coordinate the local supply of nurses by bringing them under one authority, improve the efficiency of district nursing and assist in providing small cottage hospitals with nursing services.

Early public health nurses

Public health nursing began formally in 1905 when Christine Mitchell joined Toronto's health department and became the city's first tuberculosis nurse. Manitoba was the first province to employ public health nurses paid from public funds. In 1916 the Manitoba government employed five public health nurses to investigate infant mortality in order to demonstrate the usefulness of such nursing. The public health nurses emphasized health education, especially immunization against childhood diseases. The public health work of nurses was assisted by the introduction of water chlorination and pasteurization of milk in some of the larger communities.

In 1921 the VON sponsored a programme to award scholarships at Canadian universities for postgraduate courses in public health nursing. By the end of the Second World War almost 300 scholarships had been awarded. Dalhousie University offered the first course for graduate nurses in public health nursing in 1920. The first university degree programme in nursing (in the British Empire) was started at the University of British Columbia in 1919 by Ethel Johns. A Director of Nursing at the Vancouver General Hospital, she was given a university appointment, first as lecturer and then as assistant professor.

The Red Cross

Dr George Sterling Ryerson was responsible for starting the Canadian Red Cross Society in 1896. The Society financed the employment of public health nurses and provided funds for them to take specialized university courses. Between 1920 and 1938 it had established over 60 outposts (hospital beds and public health centres) and nursing stations in the Canadian north.

Nursing and war

As in other countries Canadian nurses were much affected by recurring wars. During the Boer War the 7000 Canadian soldiers in South Africa were accompanied by Canadian nurses under the leadership of Georgia Fane Pope from Prince Edward Island. The experiences in South Africa convinced Canadian army medical officers that army nursing services were essential. During the First World War 65 army medical units and a number of military hospitals were established. At the end of the war over 2000 nurses returned to Canada to work in a variety of hospitals, outposts and mental health facilities.

During the Second World War over 4000 nurses served with the Canadian Military sisters, two-thirds of whom were overseas. Not surprisingly there had been considerable growth in the number of nurses in the first half of the 20th century. In 1911 there were fewer than 6000 nurses but by 1941 there were about 26 000 nurses listed in the Canadian Census (Gibbon and Mathewson, 1947).

NURSES ASSOCIATIONS AND JOURNALS

The first nursing alumni group was formally organized in 1884 at Toronto General Hospital School of Nursing. A number of provincial nursing associations were constituted in the early 1900s. In 1930 the Canadian Nurses Association was formed as a federation of the nine provincial associations, with about 8000 members. The forerunner of the Canadian Nurses Association was the Provincial Society of the Canadian National Association of Trained Nurses (CNATN), which first met in 1909. The Toronto General Hospital Alumnae Association also sponsored the first quarterly issue of 'The Canadian Nurse and Hospital Review' (1905). In 1916 CNATN bought the publication from a business firm; later it became the national journal of the Canadian Nurses Association – 'The Canadian Nurse'.

During the 1930s one of the most important events for Canadian nursing was the publication of the Weir Report (Weir, 1932), which was stimulated by an apparent shortage of nurses and was sponsored jointly by the CNA and the Canadian Medical Association. The report made recommendations for the development of curricula and standards for schools of nursing. Another recommendation was that schools of nursing be subsidized by government funding and incorporated into the general education system.

The continuing growth in many areas of Canadian life necessitated the formation of a federal Department of Health in 1919, later merged with the Department of Soldier's Civil Re-establishment to form the Department of Pensions and National Health. In 1944 this became the Department of National Health and Welfare, which has responsibility for all federal matters relating to health promotion and prevention, social security and social welfare (Hastings, 1985).

THE DEVELOPMENT OF NATIONAL HEALTH INSURANCE

The federal government of Canada has direct responsibility for personal health services for specific groups of people, including the armed forces, veterans, prisoners in federal institutions and Royal Canadian Mounted Police, and federal civil services for occupational health services. It also provides personal health services to Indians and Inuits in remote areas through federally run hospitals and nursing stations. Provision of all other health services is the responsibility of provincial governments.

Beginnings of health insurance

Health insurance was initiated in various provinces in the 1930s and 1940s. In 1934 Newfoundland (not part of the Confederation until 1949) developed a publicly financed Cottage Hospital and Medical Care Plan that employed nurses and doctors to provide health services to Newfoundland's sparse and scattered population (Miller, 1951). Many early attempts to pass provincial legislation in Alberta, British Columbia, Quebec and Saskatchewan failed for a variety of social and political reasons as well as because of medical opposition. In the 1940s discussion of the health sector at the national level prompted the federal government to propose to the provinces a broad programme of social security, including a cost-shared health insurance plan, although no agreements were reached at that time.

Saskatchewan led the way in 1947, introducing the Saskatchewan Hospital Services Plan that provided universal and compulsory hospitalization coverage for all residents of the province and was financed from compulsory premiums and general taxation. Within the next two or three years other provinces, including British Columbia, Alberta and Newfoundland, had developed their own hospital plans. In 1948 the federal government introduced a new programme of national health grants that provided provinces with funding for public health, hospital construction, health planning and professional training, a step intended as preparation for further development of a national health scheme. In 1957 the Federal Hospital Insurance and Diagnostic Services Act was passed, which gave provinces grants-in-aid to administer plans for all hospital beds and emergency and some diagnostic services. The cost sharing between federal and provincial governments was equal but was also based on the province's ability to pay: richer provinces such as Ontario paid more than less affluent provinces (Taylor, 1978).

During this period there was also rapid growth in medical care insurance, with about half of all Canadians buying some form of medical insurance from private companies.

Towards a national health scheme

One of the most important steps towards development of a national health scheme was the appointment in 1961 by Conservative Prime Minister John Diefenbaker of a Royal Commission to investigate health services. The Commission, chaired by the Hon. Emmett Hall, made far-reaching recommendations that not only suggested a national health scheme but also specified coverage for a wide range of medical, dental, optical, drug and other services in addition to hospital services. The Liberal Party was in power by the time the report was finished and, much to the dismay of the medical associations and insurance companies, passed legislation that led to the development of the Federal Medical Care Act, which came into effect in 1968. Some provinces initially resisted the programme because of cost sharing arrangements in which all provinces were obliged to participate but in which the richer provinces did not receive a full return of their contributions, the money going to the poorer provinces.

Purposes of the health insurance plan

The new health insurance scheme had four essential directives. First, the programme must provide comprehensive coverage for a full range of health services. Second, services should be universally accessible to all Canadians. Third, the programme should be publicly administered. Fourth, there should be portability of the insurance across the provinces. Each province was free to design its health service within these guidelines, and it is often said that there is not one system but ten provincial and two territorial systems.

For the next ten years federal and provincial governments debated cost sharing arrangements, until 1977 when the Federal-Provincial Fiscal Arrangements and Established Programs Financing Act was passed, under which the federal government gave up personal and corporation income tax points to provinces as well as providing cash block funding (Van Loon, 1978).

Rising costs of health care

There had been considerable concern about escalating health care costs throughout the 1960s (Task Force Report on the Cost of Health Services in Canada, 1969) and in the 1970s the provinces developed a number of strategies to try to control costs. These included placing stricter *limits* on hospital budgets, hospital beds, medical fee schedules, immigration of doctors and other health personnel. (Introduction of new expensive technologies, however, often diluted cost containment efforts.) These strategies along with wage and price controls held GNP expenditures on health services to about 7.5% compared to 9.5% in the US. In 1982 the percentage of Canadian GNP allocated to health services was estimated at 8.4% compared to 10.5% in the US (Hastings, 1984).

During recent years there has been growing concern that the universality of health services is threatened. Some provinces charge user fees directly to individual patients for hospital stay. Others allow physicians to opt out of direct billing of the medicare plan and charge patients directly. Still others allow physicians to charge patients over and above scheduled payment levels, i.e. extra billing. These practices skewed accessibility of certain services towards the more affluent. After considerable debate amongst governments, professional associations and consumer groups, the Canadian Health Act was passed in 1984 that reaffirmed the four directives of the Medical Care Act and financially penalized provinces that continued to allow user fees extra billing by physicians.

THE SOCIAL CONTEXT AND CHANGING ENVIRONMENT OF CANADA

The political system

Canada has a parliamentary system of government, with citizens electing a parliament at both federal and provincial levels. The political party with the majority of elected members forms the government, the leader of which is the Prime Minister at the national level and the Premier at the provincial level. Ministers are appointed to a cabinet that determines government policies. The Queen, as head of state, is represented at the federal level by the Governor-General and at the provincial level by Lieutenants-Governor.

Since health is considered a provincial matter provincial health legislation is formed in two stages. Legislation must be approved by, first, the cabinet and, second, the legislature. Before receiving cabinet approval the proposed legislation is usually further developed by a committee of cabinet under the direction of the Minister of Health. It then may be considered by the full cabinet and, once approved, is submitted to the legislature. The Bill usually goes through three readings on three different days, during which it is available to the public and expert witnesses and interested parties to provide additional information to the government. If the Bill is passed it is presented to the Lieutenant-Governor as the Queen's representative, although this is usually a formality (Soderstrom, 1978).

Demographics and nursing

Canada has a population of about 26.5 million people, the majority of whom live within 200 miles of the US border. Over 60% of Canadians live in Ontario and Quebec. Accordingly there is a large proportion of Canada that is sparsely populated, often isolated and difficult to service. Because of Canadian immigration policy and immigration patterns Canada is today characterized by high multiculturalism, especially in the larger cities. Unlike the US Canada has encouraged new immigrants to retain essential characteristics of their original cultures, creating what has been called the Canadian Mosaic. The individual cultures hold their own beliefs and attitudes towards health and health behaviours and are a special concern to nurses. In addition many people in the Eastern provinces need two languages (English and French) in order to find employment. In Quebec nurses must pass French language proficiency tests to obtain registration. Although Canada's population has been relatively young because of the large proportion of new immigrants, the proportion of very old people (over 80 years of age) is increasing, especially in rural areas.

Technology

Increasing sophistication of medical technology has resulted in more Canadians surviving serious health problems and living longer, often with chronic illnesses. As elsewhere the health services system in Canada is struggling to keep abreast of these new developments. Each may have considerable impact and often unpredictable effects on nursing practice and management. For example widespread introduction of computers into health services facilities for both clinical and managerial data handling should provide a better database for decision making over the long term.

Cost constraints

As with other countries Canada has a growing concern about increasing costs of health services. Historically although institutions such as hospitals or long-term care facilities were aware of costs, they were not under any particular pressure to contain them. A deficit incurred by a hospital was often automatically assumed by the provincial government. However in recent years provincial governments have taken stronger positions and declared publicly that deficits are the responsibility of individual hospitals. Indications of provincial governments' more serious approach to cost-containment in hospitals is illustrated by Ontario's business orientated new development (BOND) programme that provides incentives for hospitals to use business-like methods. Although there is currently no crisis for basic funding of health services, there is some unease about the future. Significant real increases in operating and capital budgets are unlikely (Thompson and LeTouze, 1984). Clearly as hospital budgets shrink so proportionally do those of nursing departments.

RATIONALIZATION OF HEALTH SERVICES

Attempts to rationalize Canada's health services system through regionalization have met with limited success, except in Quebec (Gosselin, 1984). In Ontario district health councils have regional responsibilities for health planning but no fiscal authority. Canadian hospitals are not mandated to provide the total range of health services. In the future, however, it is expected that attempts to assign priorities to programmes will be increasingly controlled by provincial governments, with pressure to limit provision of certain programmes through greater regulation. Some people predict the reintroduction of private funding of health services and there have been a few examples in Ontario of private funding of capital projects (Leatt, 1986).

In the late 1970s, stimulated by the Lalonde Report (1974), many health care providers hoped that greater emphasis would be given to health promotion and disease prevention activities. Because these changes have not materialized the focus within the health services system remains on treatment of acute episodes of illness. The hospital and institutional sectors account for about 54% of expenditure (Hastings, 1985).

TRENDS IN THE ORGANIZATION OF HEALTH SERVICES

Delivery of personal health services is fragmented and uncoordinated (Hastings, 1985). Ambulatory and hospital services are often provided by different physicians while most primary care is provided by general practitioners who work in private practices. The predominant method of payment to doctors is fee-for-service on submission of accounts to provincial medical plans. A small proportion of nurse practitioners, social workers, physiotherapists and nutritionists are in private practice; pharmacists and chiropractors practise privately in somewhat larger numbers. In an attempt to encourage a team approach to health service delivery, community health centres were developed in the early 1970s (The Community Health Centre in Canada, 1973). These primary care centres employ a range of health professionals, including physicians, and provide services to a local community. The concept has not, however, been extensively implemented, mostly because of resistance by physicians. Currently there are 112 centres in Quebec, 28 in Ontario and 19 across the rest of Canada (Hastings, 1985).

Because of pressure to contain costs and to rationalize the health services system individual health service organizations are more and more being encouraged to coordinate with other providers of health and social services. Small communities, for example, that have two hospitals with relatively low occupancy rates are encouraged to merge, share and/or eliminate certain services. Because of the ageing population acute hospital beds in small communities are being converted to chronic hospital beds. In large urban hospitals there is sharing not only of traditional hotel services such as food, housekeeping, laundry and purchasing but also of clinical areas such as medical staff. There are growing numbers of multi-institutional arrangements, with several hospitals or facilities being managed by one corporate structure (Leatt, 1986). Because of the complexity of medical technology traditional hospital organizational designs (such as functional structures) are becoming less common. It is predicted that there will be increasing tendencies towards multiple reporting relationships, mixed-matrix designs and a need for multidisciplinary approaches (Leatt, 1985).

IMPLICATIONS FOR NURSING IN CANADA

Today's environment in Canada presents an interesting challenge for nurses. In general consumers of health services are satisfied with the level of service they receive; most Canadians believe they have good health care services and have no major criticism of the system (Roemer, 1985). Nurses, as the primary direct care providers in most health services organizations, deserve much of the credit for the strong positive feelings of consumers towards the health services system.

Nurses are employed in a large variety of health service organizations, including acute general hospitals, public health units, psychiatric, rehabilitation and long-term-care facilities, home care programmes and government. For example, in the more than 1000 general hospitals it is estimated that, on average, the nursing budget accounts for over 50% of the hospital budget and two-thirds of the personnel budget. In 1983 there were approximately 250 000 registered nurses and over 38 000 nursing assistants (Canadian Health Manpower Inventory, 1984).

Because of the changing characteristics of the health services system, as well as the relative unpredictability of the larger environment, high quality nursing services in all types of health services organizations are critical. It is important that nurses assume a pro-active role as members of the health team. Traditionally nurses have tended to assume a rather reactive role; they have been subordinate to physicians because of their professional status and to other administrators bureaucratically. Past nursing leaders have not been skilful or forceful enough in articulating the needs of nursing departments to other groups. New roles are emerging for nurses but they have not been clearly identified or even broadly discussed (Leatt, 1985a).

There has been a proliferation of new health workers in recent years. Many activities that were the domain of nursing have been taken over by new groups, which is forcing a re-examination of nursing roles (Flaherty, 1985). Because of the multidisciplinary nature of health teams it is vital that nursing roles be considered in relation to other health occupational groups (Canadian Nurses Association Brief, 1984).

10
Nursing education

As noted in Chapter 9, the first hospital-based school of nursing was established in 1874 in St Catherine's, Ontario. There followed a rapid increase in the number of nurse education programmes across Canada around the turn of the century. By the 1920s all Canadian provinces were developing legislation to control standards of nursing education. The typical school programme was three years in length and the curriculum included both practical experience and lectures. During this period the provinces also passed laws requiring nurses to be registered at the provincial level. These laws accorded trained nurses permanent legal status that set them apart from untrained nurses competing for the same jobs.

ADVANCED EDUCATION

Until 1919 graduates from Canadian schools who wanted additional education found it necessary to go to the US. In 1919 the first baccalaureate programme in Canada, at the University of British Columbia, provided nurses with a liberal arts education as well as practical nursing experience. In 1920 McGill University started a course in teaching and supervision, and several universities developed diploma courses in public health. By 1926 eight Canadian universities offered courses to nurses (Lamb, 1981).

Nursing leaders in these early years were critical of hospital-based programmes and their relatively poor standards of education. The Canadian Nurses Association (CNA) and the Canadian Medical Association co-sponsored a survey of schools of nursing that resulted in the Weir Report (Weir, 1932). Of the many recommendations made about the operations of the schools the most noteworthy was the one to transfer nursing education to provincial systems of general education. As a result of the Weir report the CNA established a National Curriculum Committee to develop guidelines for the revision of curricula in nursing schools, although poor economic conditions during the 1930s prevented many of the proposals being implemented. In fact some small schools were closed.

In 1944 Nettie D. Fidler, a faculty member at the University of Toronto, expressed concern about standards of education in the schools. She felt that there was a need for more factual information about nursing requirements in Canada so that educational programmes could be tailored to meet these needs. Fidler also suggested that schools be made financially independent from hospitals and that hospital and nursing school budgets be separated (Mussallem, 1965).

In 1946 an experimental school of nursing was created that was financially independent of a hospital to investigate the feasibility of educating nurses in a two-year period. The project was supported by funds from the CNA, the Red Cross and the Ontario Department of Health.

The military requirements of the Second World War caused an acute shortage of nurses and, subsequently, of the development of programmes to prepared nursing assistants. The CNA produced a curriculum guide for a nursing assistants' education programme. Also federal grants were made available to supplement nursing education costs in a variety of ways: to recruit student nurses, administer nursing school programmes and provide bursaries for students.

During this time the CNA cooperated with the National Selective Service and the Canadian Medical Procurement and Assignment Board in a survey that found an acute shortage of general duty nurses. It was found that most nurses worked as private nurses because of shorter hours and higher salaries. The conclusion resulting from the survey was that, if the shortage of nurses were to be alleviated, nurses' working conditions and salaries would have to be improved.

The CNA continued to play a major role in promoting better educational standards during the post-war period. It sponsored the first Canadian Conference on Nursing in 1957, from which came major recommendations for nursing education and recruitment. It suggested that schools of nursing have greater control over student learning, that financing of schools be through educational institutions, that there be more qualified nursing teachers and that nursing curricula be aimed at preparing generalists rather than specialists. There was some interest during the late 1950s in developing a national accreditation programme for nursing schools but a survey by the CNA showed that only 16% of the schools met established criteria, so the programme was shelved.

The Royal Commission on Health Services (1964) reported extensively on the nursing profession, nursing education and nursing recruitment. During the time of the Commission there were 17 university schools of nursing, 171 hospital schools, 79 assistant programmes and 8 programmes for psychiatric nurses. The Commission received representatives and studies from a wide range of individuals and organizations, including 25 recommendations from the CNA in 1962. A nurse, Alice M. Girard: the immediate past-president of the CNA, was a member of the Commission.

The main recommendations of the report clearly reflected the views of nursing leaders. They are summarized in Figure 10.1. Echoing themes of the previous 20 years recommendations focused on improving standards of nursing school programmes by making them more independent of hospitals, graduating more people with baccalaureate degrees and developing master's degree nursing programmes.

Nursing education and recruitment
1. About 75% of the hospital schools do not have qualified instructors (minimum BSc) nor do 56% of the university schools (minimum Master's degree).
2. The apprenticeship approach to nursing education should be re-examined.
3. Nurses perform some functions for which they are overqualified and some for which they are not qualified.
4. The period of training (three years) in hospital schools is too long and includes too much service.
5. About 25% of the positions in nursing require a four- to five-year integrated basic university programme and the rest of the positions should be filled by clinical nurses who have taken a new type of two-year diploma programme.
6. There is no need for speciality programmes in psychiatric nursing and these should be phased out.
7. Nursing assistants are still necessary to promote the effective use of nurses.

Hospital schools of nursing
1. A Nursing Education Planning Committee should be established in each province to advise the Minister of Health about new nursing programmes.
2. In hospital schools the school of nursing budget should be separate from the hospital service budget.
3. Formal arrangements or contracts between nursing schools and hospitals should be established to enable the use of clinical facilities for practical experience.
4. A new educational curriculum leading to a diploma in two years should be established.
5. The amount of time students spend providing nursing service should be reduced and therefore there is a need for the service agencies to recruit replacements.
6. Experimentation in the provision of nursing education programmes should be undertaken with other agencies (such as Junior Colleges).
7. Financial assistance should be provided to students who cannot pay their own fees and/or maintenance.
8. More highly qualified instructors should be prepared.

University schools of nursing
1. Eight of the 14 schools offer a programme which includes two years of university instruction plus the usual three years in a hospital school of nursing. The other six schools offer integrated five-year programmes in which the university controls all the students' learning experiences. The integrated approach is the preferred model.
2. University schools must expand in order to prepare 25% of the nursing workforce.
3. At least one university school in each of Canada's four main regions should develop a Master's degree programme in nursing.

Figure 10.1 Summary of the Findings of the Nursing Royal Commission on Health Services, 1964.

REGISTRATION AND LICENSURE

Since 1943 all graduate nurses have been required to register in order to practise. In all provinces graduates of approved schools of nursing are required to pass a registration examination before receiving a certificate of registration. Initially Canada had an agreement with the National League for Nursing in the US to use its testing services until the CNA could develop its own national testing service, which it did in 1961. The service is used by all the provincial associations.

The number of licences issued to nurses in Canada from 1978 to 1988, by province, is shown in Table 10.1. Note that the number of licences issued has consistently increased in the last decade from 220 996 in 1978 to 268 674 in 1988. The largest number of licences issued was in Quebec and Ontario, these provinces accounting for 64% of them.

Most of the education programmes to prepare nurses for registration are located in diploma schools, although there are increasing numbers of nurses obtaining their educations through university programmes. Recruitment of students is usually the responsibility of individual programmes, although the CNA has developed a 'career kit' that is widely available.

Registered nurse diploma schools

Nursing legislation throughout Canada falls within provincial and territorial jurisdiction. Saskatchewan was first to locate nursing schools completely under the control of the general education system (1966), although the first nursing diploma programme conducted within the general education system was at Ryerson Polytechnical Institute in Toronto in 1964 (Allen and Reidy, 1971). It was three years in length and on completion students were eligible to take the registered nurse licensure examination of the College of Nurses of Ontario. The curriculum was broadly based, with the first-year curriculum comprising courses in psychology, nutrition, English, biology, microbiology and nursing. Second-year courses included growth and development, sociology, disease and therapy, nursing and development of Western thought. Third-year coursework included community health, disease and therapy and nursing. Overall curriculum content pertaining directly to nursing was 59% of the total.

Figure 10.2 shows the current distribution of registered nurse diploma courses across Canada. Some provinces still have hospital-based schools while others have completely transferred nursing education to the general educational system. The typical diploma programme today is six semesters over two to three years, depending on the content. Admission requirements include high school graduation. Some colleges also require courses in general science and behavioural sciences.

Table 10.1 Number of nurses registered/licensed[1] by province, Canada, 1978–88

Province	1978	1979	1980	1981	1982	1983	1984	1985	1986	1987	1988
Newfoundland	4 314	4 485	4 687	4 817	4 941	4 997	5 142	5 247	5 328	5 405	5 465
Prince Edward Island	1 060	1 077	1 074	1 127	1 136	1 139	1 181	1 234	1 256	1 393	1 319
Nova Scotia	6 630	7 476	7 755	8 172	8 400	8 570	9 043	9 336	9 498	9 637	9 722
New Brunswick	6 883	7 001	7 028	7 181	7 309	7 519	7 676	7 841	8 076	8 087	7 980
Quebec	53 111	52 474	54 941	56 178	56 393	57 316	58 505	60 647	61 217	61 895	62 821
Ontario	94 298	95 508	96 165	98 037	98 632	100 091	100 171	101 704	103 523	105 918	107 948
Manitoba	8 798	8 916	9 000	8 654	8 850	9 429	9 734	9 654	9 708	10 401	10 855
Saskatchewan	7 495	8 073	8 310	8 523	8 831	9 071	9 409	9 436	9 518	9 633	9 720
Alberta	16 611	17 707	18 892	20 104	21 049	22 078	19 967	20 666	21 427	21 875	22 124
British Columbia	21 523	22 788	24 675	26 239	26 719	26 744	27 265	27 647	28 279	29 173	30 138
Yukon[2]	–	–	–	–	–	–	–	–	–	–	–
Northwest Territories	273	274	293	306	304	340	334	341	391	454	582
Total	220 996	225 779	232 820	239 338	242 564	247 294	248 427	253 753	258 221	263 871	268 674

[1] Some nurses are registered (licensed) in more than one province. The figures also include nurses registered in one or more provinces but actually working/living abroad.
[2] No licences were issued by Yukon; therefore nurses working in Yukon are registered in other jurisdictions.

Source: Canadian Health Manpower Inventory, 1990.

The curricula include general education courses as well as courses in nursing science. The diploma courses also require a certain number of weeks (typically 45 or more) in clinical experience, which is generally supervised directly by the school except during the 'consolidation' (last semester) when students receive indirect supervision. Many diploma programmes attempt to attract mature students. The number of students enrolled in the programmes at any one time ranges from 80 to over 400.

The western provinces also have two-year programmes to prepare nurses for registration as psychiatric nurses, although these are now being phased out. There are two in British Columbia, two in Alberta and one each in Saskatchewan and Manitoba.

The number of graduates from diploma programmes from 1978 to 1988 is shown in Table 10.2. Overall there has been a small decline in the number of diploma graduates over the ten years, although not all the schools report information fully. During the period 1979–88 the ratio of diploma to degree graduates decreased steadily.

Nursing programmes in Canadian universities

There are 25 programmes in Canadian universities (or equivalent) providing baccalaureate education in nursing. Most offer a basic bachelor of science degree in nursing, equivalent to four years' full-time study. Most programmes also offer a post-registered nursing course that may be completed over two or three years' full-time work, depending on the nurse's prior academic performance. Admission requirements for a baccalaureate in nursing are the same as for any other university programme in Canada and include high school grade 12 or equivalent. For the post-basic programmes, some universities are more flexible in admission criteria for mature students as long as the nurse is eligible for registration and in good standing at the provincial level.

The curricula of baccalaureate programmes across the country are similar because standards are defined by the Canadian Association of University Schools of Nursing in Canada, through their accreditation programme. A broad liberal education is provided in the first two years, clinical nursing content is increased in third and fourth years and there is a required amount of supervised clinical experience. Although courses are offered in specialized areas such as maternal and child health and psychiatry and community health, the baccalaureate programmes typically provide a general education.

The number of graduates from baccalaureate programmes from 1978 to 1988 by province is shown in Table 10.3. Overall the number of graduates

Type of education programme	British Columbia	Alberta	Saskat- chewan	Manitoba	Ontario	Quebec	New Brunswick	Nova Scotia	Prince Edward Island	Newfound- land	Total
RN diploma											
Hospital-based schools of nursing	1*	4		5				7		4	21
Diploma in provincial education system	9	7	2	1	23	41					83
Regional independent schools							5		1		6
University											
Baccalaureate	2	3	1	1	8	5	2	2	0	1	25
Master's	1	2	1	1	2	2		1		1	11
Nursing assistants											
Registered nursing Assistants	5	2	2	4	32	50	4	7			106

* Is in the process of converting its school of nursing from a diploma to a baccalaureate programme.

Source: Nursing Programmes and Entrance Requirements at Canadian Universities (1988) Ottowa: Canadian Nurses Association, The Helen K. Mussallem Library.

Figure 10.2 Education programmes for nurses, by province.

Table 10.2 Number of nurse graduates of initial diploma programme, by province, Canada, 1978–88

Province	1978	1979	1980	1981	1982	1983	1984	1985	1986	1987	1988
Newfoundland	251	210	214	174	247	275	266	263	229	195	179
Prince Edward Island	49	48	47	52	48	54	56	50	45	47	49
Novia Scotia	302	281	299	328	328	385	374	361	343	304	236
New Brunswick	230	180	204	216	229	287	263	243	242	265	235
Quebec	2 346	2 353	2 200	1 874	1 477	1 505	1 857	1 754	1 414	1 792	1 970
Ontario	2 309	1 932	2 045	2 083	2 237	2 273	2 001	2 525	2 419	2 266	2 096
Manitoba	404	345	402	450	477	532	478	409	446	461	441
Saskatchewan	303	296	296	286	311	335	340	315	314	326	306
Alberta	585	509	478	474	609	514	622	711	700	752	755
British Columbia	624	526	500	541	658	601	614	587	610	646	714
Total	7 403	6 680	6 685	6 478	6 621	6 761	6 871	6 218	7 762	7 054	6 981

Source: Canadian Health Manpower Inventory, 1990.

of baccalaureate programmes has increased over the past ten years from 1455 in 1978 to 2265 in 1988.

POST-BACCALAUREATE PROGRAMMES

There are 11 universities in Canada that offer master's degrees in nursing or nursing sciences. Courses are two years in length and there is considerable flexibility to tailor the graduate programme to an individual student's clinical interests. For example students may specialize in maternal and child health, mental health, community health, etc., depending upon the university. There is only one graduate programme offered in French (University of Montreal); the course at McGill University is also open to non-nurses.

Graduates of the master's degree nursing programmes are usually employed as teachers in education programmes, in nursing management positions or as clinical nurse specialists. In 1968 the CNA published a policy statement on the clinical nurse specialist that described the educational requirements for this role as a master's degree with specialization in a clinical area.

A few universities offer specialized certificate or diploma courses. The Memorial University of Newfoundland gives a one-year Community Primary Health Care Nursing Diploma and a Nurse Midwifery Diploma to educate nurses for outpost nursing. Credits from these diploma courses may be applied towards a Bachelor of Nursing degree. Ryerson Polytechnical Institute and the University of Alberta also offer short certificate courses in areas such as critical care and oncological and gerontological nursing.

There is currently one programme at the University of Alberta that prepares nurses at the doctoral level in nursing. Several other universities are also preparing PhD programmes following a national conference on the issues involved (Zilm *et al.*, 1979). An earlier survey by Larson and Stinson (1979) had identified 76 nurses with earned doctorates and 72 studying at that level. Of those with doctoral degrees 54 were employed at universities. An update in 1989 found 257 nurses with earned doctorates 55 of whom held a lower degree from a Canadian university and 265 nurses were in doctoral programmes. Most (62%) of the PhDs were employed in universities but 14% were found in health agencies. Fifty-nine (23%) had obtained their degree in nursing and 122 (47) in education (Chapter 13).

Management education

Opportunities for nurse managers to obtain education for entering management positions are relatively few (Leatt, 1985b). In baccalaureate nurs-

Table 10.3 Number of nurse graduates of basic baccalaureate programmes and post-RN baccalaureate programmes, by province, Canada, 1978–88

Province	1978	1979	1980	1981	1982	1983	1984	1985	1986	1987	1988
Newfoundland	44	53	42	51	49	41	57	57	78	89	57
Prince Edward Island	–	–	–	–	–	–	–	–	–	–	–
Nova Scotia	80	84	93	79	84	96	108	109	161	135	140
New Brunswick	113	108	87	76	83	96	63	86	85	156	128
Quebec	224	228	185	308	269	285	272	437	330	430	485
Ontario	499	433	537	473	517	528	636	621	719	648	699
Manitoba	89	62	68	61	61	67	85	74	82	75	118
Saskatchewan	83	86	101	77	88	89	78	92	92	94	90
Alberta	178	133	172	157	239	295	261	277	297	338	342
British Columbia	145	143	168	143	200	189	169	204	193	256	206
Total	1 455	1 330	1 453	1 425	1 590	1 686	1 729	1 957	2 037	2 221	2 265

Source: Canadian Health Manpower Inventory, 1990.

ing programmes there are usually only one or two courses in leadership or nursing administration. Three master's programmes offer a minor or major in administration.

The CNA and the Canadian Hospital Association jointly sponsor an introduction to nursing management (formerly nursing unit administration) programme for nurses interested in or already working as nurse managers in a variety of settings. The course, one year in length, is conducted mainly by correspondence. The Canadian Hospital Association sponsors a two-year programme in health services management as well as one in long-term care management, open to all health administrators. The majority of these are correspondence courses and participants receive a certificate upon graduation.

Two undergraduate programmes with health administration majors are part of the Association of Universities and Colleges of Canada (AUCC). The University of Saskatchewan offers a distance learning programme for students already employed in the field, leading to a Bachelor of Commerce degree with a major in health administration. York University in Toronto offers a Bachelor of Commerce degree, with a specialization in health administration, that may be taken on a part-time basis.

There are six graduate programmes in health administration, five of which are located in faculties of medicine (or health sciences) and the sixth in a faculty of business and commerce. These programmes are open to all who are interested in health administration and, although the numbers vary by programme and year, it is estimated that approximately one third of the students have a nursing background. On average there are approximately 40–45 people with nursing backgrounds who graduate from this programme each year. Only one health administration programme (University of Alberta) offers a specific course in nursing administration as part of the curriculum (Stinson, 1978).

Nursing assistant programmes

The registered nursing assistant category was introduced in Canada because of a shortage of nurses following the Second World War. Historically most nursing assistants have been employed in hospitals, especially on medical and surgical units (Imai, 1981). Most recently registered nursing assistants are finding employment in home care schemes and in long-term care facilities. The number of licensed nursing assistants from 1978 to 1988 is shown in Table 10.4. There has been an overall increase in the number of licensed nursing assistants over the past ten years. The largest number are in Ontario and Quebec, these provinces accounting for 64% of the total in 1988.

Table 10.4 Number of licensed nursing assistants by province licensure, Canada, 1978–88

Province	1978	1979	1980	1981	1982	1983	1984	1985	1986	1987	1988
Newfoundland	1 716[b]	1 764[b]	1 813	1 980	1 940	2 400	2 340	2 411	2 450[c]	2 379	2 496
Prince Edward Island	558	526[d]	483	450	487	503	481	509	494	523	582[e]
Nova Scotia	2 369	2 474	2 848	3 038	3 232	3 289	3 376	3 298	3 360	3 388	3 307
New Brunswick	2 157	2 138[f]	2 169[f]	2 252[f]	2 187[f]	2 267[f]	2 206[f]	2 239[f]	2 192[f]	2 172[f]	2 180[f]
Quebec	16 908	17 521	18 567[e]	18 355[e]	18 519[e]	18 823[e]	19 040[e]	18 917[e]	17 843[e]	20 029[e]	19 860[e]
Ontario	32 030	33 659	33 551	33 861	33 931	34 501	34 080	33 999	34 237	34 491	34 815
Manitoba[h]	3 865	3 932	3 787[i]	3 341[i]	3 676[i]	3 868[i]	3 770[i]	4 140[i]	4 216[i]	3 877[i]	3 807[i]
Saskatchewan	2 499	2 452	2 393	2 520	2 366	2 420	2 317	2 536	2 549	2 477	2 412
Alberta	6 442	5 817[j]	7 140[j]	7 386[j]	7 254[j]	7 875[j]	8 251[j]	8 168[j]	8 643	7 894	7 225
British Columbia	6 809	7 128	7 370	7 593	7 554	7 409	6 977	6 664	6 457	6 189	5 949
Yukon[k]	69	80	76	70	61	59	56	59	61	67	69
Northwest Territories	119	112	100	108	103	125	156	123	106	124	124
Total	75 541	77 603	80 297	80 954	81 310	83 539	83 050	83 063	82 608	83 610	82 826

Source: Canadian Health Manpower Inventory, 1990. Limitations in reporting accurate data because of variations in reporting the information by provinces: note in original.

Distribution of educational programmes for registered nursing assistants, by province, is shown in Figure 10.2. The majority of these programmes are in Ontario and Quebec. They are offered by hospitals, community colleges and secondary and regional schools. Approximately ten months long, the curriculum includes nursing skill development, basic sciences and human growth and development. In Ontario, for example, the Ministry of Colleges and Universities requires about two-thirds of the curriculum content to be used for clinical experience and the other third for theory and biological and social sciences (Ontario Association of Registered Nursing Assistants, 1985).

The number of approved nursing assistant programme graduates from 1978 to 1988 is shown in Table 10.5. There has been an overall decline in number of graduates of nursing assistants during the period 1978–88.

Entry to practice

In February 1982 the Board of the CNA made a rather progressive but controversial policy decision 'that by the year 2000 the minimal educational requirement for entry into the practice of nursing should be successful completion of a baccalaureate degree in nursing' (Registered Nurses Association of Ontario, 1982). The rationale for this proposed change was the perceived health needs of Canadians, changing concepts of health and illness and changes in nursing practice. The characteristics of a proposed model baccalaureate programme of the future are summarized as follows. It should:

1. Provide a primary basis in physical, biological and social sciences;
2. Recognize nursing as a discipline including nursing research and ethics;
3. Emphasize all aspects of health, including health promotion, generation and development, protection, maintenance, restoration and palliation;
4. Emphasize critical, analytic thinking;
5. Emphasize nursing of individuals, families, groups and communities, taking into consideration the multicultural nature of the Canadian population in a variety of settings;
6. Promote individual self-care;
7. Emphasize flexibility and competence;
8. Focus on health policy and resource allocation;
9. Emphasize professionalism through knowledge, service to society, integrity, accountability and continuous learning.

The CNA policy statement has received mixed reactions, especially from governments concerned about cost implications.

Table 10.5 Number of graduates of provincially approved programmes for nursing assistants, by province of graduation, Canada, 1978–88

Province	1978	1979	1980	1981	1982	1983	1984	1985	1986	1987	1988
Newfoundland	183	191	172	164	172	164	72	70	52	49	107
Prince Edward Island	–	34	25	25	26	29	22	30	28	26	23
Nova Scotia	219	283	232	239	250	240	236	213	197	215	198
New Brunswick	71	65	75	82	74	81	68	68	58	62	49
Quebec	1 402	980	715	596	700	590	604	435	493	402	311
Ontario	1 375	1 312	1 190	1 271	1 392	1 507	1 350	1 293	1 317	1 293	1 304
Manitoba	277	256	230	233	232	275	199[a]	173	154	174	173
Saskatchewan	196	201	178	179	181	175	157	134	127	125	103
Alberta	157	149	312	220	285	216	267	282	290	258	140
British Columbia	336	335	335	244	268	211	179	223	221	232	169
Yukon	12	12	10	12	14	6	8	8	6	–	8
Northwest Territories	6	–	5	11	4	4	5	4	7	–	4
Total[1]	4 234	3 818	3 479	3 276	3 598	3 498	3 167	2 933	2 950	2 836	2 589

[1] Enrolment in schools was reduced because of a perceived surplus of nursing assistants.

Source: Canadian Health Manpower Inventory, 1990.

The potential change in entry to practice requirements has sparked activities from many different groups and interested parties at the provincial level. For example the Ministry of Education in British Columbia (UBC) conducted a comparison of the eight college- and institution-based diploma programmes in the province with the one baccalaureate programme at the University of British Columbia (UBC). In general the findings showed that the UBC programme was more generic and provided a broader knowledge base. The degree programme had about twice the amount of theoretical content as practical content whereas the diploma programme was equally split between theory and practice. The degree programme provided more community orientated experience. The diploma programmes had fewer academic requirements for admission and had only 20% general education courses whereas the baccalaureate programme had 36%. No conclusions were drawn about the quality of the graduates and their abilities to practice (Ministry of Health of British Columbia, 1983).

The Registered Nurses Association of Ontario has identified some of the most important issues in bringing about the change to a baccalaureate degree as the requirement for entry to practice. Two of the most critical issues are: first, differentiation between and articulation of diploma and baccalaureate programmes; and, second, accessibility of baccalaureate programmes in different regions (Registered Nurses Association of Ontario, 1982, 1985). By 1986 the CNA position on entry to practice had been endorsed by the majority of the provincial associations.

FINANCIAL AND HUMAN RESOURCES FOR NURSING EDUCATION

Since 1951 the government of Canada has provided financial support for the operation of universities and colleges. Financing is shared by federal and provincial governments: approximately 40% is from income taxes (about $2 billion), about 40% from federal cash payments ($2 billion) and the remainder from provincial revenues (about $1 billion). The amount of funding received by individual universities or colleges can vary according to the priority given to post-secondary education by the provincial government. The proportion of the gross national product made available by the federal government to universities and colleges for core operations has declined from 1.35% in 1977/78 to 1.24% in 1984/85. During the same time period, however, enrolment in universities increased by 27% and in colleges by 36% (CNA Entry to Practice, May 1985).

It is difficult to estimate actual costs of educational programmes specific to nurses. Often the budget for the nursing department within a college or university may be used; however this estimate typically does not include indirect costs such as libraries, buildings, land, equipment and administration where costs are shared with other programmes. Accounting systems in colleges and universities are not sufficiently well developed to allow derivation of costs per student year. Lack of ability to define costs in a standardized way provides further barriers to assessing the potential effects of implementing the CNA position on entry to practice (CNA Entry to Practice, August 1984).

Total established programme financing of post-secondary education, by province, in 1984/85 in thousands of dollars is shown below.

Newfoundland	97 945
Prince Edward Island	20 950
Nova Scotia	145 057
New Brunswick	119 448
Quebec	1 100 809
Ontario	1 493 578
Manitoba	177 236
Saskatchewan	168 588
Alberta	398 937
British Columbia	477 675
Yukon	3 654
Northwest Territories	8 363
Total	$4 212 240

Variations in amounts by province reflect differences in the size of the population of each province and the number of universities and colleges.

Nurse educators

Statistics Canada provides statistical information on the number of registered nurses in Canada employed in nursing educational institutions, including nurse educators for diploma courses, universities and nursing assistant programmes. In 1980 there were 4646 nurses employed in all nursing educational programmes and by 1984 this number had increased to 5113. In 1984 49% of nurse educators had a baccalaureate degree in nursing as their highest level of educational preparation, whereas in 1988 51% did and 10% had a master's degree in nursing. The registered nurse diploma was the highest qualification for 43.5% in 1980 and 41% in 1984. Many of these nurses had degrees in other disciplines although about 17% of nurse educators in 1988 did not have a university degree.

Financial and human resources for nursing education 145

Table 10.6 Full-time and part-time nurse faculty members in schools of nursing, by type of programme and level of education, Canada, 1984–88

Programme and level of education	1984 Full-time n	1984 Full-time %	1984 Part-time n	1984 Part-time %	1988 Full-time n	1988 Full-time %	1988 Part-time n	1988 Part-time %
University								
Doctorate	100	15.3	9	4.0	153	22.7	14	3.0
Master's	435	66.8	40	17.8	441	65.4	195	42.0
Baccalaureate	84	12.9	175	78.0	40	5.9	167	36.0
No degree	–		–		–		–	
Not stated	32	4.9	55		40	5.9	84	18.0
Total	651		224		674		460	
Diploma school								
Doctorate	6	0.2	–	–	23	0.8	3	0.5
Master's	320	13.0	24	6.6	587	21.4	60	10.7
Baccalaureate	1 668	67.8	237	65.6	1 717	62.6	311	55.5
No degree	421	17.0	98	27.0	352	12.8	149	26.6
Not stated	43	1.7	2	0.6	62	2.2	37	6.6
Total	2 458		361		2 741		560	

Table 10.6 shows data on faculty qualifications for diploma and university programmes *only* in 1984 and 1988. There does appear to be a pattern, with university programmes having more highly educated nurse educators than diploma programmes. Also included in the table is the distribution of nurse educators with various levels of preparation. In 1984 about 61% of both part-time and full-time educators had a baccalaureate degree as their highest level of education in nursing, and 21% had a master's degree in nursing while 15% did not have a baccalaureate degree.

Between 1984 and 1988 there was, in the university sector, a 3.5% increase in the number of full-time staff compared with a 48.6% increase of part-time educators. The number of full-time educators with doctorates increased by 65% whereas the number of full-time educators with baccalaureate degrees decreased by 47%. In diploma programmes there was a three-fold increase in educators with doctorates although they still only represented 0.8% of the educators in that sector. However there was an 83% increase in educators with master's degrees.

11

The practice of nursing

Louise Lemieux-Charles

Nurses are witnessing dramatic developments in treatment methods used to manage individuals with specific disease entities and in the way health care is delivered. As a result of pressures to contain costs and to rationalize services the health care system is becoming more business-like. Such developments are raising issues about nursing's role within the health care system's hierarchy and its relationship with other health team disciplines. The changes are affecting the environment in which nurses deliver patient care and are having a profound effect on their practice.

THE PRACTICE SETTING

Demographic characteristics

Nurses in Canada work in a variety of practice settings. Table 11.1 outlines the number of registered nurses employed in Canada, by place of employment, for the years 1980 and 1988.

In comparing the 1988 numbers with those of 1980 two areas show an increase of some importance – nursing home and community health –

Table 11.1 Registered nurses employed, by place of employment, Canada, 1980 and 1988.

Place of employment	1980 n	1980 %	1988 n	1988 %	Percentage increase
Hospital	114 230	73.6	153 932	73.1	34.7
Nursing home/home for the aged	9 667	6.2	14 579	6.9	50.0
Community health	13 739	8.9	20 890	9.9	52.0
Physician's office/family practice unit	4 346	2.8	5 363	2.6	23.0
Educational institution	4 646	3.0	5 693	2.7	22.0
Other	5 168	3.3	8 195	3.9	58.0
Not stated	3 382	2.2	1 854	0.9	
Total	155 178	100.0	210 506	100.0	

Source: Revised Registered Nurses Data Series, Statistics Canada, Health Division.
Prepared by: Data Centre, Canadian Nurses Association, March 1989.

with 50% and 52% increases respectively, followed closely by hospitals (34%) physicians' offices (23%) and, lastly, educational institutions (22%). However, percentage distribution among all settings has remained relatively constant over the eight-year period.

The educational level of nurses working in the above settings is described in Table 11.2. The number of nurses with a bachelor's degree in nursing has grown from 14 559 (9.4%) in 1980 to 27 388 (13%) in 1988. The number of nurses holding a master's or higher degree has increased from 1017 (0.7%) in 1980 to 2120 (1.0%) in 1988.

Table 11.2 Percentage of registered nurses employed by place of employment and highest level of education in nursing, Canada, 1988.

Place of Employment	Registered nurses diploma %	Post-basic diploma %	Baccalaureate degree %	Master's degree of higher %
Hospital	72.6	16.5	10.2	0.7
Nursing home/home for the aged	76.5	17.2	5.9	0.4
Community health	45.7	23.6	29.5	1.2
Physician's office/family practice unit	80.1	13.2	6.4	0.3
Educational institute	26.0	13.1	50.6	10.3
Other	62.6	19.4	15.8	2.2
Not stated	74.2	14.8	9.7	1.3
Total	68.7 (144 804)	17.0 (36 194)	13.0 (37 388)	1.0 (2 120)

Source: Revised Registered Nurses Data Series, Health Division, Statistics Canada.
Prepared by: Data Centre, Canadian Nurses Association, January 1990.

As noted in Chapter 10 nurses are becoming increasingly concerned that educational opportunities be available, first, to obtain a baccalaureate degree in nursing and, second, for nurse managers to obtain education for entering nursing management positions. Table 11.3 describes the highest level of education in nursing, by position, of nurses employed in Canada in 1988. Of the approximately 30 000 nurses in administrative positions a baccalaureate degree was the highest level of preparation for 18%, while 1% had a master's or higher degree. Another 25% had a diploma or certificate beyond basic preparation in nursing but it is not known how many of these were in nursing administration. A large number of nurses in first-line management positions have taken the

Nursing Management Program, a one-year distance education programme co-sponsored by the CNA and the Canadian Hospital Association. It has been a major source of preparation in nursing administration for nurses who cannot leave their jobs for full-time study and who are either in nursing administration positions or who want to prepare for them.

Table 11.3 Percentage of registered nurses employed, by position and highest level of education in nursing, Canada, 1984

Position	Highest level of education				
	Total	Registered nurses diploma	Post-basic diploma	Baccalaureate degree	Master's degree or higher
	%	%	%	%	%
Director/Assistant/ Associate Director	2.5	44.2	23.6	25.8	6.4
Supervisor/Co-ordinator/Assistant Supervisor/Co-rd.	5.2	54.2	23.5	20.6	1.7
Clinical specialist	0.6	46.0	16.5	22.1	15.4
Head nurse	7.5	63.6	23.5	12.0	0.9
General duty/staff nurse	72.5	74.0	15.9	9.8	0.3
Instructor/professor	2.6	21.5	12.7	56.1	9.6
Other	6.5	56.5	20.3	21.2	2.0
Not stated	2.6	74.1	13.6	10.8	0.9

Source: Revised Registered Nurses Data Series, Health Division, Statistics Canada.
Prepared by: Data Centre, Canadian Nurses Association, January 1990.

Data to determine the type of clinical specialty courses nurses have taken are not available, although the category 'post-basic diploma' suggests that 36 194 (15.9%) staff nurses have taken courses beyond the diploma level.

Nurses' relationship to other health care workers

A wide variety of personnel undertakes specific nursing activities under supervision of the registered nurse (RN). Nursing assistants, nursing aides and nursing orderlies are the health care workers who most commonly assist nurses.

Recently concern has been expressed by nursing assistants about a perceived shift in employment practices leading to a loss of positions, especially in tertiary care settings and in specialty units of active treatment hospitals. In Ontario the Ontario Association of Registered Nursing Assistants commissioned a study to examine the extent, rate and location of attrition of RNA positions in Ontario health care and to obtain information on the rationale supporting the change in employment practices (Woods, 1985).

The study found that even though chronic and rehabilitation hospitals have added positions these have not been sufficient to offset losses in active treatment hospitals. The most frequently stated reason for replacing RNAs with RNs was that RNs were perceived to be more economical because fewer, more qualified staff could provide patient care on all types of patient units and nursing shifts. The authors concluded, first, that the economics of employing RNs and RNAs needs additional research, second, that current RNA programmes need to be evaluated in the light of employers' perceptions and expectations and, third, that management should be open-minded when making decisions about staffing mix until results of further research are known. The report states that 'the gradual attrition of RNA positions in Ontario hospitals is a symptom or by-product of the nursing professionalization movement'.

To further understanding of the issue five other provinces commissioned studies. They included associations in Alberta (Jacobsen, 1986), New Brunswick (The DPA Group Inc., 1987), Newfoundland (Council for Nursing Assistants, 1987) and Saskatchewan (NGA Research Committee, 1986) and the government of Manitoba (Manitoba Association of Licensed Practical Nurses, 1989). Also the Canadian Association of Practical and Nursing Assistants conducted their own study in 1984. Similar findings were reported in all studies, with a decline in RNA utilization in acute care settings due to increased acuity and instability of patients and an increase in demand for RNAs in long-term care settings representing the overriding pattern of utilization. Table 11.4 compares the supply of registered nurses and nursing assistants from 1965 to 1988.

Table 11.4 Supply of registered nurses (RNs) and registered nursing assistants (RNAs), Canada, 1965–88

	1965	1970	1975	1980	1986	1988
Registered nurses						
Number	104 349	135 047	177 182	203 549		210 506[1]
Percentage increase	–	29.4	31.2	15.1		3.4
Population/RN	159	159	129	119		123
Nursing assistants						
Number	30 172	46 184	69 475	80 297		82 826[2]
Percentage increase	–	53.1	50.4	15.6		3.4
Population/RNA	658	465	329	302		312
Ratio RN:RNA	3.5 : 1	2.9 : 1	2.6 : 1	2.5 : 1	2.9 : 1	2.5 : 1

[1] Nursing in Canada – 1988. Statistics Canada, January 1990.
[2] Health Personnel in Canada, Health and Welfare, Ottawa, January 1990.

Nursing assistants in Ontario are also advocating a change in title from 'registered nursing assistant' to 'licensed practical nurse'. This title is used in British Columbia and Manitoba and has been suggested by Saskatchewan (College of Nurses, 1986). They believe that the current title implies an assistant relationship to the RN when, in reality, the RNAs, while working under the direction and general supervision of the RN, are accountable for their own practice. Ontario is the only province where RNAs are registered through the same body, i.e. the College of Nurses, as RNs.

Clarification of nursing's role is occurring not only among personnel involved in nursing activities (Table 11.4 above) but also among other health professionals. With the progress in medical science and technology during the last three decades, there has been a proliferation of allied professional and technical workers, each competing for the patient's time and each constituting a pull on the health care dollar. Many duties previously under the jurisdiction of nursing have been taken over by new groups, at least during day-time hours (CNA Entry to Practice, 1982). The CNA, in its statement on the physician's assistant (CNA, 1982), believes that the proliferation of health care workers leads to fragmentation of services to individuals and families, that the nurse is able to undertake, with little or no additional preparation, functions described for paramedical and physician's assistants, and that special programmes for the education of these categories of workers are expensive and lead to dead-end careers.

Recently in the face of resident cutbacks in Ontario expanded role nurse (ERN) positions were instituted in orthopaedics, cardiology and cardiovascular surgery in two major health sciences centres. Master's level preparation is a prerequisite (Rubin, 1988).

The management of nursing services

As changes occur in the health care system the nursing profession must identify nursing's unique contribution to the care of patients or clients and their families. Application of nursing theories in the clinical setting is one way in which the practice of nursing can become goal directed. Several health care agencies in Canada have decided to use nursing theory as the basis for development of their nursing standards. Currently they are all at different stages of implementation. Because the major nursing theories do not contain blueprints for their applications in the clinical settings their introduction has been slow.

The Standards for Nursing Practice developed by the CNA support the use of a conceptual model to guide practice (CNA, 1980). Four interrelated and interdependent standards and related behaviours were developed. They reflect the belief that nurses use the nursing process as their method of practice and as a conceptual model for nursing practice. Because the nature of interaction with the client is a helping one, one standard on the helping relationship is included. The fourth standard addresses the nurses' professional responsibilities.

Since 1980 several national conferences have addressed the use of nursing theories in practice and each conference has been extremely well attended. In August 1986 a Nursing Theory Congress entitled 'Theoretical Pluralism: Direction for a Practice Discipline' was held. The question of whether an agency should adopt a specified identified theoretical model or whether the nurse should be permitted to apply the theoretical model appropriate to the situation (theoretical pluralism) is being raised by nurse administrators and practitioners.

Development of practice standards is the responsibility of each provincial jurisdiction. The Standards for Nursing Practice guidelines developed by the CNA have been one way of providing leadership at the national level. Support for the development of national Standards for Public Health Nursing was endorsed in June 1986 at the Canadian Public Health Association annual meeting. National and provincial standards tend to be general in nature and do not address specialization.

Specialization

Although nurses work in a variety of specialty areas there was no formal mechanism to recognize specialization until recently. Specialization will be recognized through a certification process that the CNA will coordinate. Now occupational health nurses have a certification examination in collaboration with the CNA's Testing Services; the neuroscience nurses will be the next group to develop one.

Interest groups

Midwifery as a specialty has received considerable attention in past years. Although it is formally recognized in one Canadian jurisdiction there is a lobby in several provinces that it be regulated as an autonomous profession. A survey of all provinces regarding the status of midwifery (Clark, 1986) reveals that six out of 12 jurisdictions have not taken a position in relation to midwifery, advanced levels of maternal–infant nursing or other related issues. Among the other six nursing associations there is a consensus that the practice of midwifery belongs within the scope of nursing. The CNA defines two specialist roles in maternal–infant nursing: those of primary care and high risk care. The role of the nurse–midwife is incorporated into the primary care specialist category.

In four provinces (British Columbia, Quebec, Alberta and Ontario) there are active lobbies for the credentialling of midwifery. The Task Force on the Implementation of Midwifery in Ontario (1987) recommended that midwifery be considered a self-regulating profession with multiple routes of entry. Midwifery is now one of 24 health professions which will be regulated by the Regulated Health Profession Act. In all other provinces the future role of midwifery and maternal–infant nursing remains unclear.

ETHICS AND NURSING PRACTICE

Rapid changes in the delivery of health care, including the introduction of new technologies, has increased the number of treatment options. Decision making regarding the most appropriate option has created new ethical dilemmas that must now be resolved. In an editorial on the role of the nurse as patient advocate, Schaffer (1985), Director of the Centre for Professional and Applied Ethics at the University of Manitoba, notes that the CNA Code of Ethics makes no mention of loyalty to doctors or unquestioning obedience. He contrasts the Code with the Nightingale Pledge in which nurses state that 'loyally will I endeavour to aid the physician in his work' and observes that the model of the nurse as an obedient foot-soldier has been replaced by the model of the nurse as patient advocate. The pledge of loyalty to physicians has been replaced by the 'obligation to ensure that the patient receives competent and ethical care' (CNA, Ethics, 1985). The Code expresses and seeks to clarify those ethical principles that are definitive of nursing activity and distinguishes between ethical violations and ethical dilemmas.

Nurses are not the only professionals faced with ethical dilemmas for which there are no clear answers. With advanced technology new treatment and life-and-death dilemmas must now be faced by professionals, patients and families. Hospitals have reacted to this focus on ethics by renewing discussions of their philosophies, developing moral codes, forming ethics committees and offering staff educational sessions on topics related to ethics (Youell, 1986).

A survey of Canadian hospitals over 300 beds in size was conducted to assess the existence, function and composition of ethics committees. Results revealed that 18% of the committees had been established in the past three years (Award *et al.*, 1985). The study definition excluded committees whose sole purpose was to review biomedical research proposals and therapeutic abortions. Ethics committees were most likely to be found in hospitals with more than 700 beds. The majority of respondents reported that the ethics committee:

1. Reviewed and recommended policies that governed ethical choices;

2. Educated hospital personnel and/or patients on ethical matters and counselled physicians;
3. Counselled other health professionals;
4. Made decisions about continuing life support.

Nurses were represented on the ethics committee of 81% of hospitals surveyed. The authors note that there is a general feeling that ethics committees are considered good but that their value has not been evaluated and their use by the public and professionals is not well understood.

It is often assumed that nurses involved in clinical practice are the only ones faced with ethical dilemmas. However the CNA Code of Ethics states that nurse administrators have a role in promoting ethical conduct by conveying the values and standards of the Code to newly hired employees, by conducting accurate performance appraisal and by ensuring that staff are competent. A study of ethical dilemmas faced by nurse administrators revealed that they experienced problems with resource allocation, technology, conflicting loyalties and values, staff relationships, conflict between nursing staff and physicians and promotion of quality of care (Youell, 1986). The author notes that the ethical problems faced by the nurse administrator reflect a combination of both clinical and administrative issues. Many of these ethical dilemmas are exacerbated by the trend of computerization and the application of business practices.

COMPUTERIZATION AND THE APPLICATION OF BUSINESS PRACTICES

Control of the rapidly escalating costs of health care have led to efforts to monitor and analyse hospital performance more effectively and to the development of patient groupings based on similarities of treatment and resource use. Based on the Canadian International Classification of Diseases, they are known as Case Mix Groupings (CMGs) and are similar to the Diagnostic Related Groups (DRGs) used in the US. At present they are used as a measure of productivity and as a way to examine the mix of cases handled by a hospital or institution. CMGs are not used for funding but the trend to private sector management of hospitals to boost 'productivity' and streamline efficiency is evident.

The Hospital Medical Records Institute, a non-profit making, federally chartered company that specializes in processing information for health care institutions, is testing the use of CMGs in nine hospitals across the country. In public health there has been a trend towards the development of programmes for specific target groups.

The MIS project, sponsored by the Canadian Hospital Association, has developed guidelines for the implementation of management information systems. It is expected that one outcome of the project will be development of standard methodologies to identify and cost resources utilized on a patient specific basis. Nurses have been involved in the development of guidelines related to workload management systems for nursing.

The above projects provide excellent ways for organizing data essential to planning and decision making. However the key to making those data accessible is a sophisticated computerized information system in which clinical, financial and administrative information is integrated. There are presently no such systems in Canada, although there are plans underway to install them in several large teaching hospitals (Clark, 1985). The majority of computerized systems presently in use in Canada deal with one or two functions, mainly in the financial and administrative areas, for example budget information, productivity indicators and staffing functions.

In nursing, patient classification systems link patient characteristics and the administrative or financial system. There are many different classification systems in use across Canada. As pressure to control costs has increased in hospitals patient classification systems have been implemented to plan nursing budgets and make staffing decisions that match patient needs with available nursing resources (Keddy and Wolnik, 1985). The most frequently used classification systems include the Saskatchewan System (HSSG), the PRN System, the GRASP system and the MEDICUS system. Many facilities have designed their own patient classification systems. Although there has been interest from funding agencies in the use of the systems to determine appropriate funding levels, the number of different patient classifications in use has made it difficult to do so. There are few systems for other types of health care organization.

ACCREDITATION AND QUALITY ASSURANCE

The Canadian Council on Hospital Accreditation is responsible for accreditation of Canadian hospitals and long-term care centres. It is primarily interested in establishing standards for health care facilities in Canada and assisting such facilities in monitoring and improving the quality of care they provide by voluntary means. The history of such activity dates back to 1918 when the American College of Surgeons established the Hospital Standardization Program. This was followed by the establishment of a Joint Commission on Accreditation of Hospitals in 1951. The Canadian Medical Association was one of its sponsors. In 1958 the Canadian Council on Hospital Accreditation was incorporated, with responsibility for accreditation in hospitals in Canada (Canadian Council on Hospital Accreditation, 1983).

The 14-member Board of Directors is composed of representatives from the Canadian Hospital Association, CNA and Canadian Long Term Care Association. The CNA has had two members on the board since 1976. The Canadian Long Term Care Association was added in 1982 in order to represent the interests of long-term care facilities in Canada.

Recognizing an increase in specialization and a continuing cross-over of demarcation lines between one type of health, hospital or social care centre and another, the council has moved towards the accreditation of health care facilities other than hospitals, focusing on general hospitals, mental health services and extended care centres (Keddy and Wolnick, 1985).

The accreditation of public health units in Canada dates back to 1980 and occurs only in the province of Ontario, under the auspices of the Ontario Council on Community Health Accreditation. Interest has been expressed by other provinces in a national accreditation system but little has been done to date (Nason, 1986).

The Canadian Council on Hospital Accreditation has recently included in its Standards the requirement that each hospital and long-term care centre have an overall quality assurance programme. The use of CMGs will provide standards that can be applied to quality as well as cost, thus providing the basis for a system of quality assurance. However the system is based on outputs and fails to measure outcomes (Hodgson and Ormerod, 1985). Robert Evans, a well-known Canadian economist, supports the need for more outcome measures and cites studies that show enormous variation in utilization rates without any noticeable difference in outcome (Evans, 1984).

ROLE AND FUNCTION OF NURSE ADMINISTRATORS

During the 1980s, many health care settings adopted an organizational structure based on the corporate model. Such nursing titles as Associate Administrator Patient Care Services, Vice-President Nursing or Associate Executive Director Patient Care Services reflect corporate responsibility. Presently hospital accreditation standards state 'that nursing services shall be under the direction of a legally and educationally qualified nurse who is responsible to the Chief Executive Officer for the nursing care programs' (Canadian Council on Hospital Accreditation, 1984). However nurses in senior positions are often responsible for other departments and there has been growing concern that in the future these new positions will not be filled by nurses.

As nursing is increasingly being held accountable for resources used, nurse managers in Canada have need to increase their knowledge of workload management systems, budgeting processes and computerization. Accountability is being achieved partially through the decentralization of management responsibilities to the nursing unit level. Head Nurse titles are being changed to Unit Administrator. Nurse Manager, etc. in order to reflect these new responsibilities. For head nurses who have derived their major work satisfaction from clinical involvement addition of management responsibilities has been a difficult transition. The emerging Personal Health Care Managers in public health units are experiencing the same transition.

The need for better qualified nurse managers has been underscored by the results of a Canadian Health Administrator study (Hastings, 1981) that described the increasing complexity of health administrator positions and the need for better preparation for such positions. The CNA has attempted to clarify roles for various levels of nurse administrator as there has been no consistent definition or interpretation of expectations, relationships and skills inherent in the role. A Position Paper on the Role of the Nurse Administrator and Standards for Nursing Administration was developed and adopted by the Board of Directors in 1983 and revised in 1988. Ongoing discussions with the Canadian Hospital Association, the Canadian College of Health Service Executives, the Canadian Association of University Schools of Nursing, the Canadian Public Health Association and the CNA have resulted in the publication of a Joint Statement that supports the need for graduate level education for nurse administrators.

RELATIONSHIP TO OTHER HEALTH PROFESSIONALS

Increased focus on cost-containment and resource allocation has led to the involvement of physicians in the management process. As physicians do not have special training in management special programmes (begun in 1984) have been developed by the Canadian College of Health Service Executives and the Canadian Medical Association in order to assist them in assuming responsibilities.

The implications of introducing such a role have required that nurses and physicians collaborate in preparing, reviewing and revising annual budgets of nursing units. They must also cooperate to review and deploy resources during each fiscal period, to develop appropriate action plans and to analyse the impact of the addition and deletion of personnel and programmes on resources. It is anticipated that collaboration will also take place in developing patient care and that quality assurance processes will be developed and implemented. Although there has been much discussion about the above relationships there have been few changes in hospital structure, still mainly based on a functional model, although some have implemented a programme management approach to the delivery of care.

12

The nurse at work

Louise Lemieux Charles

The nurse now practises in a workplace characterized by increased decentralization, cost-containment and application of business practices, specialization and technological development, quality assurance and risk management. Increasing computerization and the sharpened focus on legal and ethical issues permeate many of these trends. Set against all the trends are increased expectations of a workplace that will acknowledge the profession's unique contribution to the care of patients and families.

SOCIAL AND DEMOGRAPHIC CHARACTERISTICS

The registered nurse in Canada in the 1980s was most likely to be female (98%) and employed in nursing (84%) in an institutional setting (73%). Table 12.1 shows the number of registered nurses, by employment status and age group.

The majority of nurses (54%) are under the age of 39. A small percentage (5%) are not employed in nursing and are not seeking employment in the field. In 1988, 57% of registered nurses were working full time whereas 34% were working part time. Although the definition of part-time work is not consistent throughout Canada (Table 12.2) the percentage, excluding Quebec, ranges from 16% (in Newfoundland) to 46% (in Alberta). Implications of nurses working part time are elaborated in the section 'Quality of Working Life', below.

The number of nurses (152 516) working at the general staff level in 1988 represents a 48% increase over 1980 when 103 179 were employed as staff nurses. Table 12.3 outlines the number of registered nurses employed, by position. The high percentage in 'other' and 'not stated' categories may reflect the fact that present statistical methodology does not allow the Canadian Nurses Association (CNA) to determine whether there has been expansion to other roles and positions. For example it is very difficult to determine the number of nurses working in non-traditional roles. Another example is the difficulty in identifying nurses in clinical nurse specialist positions. Statistically this position refers to nurses who self-report their position as clinical specialist despite their educational qualifications. The CNA position statement describes the clinical specialist as having a master's degree in a clinical nursing specialty

Table 12.1 Registered nurses, by employment status and age group, Canada, 1988

Age group	Total	Employed in nursing	Total	Not employed and seeking employment in nursing	Not employed and not seeking employment in nursing	Not stated
Under 25 years	12 338	10 155	384	282	102	1 799
25–29	33 147	29 155	1 340	753	587	2 652
30–34	42 406	36 712	2 754	1 013	1 741	2 940
35–39	46 035	39 687	3 254	1 037	2 217	3 094
40–44	39 276	33 771	2 961	989	1 972	2 544
45–49	30 072	25 773	2 287	791	1 496	2 012
50–54	19 927	16 662	1 716	537	1 179	1 549
55 years and over	25 775	18 243	4 554	915	3 639	2 978
Not stated	697	348	99	38	61	250
Total	249 673	210 506	19 349	6 355	12 994	19 818

Source: Nursing in Canada – 1988, Canada Centre for Health Information, Statistics Canada, January 1990.

Table 12.2 Registered nurses, employed in nursing by full-time or part-time status, type of employer and province of employment, Canada, 1988[1]

Type of employer employment status	All Canada	Newfoundland	Prince Edward Island	Nova Scotia	New Brunswick	Quebec[2]	Ontario	Manitoba	Saskatchewan	Alberta	British Columbia	Yukon and Northwest Territories
Full time	120 860	2 987	509	5 318	3 903	24 484	48 219	7 534	3 344	10 912	13 420	230
Part time	71 095	675	555	3 048	1 429	17 960	26 897	1 015	2 502	9 259	7 718	37
Not stated	18 551	642	–	–	1 066	11 388	–	447	2 385	–	2 590	33
Total	210 506	4 304	1 064	8 366	6 398	53 832	75 116	8 996	8 231	20 171	23 728	300

[1] The cut-off for Statistics Canada for full-time work is 35 hours per week and above.
[2] Positions are considered full time if nurses work 32 hours or more per week.

Source: Nursing in Canada – 1988, Canada Centre for Health Information, Statistics Canada, January 1990.

Table 12.3 Percentage of registered nurses employed, by position held, Canada, 1980 and 1988

Position	1980 n	%	1988 n	%
Director/Assistant Director	3 792	2.0	5 160	2.5
Supervisor/Co-ordinator Assistant Supervisor	7 672	5.0	10 834	5.2
Clinical specialist	2 676	2.0	1 382	0.6
Head nurse	16 263	10.0	15 872	7.5
General duty/staff nurse	103 179	67.0	152 516	72.5
Instructor/professor	4 360	3.0	5 613	2.6
Other	9 881	6.0	13 694	6.5
Not stated	7 355	5.0	6 435	2.6

Source: Revised Registered Nurses Data Series, Health Division, Statistics Canada. Prepared by Data Centre, Canadian Nurses Association, January 1990.

Table 12.4 Clinical nurse specialists employed, by highest level of education in nursing, Canada, 1980 and 1988

Clinical specialist	1980 n	%	1988 n	%
RN diploma	1 865	70	636	46.0
Post-basic diploma	436	16	228	16.5
Baccalaureate	167	6	305	22.1
Master's/higher degree	50	2	213	15.4
Not stated	158	6	–	–
Total	2 767	100	1 382	100

Source: Revised Registered Nurses Data Series, Health Division, Statistics Canada. Prepared by Data Centre, Canadian Nurses Association, March 1985.

(CNA, 1978). There has been increasing acceptance in the nursing community that these qualifications are appropriate, although confusion about the meaning of clinical specialization and the necessary educational qualifications required continues. Table 12.4 illustrates this point.

The number of master's level prepared nurses identifying themselves as clinical specialists has increased from 2% in 1980 to 15% in 1988 whereas the number of diploma prepared nurses who identified themselves as clinical specialists has decreased from 70% to 46%.

As Baumgart (1988) notes the nursing workforce has grown by almost 175% over a 20-year period, compared to an increase in population of just 25%. In contrast to the more than 300 000 nursing personnel the next three largest groups of health care personnel consist of some 50 000 physicians, 16 000 medical laboratory technologists and 15 000 pharmacists. However there are concerns about the potential for decreasing numbers of students entering nursing programmes due to other career avenues now open to women, although a strong trend has not yet been noted.

LICENSURE AND MEMBERSHIP OF PROFESSIONAL ASSOCIATIONS

In order to practise as a registered or licensed nurse an individual must be registered or licensed by the appropriate body. Each province and territory has its own nursing association that is responsible for both registration or licensure of nurses as described in its Nurses' Act and professional functions, which include, among others, continuing education, career development and political activities. The province of Ontario is the exception because regulatory and professional functions are separate and are the responsibility of two different organizations. Nurses in Ontario may choose to become members of their professional association but must possess a certificate of competence issued by the regulatory body if they are to practise as RNs.

Graduates of nursing education programmes must pass written examinations for initial registration. Comprehensive examinations in English and French have been developed by the CNA in collaboration with all user groups. Graduate nurses who pass the examinations and meet provincial or territorial licensing requirements may practise anywhere in Canada. In 1986–7, 10 000 graduate nurses took the examination. An examination has also been developed for nursing assistants, 12 000 of whom took the examination in 1986–7.

As members of their professional associations nurses are also members of the CNA. The CNA, founded in 1908, is, at the national and international level, the only body representing and speaking for organized nursing in Canada. It is a federation of provincial and territorial nurses' associations financially supported by membership fees collected by constituent members. Until December 1985 it represented all provinces and territories and spoke for 169 000 members. As of January 1986 the province of Quebec is no longer a member of the CNA. Members of l'Ordre des Infirmières et Infirmièrs du Quebec voted in November 1984 to withdraw from the national body. They stated that membership of the CNA through mandatory membership of the provincial association was an obsolete concept and that individual members should be free to choose whether they wished to belong to the national association. With Quebec's disaffiliation the CNA now represents 105 000 members.

UNIONISM

In Canada unions are legally certified under a provincial labour relations act that accords them sole and exclusive right to represent a defined body of employees for collective bargaining purposes. Although collective bargaining is a provincial responsibility the CNA recognized it as one means of improving the social and economic status of its members and played an active role in publicly approving the principle in 1944. However with the exception of British Columbia, where in 1946 provincial government recognized the nurses association as rightful agents to bargain collectively for its members, labour organization among nurses was not a major movement until the 1960s (Roswell, 1982).

Between 1944 and 1960 the nurses associations published, on a yearly basis, employment standards and recommended salaries that could be used to support negotiations for better working conditions and wages. As these policies brought little change provincial associations began to develop collective bargaining structures and prepare for negotiations with employers. The decision of whether or not to include nurses in management positions in bargaining units has been difficult. The problem of deciding at what level a nurse becomes management (within the meaning of the Labour Act) has also plagued employers and provincial labour boards. This issue has resulted in a variety of decisions across Canada. For example British Columbia, New Brunswick and Prince Edward Island include all positions except director and assistant director of nursing. Alberta, Saskatchewan, Manitoba, Nova Scotia and Newfoundland include head nurses in their bargaining units, and Quebec has two separate units, one including general staff nurses and a second including head nurses and supervisors. In Ontario panels of the labour board have handed down awards that include supervisors in a few units and head nurses in others, with the majority including only assistant head nurses and general staff nurses (Roswell, 1982).

Collective bargaining

Early in 1970 the professional associations' role in collective bargaining began to change. Questions were raised by the labour boards about the management domination of the boards or councils of the nurses associations. The turning point came when the Service Employees International Union opposed the application of the Saskatchewan Registered Nurses Association for certification of a nursing unit and alleged that the Association was not a trade union because it was company dominated. The Supreme Court of Canada concurred. This resulted in the provincial labour boards reviewing their own labour legislation relative to the certification of nursing units for the purpose of collective bargaining rights.

Under the Prince Edward Island Nurses' Act control of collective bargaining was removed from nurses associations and provincial nurses unions were established (Roswell, 1985). In general nurses unions have been controlled and operated by nurses.

Provincial nursing unions represent 64% (121 000) of nurses working in nursing (CNA, 1985). This number does not include public health nurses and nursing school instructors who belong to the civil service union in their province. Unionized nurses employed in the Yukon and Northwest Territories belong to either the union, which bargains for other employees of the territorial government, or the Professional Institute of the Public Service of Canada. Of note is that membership is drawn from the same population of nurses who belong to a professional association. Accordingly the two organizations engage in many similar activities, sharing the same interests, values and attitudes on many issues (Conroy and Hibberd, 1983).

In 1981 the National Federation of Nurses Unions was founded to give nurses a voice in matters of national concern. Its membership includes five provincial nursing unions and one institutional union, which represent approximately 24 000 nurses. It liaises with the CNA and has been especially active in its involvement in development of the Code of Ethics as well as in lobbying efforts concerning the Canada Health Act.

Economic conditions

In the early 1970s nurses made significant gains in salary increase. Table 12.5 compares 1974 and 1988 salaries. Increases between 10% and 30% were not unusual. Salaries shown do not include shift differential payment, which may be as high as $1.00 per hour.

In October 1988 the minimum salary for a general staff nurse was $25 289 (in Quebec) and the maximum was $41 286 (in Alberta). The lower wages in Quebec reflect a provincial government decree that effectively rolled back wages in the public sector throughout Quebec. Nurses took a 20% cut but will regain lost wages by means of a cost of living adjustment intended to protect wages against erosion by inflation. Wages in Quebec were the highest in Canada before the decree and considerable ground has been lost since that time (Sethi, et al., 1986).

Higher wages in Alberta and Saskatchewan reflect significant percentage increases in contracts that came into effect in 1982. The Alberta contract gained a 29% wage increase over a two-year period while Saskatchewan gained 26%. Since 1982 yearly increases in other provinces have ranged from 1.2% to 10%. Although salaries compare favourably with current salaries reported by full-time employed 1985 graduates of Ontario universities in the summer of 1986 (Baumgart, 1988), a major

Table 12.5 Comparison of staff nurse annual salaries, 1974 and 1988

Provinces	1974 Annual salaries		1988 Annual salaries	
	Minimum	Maximum	Minimum	Maximum
Newfoundland	6 900	8 810	25 584	32 311
Prince Edward Island	7 488	8 688	25 650	34 205
Nova Scotia	7 817	9 230	26 493	31 345
New Brunswick	7 488	8 688	25 349	32 494
Quebec	6 691	10 776	25 289	41 083
Ontario	9 600	10 920	31 531	40 203
Manitoba	6 996	8 760	26 336	34 860
Saskatchewan	8 484	9 960	28 140	38 060
Alberta	7 500	9 420	31 170	37 097
British Columbia	10 200	12 240	33 316	41 268

Source: National Federation Nurses Unions, Ottawa, Ontario, Canada, 1989.

concern of unionized members continues to be the small difference between minimum and maximum salary levels. In conjunction with this minimum differential is the lack of pay differential for added expertise and education.

Right to strike

Nurses in all provinces except Prince Edward Island, Ontario and Alberta may resort to strike action to force an issue. In Ontario the Hospital Labor Disputes Arbitration Act prohibits strikes and lockouts in the hospital sector and provides for arbitration. Nurses working in hospitals do not have the right to strike whereas nurses working in public health and other community settings do. In 1988 nurses in Alberta defied the law to go on strike (as did nurses in British Columbia and Quebec) but they maintained essential services.

Nurses' major concerns centred around fears that cost-containment was jeopardizing quality of patient care and that remuneration did not reflect the nurse's level of responsibility. In those provinces where strike action is allowed certain essential facilities, productions and services can be ordered to be maintained or employees may be designated as 'essential' and not allowed to strike.

Future issues

Presidents and chief executive officers of nursing unions across Canada were surveyed in order to identify trends and issues in collective bargaining for nurses in Canada (Sethi, *et al.* 1985). The following trends were identified:

1. Union solidarity as an emerging area of importance;
2. 'Zero-point' increases as a fact of life in existing and future negotiations;
3. An increase in job sharing and part-time work;
4. More access to short-term upgrading courses and more emphasis on career development issues;
5. An increase in social development packages;
6. Separate bargaining units for supervisory staff;
7. Higher compensation for nurses in specialist areas;
8. Legal professional accountability.

The majority felt that budget constraints had limited the possibility of bargaining. They noted that most employers came to the table unprepared to bargain, stating that they 'cannot give more'.

OTHER ISSUES

As nurses have improved their economic conditions they have recently been concerned with work-related issues that may affect patient care. An example is the professional responsibility clause in Ontario Nurses Association negotiated contracts that gives nurses a forum to express concerns should they believe that their work load assignments will jeopardize proper patient care. Where hospital and nurses fail to resolve complaints through their union or management committee, an Independent Assessment Committee is appointed. The committee is composed of three registered nurses, one chosen by the union, one by the hospital and one from a roster of independent registered nurses who are well respected within the profession. The latter acts as chairperson. Some of the professional responsibility clauses permit nurses to bring the case to binding arbitration if the employer does not implement the recommendations of the Assessment Committee. This clause has been controversial among nurse administrators who believe that it sets up an adversarial situation that makes it difficult to create an environment in which high quality patient care can be delivered.

Computer technology has increased interest in occupational health and safety issues. As a response to technological development and change the Public Service Alliance of Canada (1982) has suggested that:

1. All collective agreements include a comprehensive definition of technological change to cover changes in work methods and the introduction of new and different equipment;
2. Advance notice be given in all collective agreements of the introduction of technological change and a description of foreseeable effects on employees;

3. A provision be stipulated in all collective agreements for adequate training and career development of employees affected by technological change;
4. Protection of the health and safety of nurses be ensured by negotiating appropriate working conditions;
5. Efforts be continued to decrease working hours and increase paid leave as a means of sharing in increased productivity as a result of automation.

The above are issues that probably will be raised in the health care sector. Also there will be increased demand by nurses for continuing education programmes that will enable them to stay abreast of technological changes. As noted above increased specialization resulting from these changes will necessitate that the nursing profession define its specialties and that employers understand the needs of the patient population.

The principle of 'equal pay for work of equal value' is receiving increasing attention. McKervill (1985) recently reviewed the legislation and cases involving nurses. All provinces and territories now have laws that require paying men and women 'equal pay for equal work'. However there are limitations to the legislation, which uses terms such as 'similar work' or 'substantially the same work'. Critics state that it is difficult to measure objectively differences in jobs.

The first federal 'equal pay for work of equal value' human rights case, resolved in 1980, involved nurses working in federal penitentiaries who were paid less than male technicians who had traditionally rendered health care services in this setting. It was determined that, as the jobs were identical, the pay should be equal.

On January 1st 1988 the Pay Equity Act came into effect in Ontario. The intention is that employers pay women equal wages for work of equal or comparable value, even though the jobs may be substantially different. 'Value' of work is defined as 'value to the employer' and is measured by a gender neutral comparison system using four criteria; skill, effort, responsibility and working conditions (Ministry of Labour, 1990).

Pay Equity applies to workers within a single establishment and respects the employer/employee relationship. During the implementation phase there have been complaints about inadequate preparation of job descriptions, gender and management-biased evaluation tools and the exclusion of women without male equivalents.

In July 1988 the Registered Nurses Association of Ontario (RNAO) presented a brief to the Pay Equity Commission on Gender Discrimination in Female Dominated Establishments with No Male Comparison Groups. The following points were made:

1. Nurses should not be treated as a homogeneous group. Rather diversity of requirements with respect to such factors as education, skills, training and knowledge must be recognized. That may require different comparison groups for different nursing groups and recognition of subtle and less visible tasks often done by the more skilled levels of nurse. For example head nurses, supervisors and nursing administrators have key positions and are responsible not only for patient care but also for large budgets and decisions that have an impact on the workplace as a whole.
2. Where there are no male equivalent job comparisons on a proportionate basis should be established so that groups can be paid in proportion to their value as determined through job evaluation.
3. Comparisons should be allowed on a province-wide basis in the cases of hospitals where salaries tend to be set on a province-wide basis.
4. Arbitrators should be required to consider pay equity adjustments in their awards.
5. If solutions cannot be found in female-dominated establishments with no male comparison groups the maximum of 1% of payroll allocated for pay equity adjustments should become an actual amount paid towards that end.
6. In the search of alternative solutions and in the implementation of any solutions the variety of different nursing groups must be involved in the process at all stages. There is concern that evaluation tools will not measure the 'value of nurses' work'.

In October 1989 the Pay Equity Commission recommended to the Minister of Labour that the Act be amended for female job classes without male equivalents. The Commission suggested three approaches to be tried in succession: proportional value, proxy comparison and average adjustment.

In February 1990 the Ministry of Labour released a discussion paper 'Policy Directions Amending the Pay Equity Act' recommending 'proportional value' comparisons in order to include more women under the Act (Ministry of Labour, 1990). Proportional value permits relative comparisons to be made for all female jobs in an establishment where there are certain minimal numbers of male jobs, even though some or all of the male jobs would be inappropriate comparators for job-to-job comparisons under the present Act. There must be some male job classes in the organization to calculate proportional value. The selection of only one of the Commission's recommendations still excludes 105 000 women in Ontario from pay equity.

QUALITY OF WORKING LIFE

In a Canada-wide survey of hospitals (Kahn and Westley, 1984) employees expressed dissatisfaction with traditional jobs that were production line, highly supervised and over-specialized and that lacked the important qualities of autonomy, learning mobility and meaningfulness.

Directors of nursing, union officers and directors of personnel were asked about their perception of change in employee behaviour over the previous three years. Directors of nursing thought that there had been little or no change over that time, with the exception of a major improvement in nurses' adherence to nursing standards. Specifically results obtained from the directors of nursing in relation to job needs and complaints included the concern of nurses from large urban areas that they lacked opportunities to make decisions as well as lacking opportunities for learning and advancement. A high percentage of directors of nursing also reported an increase in grievances among nurses. The authors suggest that this may be due to dissatisfaction in the workplace or lack of clarity in the collective agreement.

Hospitals were then asked to report on innovations begun in their organizations to deal with external influences and/or staff problems and needs. Some of the innovations exemplified such quality of working life principles as union-management collaboration, role enrichment, multiskill and multidisciplinary and multilevel activities.

The authors drew several conclusions, one of which was that the revolution of rising job expectations is well advanced in hospitals and that most employees see it as legitimate to complain if the job does not meet their expectations. Results obtained in the survey were not dissimilar to those obtained in a large teaching hospital where two major surveys were conducted to determine the level of satisfaction among nurses (Lemieux-Charles, 1983). Retention strategies were instituted following the first survey and their effectiveness was evaluated in the second. Retention strategies perceived to be most important were those developed to increase the effectiveness of communication, management and educational practices.

Another research endeavour that addresses quality of work for nurses in hospitals was conducted by Attridge and Callahan (1987). Their data again highlight the 'importance of management personnel in improving the quality of personnel selection and placement, implementing effective communication systems and providing appropriate salaries, benefits and forms of professional recognition and advancement' (Baumgart, 1988).

PART-TIME WORK

Flexibility in scheduling has been important not only in accommodating the needs of full-time staff but also in recognizing the requirements of the nurse working part time. As noted in a brief submitted to the Federal

Commission of Inquiry into Part-Time Work by the Registered Nurses Association of Ontario (RNAO) (1982) part-time work is not only restricted to nurses in the child rearing group who have increased family commitments but is also seen in the post-child rearing group. The Ontario Nurses Association (ONA), the nurses union in Ontario, reported in 1982 that the proportion of part-time nurses in their membership had increased by 55% in just seven years. They noted that, in a significant number of hospitals, the part-time nursing staff were in the majority yet received lower pay than the full-time staff and lacked fringe benefits and job security. Both the RNAO and the ONA concluded that part-time nursing employment is an accepted and viable proposition for both employer and employee, although not without significant costs and benefits to both parties. The RNAO recommended that:

1. Regular part-time nurses should have the option of accessing fringe benefits and pensions or receiving payment *in lieu* of these benefits on a pro-rated basis;
2. Canada Pension Plan should include the child rearing drop out provision in order to increase the retirement income of nurses who choose part-time work due to child rearing responsibilities;
3. The feasibility of job-sharing should be encouraged by both federal and provincial governments as one means of increasing access to fringe benefits and pension plans for part-time nurses.

The Commission, in its final report, noted that nurses unions, among others, have made the most progress in achieving equitable treatment for part-time workers.

CLINICAL LADDERS

Offering rewards and incentives for different levels of clinical skill have been of special interest to nurse administrators. The method most frequently reported in the literature is that of career ladders although there is no documented evidence in Canadian literature that such a system has been implemented in any health care agency. However a major project entitled The Clinical Promotion Project, in two large tertiary care settings in Alberta and Nova Scotia, was funded through the National Health Research and Development Program. It sought to answer the question, How does a system of promotion for clinical nurses based on identified competencies make a difference in patient care in tertiary care hospitals? Its purposes were: first, to address concerns related to the provision of quality of patient care in times of economic constraint; second, to develop four levels of clinical nursing competence, including performance appraisal tools; and, third, to demonstrate the feasibility of conducting a collaborative demonstration and evaluation project in order to share information, ideas and expertise. It is a longitudinal study now being conducted on only one of the sites.

In summary, there is a need to examine the organization's response to changes in technology, to demands of an increasingly complex environment and to expectations of employees. Nurses now expect an environment that makes their work effective, challenging and involved.

POLITICS OF NURSING: NURSING'S INFLUENCE ON NURSING AND HEALTH POLICIES IN GENERAL

Canadian nurses not only expect a challenging work environment but are also willing to challenge the 'system' when patient care concerns arise. In questioning the system they have become more involved in the political process, both at provincial and national levels.

National level

The CNA has historically assumed an active role in responding to social concerns of the time and has been particularly involved in matters relating to health and welfare. A powerful example of the CNA's commitment occurred when plans were announced to restructure the Acts that governed Canada's national health insurance system. The CNA decided to put extensive human and financial resources into a campaign to influence changes in the new act, which was entitled Canada Health Act.

The need for reform arose because the system was characterized by physician-controlled and hospital-based services, with an emphasis on cure instead of prevention. The Canada Health Act, designed to consolidate and update the federal–provincial cost-sharing arrangements and eliminate extra billings and user fees, failed to address the need for basic reforms. The CNA position addressed four main points towards reform of the system (Dick, *et al.*, 1985):

1. The need to assess, monitor and control health care costs and further develop multidisciplinary community and home-based care;
2. The need to give Canadians the right to consult the health care professional of their choice, with nurses and others as points of entry to the system for assessment, care or referral;
3. Billing for an insured health service rendered to an insured person in an amount over the amount paid for that service by the health insurance plan of that province;
4. A charge for an insured health service that is authorized or permitted

by a provincial health care insurance plan and payable by an insured person.

The power of the CNA's lobby is in its involvement of nurses across the country. The major amendment it sought was to remove the terms 'medical practitioner' and 'dentist' from the Act and replace them with the term 'health care practitioner'. This significant agreement was to acknowledge all health care practitioners as equal partners in the provision of care and signal the need for redirection of health care away from physician and hospital dominance (Dick, *et al.*, 1985). In the final amendment the concept of the health care practitioner was accepted but the terms 'medical practitioner' and 'dentist' also remained. By including this concept the Canada Health Act acknowledged the need for reform. However since health is a provincial responsibility federal legislation could neither address nor implement basic reform.

Involvement of provincial nursing associations is essential in that it is these organizations that continue to lobby provincial politicians for basic reforms. The Canada Health Act identified the elimination of extra billing as a national priority. Three provinces continued to bill additionally but were penalized in that for every dollar extra billed one dollar was withheld by the federal government in transfer payments (but was to be returned when the provinces banned extra billing). To protest the introduction of the bill doctors went on strike. It was the first doctors' strike in Canada since 1962 when the doctors in Saskatchewan walked out in protest of the introduction of the Medical Insurance Bill. By 1987 all provinces had banned extra billing.

Provincial level

Nurses' involvement in decision making at Vancouver General Hospital

In 1977–8 a controversy arose at the Vancouver General Hospital (VGH), a 1000-bed teaching hospital in British Columbia, over the level in the administrative hierarchy at which nurses would participate in decision making. Within the nursing profession the controversy came to light when nurses employed there forwarded to the Registered Nurses Association of British Columbia (RNABC) approximately 60 documents illustrating unsafe patient care. It escalated when a self-appointed delegation of nurses employed at VGH articulated their concerns to the hospital administration and simultaneously approached their professional association, the media and the provincial government.

The delegation called themselves the Committee of Concerned Nurses. They claimed that recent changes in administrative structure and management style at the hospital jeopardized their ability to give safe nursing care. They also claimed that nursing's attempts to discuss quality of patient care with the hospital's newly appointed administrators were being blocked. They believed that nurses should be directly involved in decisions affecting nursing care. Their demand was endorsed by the nurses employed in VGH, the RNABC, the CNA and the International Council of Nurses. The controversy reached a climax when the Ministry of Health appointed a public administrator to take over management functions of the hospital. It was considered to be resolved when the Committee of Concerned Nurses and the RNABC were given assurance by the Ministry of Health that their demand for nursing's participation in decision making would be met. Verna Lovell analysed the events and their meaning for nursing and the health care system in her book entitled 'I Care that VGH Nurses Care'.

The Hospital for Sick Children's baby deaths

Investigation of 30 baby deaths that occurred on the cardiac ward at the Hospital for Sick Children in Toronto, Ontario, served to unite Ontario and Canadian nurses. It was determined that the babies had died of high digoxin levels, the deaths having occurred between July 1st 1980 and March 22nd 1981. Efforts to solve the mystery included the following:

1. An initial investigation resulted in the arrest on March 27th 1981 of Susan Nelles, a nurse from the cardiac ward, for the murders of four babies.
2. Susan Nelles was discharged on May 21st 1982 owing to insufficient evidence.
3. A request was made by the Hospital for Sick Children for a special investigation that was conducted by epidemiologists of the Atlanta Center for Disease Control.
4. A Review Committee was established under the Public Hospitals Act to report on the quality of the hospital's management and administration and the quality of care and treatment of patients. The report was released in January 1983.
5. In April 1983 the Royal Commission into Certain Deaths at the Hospital for Sick Children and Related Matters (known as the Grange Inquiry) was set up by the Attorney General of Ontario to examine the 36 deaths that had occurred during the 'epidemic period', in an effort to determine 'how and by what means the children came to their deaths' and to examine the way in which the police had conducted the investigation and how it had happened that Susan Nelles was first charged and then dismissed. It was felt that the Commission would

satisfy the public's right to know what had happened. Their report was released on December 28th 1984.

The RNAO decided, in the spring of 1983, that it was important that they gain standing at the Commission to speak on behalf of nurses as it became apparent that nurses and nursing would be closely scrutinized.

A major concern was expressed by the RNAO when the Commissioner implied that he might draw conclusions regarding criminal responsibility. Although the Royal Commission was established as a fact-finding mission it was conducted as a trial without the safeguards of the trial process. As it became evident that nurses were being treated differently from other classes of professional, Canadian nurses began to show support. They donated funds to the RNAO Foundation to help defray RNAO's legal costs. Over $100 000 was collected. A motion was passed by the membership at the CNA's Biennial Meeting (1984) in support of the RNAO's actions to protect the profession of nursing.

The enquiry raised many concerns about nurses and nursing. Nurses had initially registered their concerns to nursing administration and staff physicians, including the chief of cardiology, about the number and nature of baby deaths on their ward. They were, in effect, the early warning system yet, perhaps because of their lack of authority, influence and power, they were unable effectively to represent their own and their patients' interests to physicians and organizations. Although nursing was not on trial it was evident that many of the questions addressed professional issues and responsibilities. Nurse experts were called upon to interpret events and describe expected standards of nursing care. The question of whether nurses are treated differently because they are predominantly women was frequently raised. One prominent Canadian nurse stated, 'The enquiry was the highest priced, tax supported, sexual harassment exercise I've ever encountered' (Baumgart, 1988). Patycuk and Galey stated that the inquiry brought out the 'contradiction between nurses' responsibility for human life and their lack of power in making key decisions related to patient care and that a mystique surrounds the male medical professions ... that insulates and encourages respect and reverence ... nurses, mainly women, enjoy no such privilege and protection'. The report provided no answers. The Commissioner attached no great blame to anyone and concluded that the system had worked.

The above two examples illustrate the level of risk nurses and their professional associations have been willing to take in order to interpret nursing's role in the delivery of health care services. Inclusion of nursing in decisions affecting patient care is the theme running through both cases. Of note is the way the formal organizational structure can enhance or impede that involvement. The role of the professional association in publicly supporting its members illustrates the power of nurses when they choose to support a cause and also demonstrates the courage required to become involved in processes with which the majority of nurses are unfamiliar.

Collaboration with other groups

Collaboration with other groups has become essential as health care issues have become more complex and responsibility for their resolution does not rest with only one group. The CNA liaises with groups at national (governmental and non-governmental) and international levels. The 1988 Biennium Report (CNA, 1988) lists activities with nine government departments and over 50 non-governmental agencies, and involvement in eight projects that have been funded by the Canadian International Development Agency.

Examples of where CNA has engaged in collaborative activities include informal alliance during the Canada Health Act lobby with the Canadian Health Coalition, which represents a broad-based coalition of consumers, labour organizations and provider groups, and the development of a joint statement on terminal illness issued by the CNA, Canadian Hospital Association and Canadian Medical Association in consultation with the Canadian Bar Association, Law Reform Commission and Catholic Health Association. This statement presents a protocol for health professionals regarding resuscitation of the terminally ill. A joint statement has also been issued with the Canadian Medical Association requesting that the federal government set up a committee to deal with problems related to administration of drugs to the elderly, particularly as it relates to appropriate dosage. A joint committee of the Canadian Medical Association and the CNA to discuss clinical issues of mutual interest was established in 1984 and meets on a yearly basis.

The status of nursing

The 1980s have been for Canadian nurses a time of greater involvement in social and political issues. Nurses have become increasingly aware that the power of their views is often affected by the image they project. Consequently there has been heightened activity in ensuring that the image projected is that of a competent professional concerned with the consumer's health. The effectiveness of a recent CNA lobby in convincing the Department of Tourism to withdraw a television advertisement that depicted nurses in a perjorative way demonstrates nursing's increasing influence.

Throughout Canada nurses are recognizing that, in order to be 'heard' by various groups, they must ensure that their briefs are well researched and based on principles shared by all nurses. Collaboration with other professionals is also believed to be one of the important routes to change.

13
Nursing research

This chapter provides an overview of nursing research development in Canada. We begin with a description of the context of such development and then focus on factors that are key to the conduct of nursing research: nurse researchers, research literature and libraries, research networks and research funding. We conclude with comments on the future of nursing research in Canada.

THE CONTEXT OF NURSING RESEARCH DEVELOPMENT

The Canadian constitution provides for a division of powers between the federal government and provincial governments, giving provinces (and territories) authority in the domains of education and health. Through funding the federal government has played an important role in the development of health care and education in Canada; however there is no federal structure for the provision of health care or for the development of nursing research. A second feature of Canada is the provision for two official languages: English and French.

National research organizations

At the national level the major structures established for research in the health care field are the Medical Research Council (MRC) and the National Health Research and Development Program (NHRDP) under the Department of National Health and Welfare (NHW). The MRC was originally a division of Canada's National Research Council (NRC) but became established as a separate council in 1969 (Wilmot, 1986). Total funding for the MRC in 1989–90 was approximately $197 million, most of which was provided by the federal government (Medical Research Council, 1990). Some additional funding is generated through the MRC's University – Industry Programs, which began in 1986. The focus of the MRC has traditionally been biomedical research, and, while not explicitly excluded, nursing research has not generally received support from the Council. Recently however there have been some indications of a policy change. Since 1986 guidelines for MRC funding do include support for nursing research. In addition a joint MRC–NHRDP programme to provide support for the development of nursing research resulted in salary support awards for three nurse researchers in 1989 (Stinson et al., 1990) and two more in 1990 for a three-to five-year period.

The NHRDP was established to further national goals in health care and foster research related to topics that the federal government considers to be priorities. The basic research awards budget for this agency is approximately 12% of that of the MRC, with occasional additional amounts, such as those given by the NHRDP in special grants for AIDS research. Although NHRDP is not a funding council and does not have a mandate to develop Canadian health research *per se* (as does the MRC), it has been a key agency in the support of nursing research, especially through support of nursing research projects, training and conferences.

The research funding programmes of the Social Sciences and Humanities Research Council (SSHRC) and the National Science and Engineering Research Council (NSERC) offer no support for nursing research. Although some nurses have received grants or training awards from SSHRC such support has primarily been for training in other disciplines or for projects that do not have nursing or health care as a major focus.

National nursing organizations

There are three national nursing organizations that have played key roles in the development of nursing research in Canada: the Canadian Nurses Association (CNA), the Canadian Association of University Schools of Nursing (CAUSN) and the Canadian Nurses Foundation (CNF). The CNA was established in 1908 and is a federation of nine provincial and two territorial nursing associations. Over the years CNA had a number of *ad hoc* committees on nursing research and then, in 1971, it established a Special Committee on Nursing Research as a committee that met regularly; it became a Standing Committee in 1976. The role of this committee has been to advise the CNA Board on a wide variety of research policies and issues. Since the early 1970s the CNA has promoted the establishment of doctoral programmes in nursing (Zilm et al., 1979), often in conjunction with the CAUSN and CNF, and it worked with the CAUSN to press the MRC pro-actively to support nursing research, an effort that resulted in the MRC convening an *ad hoc* working group in nursing research (Medical Research Council, 1985). Over the past decade the CNA has supported and published the results of four surveys of nurses in Canada with earned doctoral degrees and Canadian nurses enrolled in doctoral programmes (Lamb and Stinson, 1991; Larsen and Stinson, 1980; Stinson et al., 1984; Stinson et al., 1988), developed ethical guidelines for nurse researchers (Canadian Nurses Association, 1983) and produced a five-year plan for the development of nursing research in Canada (Canadian Nurses Association, 1984) and guidelines for the development of nursing research in Canada (Canadian Nurses Association, 1990).

The CAUSN was established in 1942 and is composed of members from 27 of the 31 university faculties and schools of nursing with baccalaureate in nursing programmes (11 of which also have master's in nursing programmes). The major focus of the CAUSN has been the improvement and expansion of university degree courses in nursing. Although the CAUSN's terms of reference provide for an emphasis on research its resources have been small and the pressing need for the development of undergraduate programmes in Canada has been a priority. Increasing attention has been given to research over the past 20 years, however, especially in relation to the development of graduate education and efforts to establish PhD in nursing programmes. The mutual support provided between the CAUSN and Deans and Directors has been beneficial in encouraging universities to support the development of nurse researcher posts on faculty.

The CNF was created by the CNA in 1962 for the purpose of providing research and educational support for nurses. Most of its awards over the years have been given to support nurses enrolled in graduate programmes, although some smaller grants are now given for nurses in post-RN baccalaureate programmes and for nursing research projects.

Provincial and territorial nursing associations

The mandate of professional nursing associations in the provinces and territories is to protect the public and to promote high standards of nursing practice and education. The promotion of nursing research may or may not be made explicit in the objectives of these associations but there is considerable evidence that they are committed to the development of nursing knowledge through research. That evidence includes some of the following activities carried out by these associations: nursing research committees (Canadian Nurses Association, 1985a); provincial foundations established for scholarships, loans and research grants; support for the national nursing research conferences; provision of provincial conference or annual meeting time for sessions on nursing research; inclusion of nursing research abstracts or reports in journals; collection of provincial members' theses and provincial and institutional nursing research reports for association libraries; lobbying provincial governments to support nursing research; and joint establishment and financing of nursing research units in collaboration with university schools of nursing in the province, as was done by the Saskatchewan Registered

Nurses Association (SRNA) and the Manitoba Association of Registered Nurses (MARN).

NURSE RESEARCHERS

There are no current national data on the number of full-time nurse researchers in Canada but earlier studies suggest that the number is low but growing slowly. A 1976 survey of nurses engaged in research indicated that there were six (Storch *et al.*, 1977). In a 1986 study Faux identified 16 nurses whose appointments involved a major emphasis (more than 50%) on the conduct or development of nursing research. In 1990 it was estimated that 15 nurses in universities had funding that protected at least 50% of their time for nursing research (Oulton, 1991). To this total can be added the unknown number of nurses in research positions in health care agencies. A number of the provincial and territorial nursing licensing bodies are now collecting data on the number of registered nurses who devote some or all of their time to nursing research but, as yet, there is no national data set.

Education for nursing research

Approximately 70% of Canada's more than 252 000 registered nurses have their initial two- or three-year nursing diploma programme as their highest level of educational preparation in nursing (Statistics Canada, 1990). These programmes do not offer course work in nursing research or introduce students to quantitative or qualitative research. Approximately 13% of registered nurses have completed a four-year baccalaureate programme in nursing or a two- to three-year post-RN programme. By the 1980s most of Canada's 31 university faculties and schools of nursing required of all undergraduates an introductory statistics course and an introductory course in nursing research.

Approximately 1% of registered nurses in Canada have at least a master's degree as their highest level of education in *nursing*. There are 11 nursing master's degree programmes in Canada and each of these stresses research in all course work. A thesis is required or optional, with the exception of one programme, that does not offer a thesis option (Field and Stinson, 1986). These courses have undergone considerable changes over the years in terms of focus and research emphases (Allen, 1986). Prior to 1965 most graduate nursing programmes focused on preparing nurse educators and administrators. Between 1965 and 1980 clinical specialization was emphasized. Currently graduate programmes focus on nursing theory, practice and research. Similarly research emphases evolved over time from a pre-1965 emphasis on 'problem solving, descriptive and evaluative research', to 'application of knowledge from other disciplines' and 'descriptive and evaluative' research between 1965 and 1980, and to a post-1980 focus on 'seeking knowledge from problems and situations arising in [nursing] practice', and emphasis on the 'scientific approach'.

Nurses with doctoral preparation

By 1989 Canada had 257 nurses prepared at the doctoral level (see Table 13.1). Of this number 23% had undertaken doctoral degrees focused primarily on nursing (Lamb and Stinson, 1991). These figures reflect the fact that Canadian nurses have had to study abroad to complete a doctoral programme in nursing. The first PhD in nursing programme in Canada was established in January 1991 at the University of Alberta (Alberta, 1991). The first nurse to graduate with a PhD in nursing from a Canadian university was Francine Ducharme, who obtained her degree in 1990 from McGill University after completing a programme as a 'special case' student.

Table 13.1 Clusters of disciplines undertaken by nurses with earned doctoral degrees, Canada, 1989[1]

Clusters	n	%
Education	122	47
Nursing	59	23
Other health related	38	15
Social sciences	30	12
Arts and humanities	8	3
Unknown	1	0
Total	258[2]	100

[1] Source: M. Lamb and S.M. Stinson. (In press) *Canadian Nursing Doctoral Statistics: 1989 Update.* Used with the permission of the Canadian Nurses Association.
[2] One nurse holds two PhDs: one in Nursing, the other in Anthropology.

Of the 257 nurses with earned doctoral degrees 55% had obtained a degree from a Canadian university. Compared to women scientists in other fields the median age at completion of the doctoral degree was high: 42 years. The majority of these nurses (62%) were employed in universities while 14% were employed in health agencies. The health agency sector is a growing one in terms of nursing research. In a survey of nursing research in Canadian teaching hospitals Thurston *et al.* (1987) identified more than 120 projects focused on patient care, despite the early stage of nursing research development in that sector.

In a recent survey (Lamb and Stinson, 1991) 265 nurses were identified as being enrolled in doctoral programmes in 1989. Of those whose discipline of study was reported the largest group (29%) was enrolled in education, followed by nursing and other health related disciplines. More than 50% were enrolled in Canadian universities, 23% in US universities, 6% in UK programmes and less than 1% at European universities. The location was not reported for 20%.

Efforts by the nursing profession to establish PhD in nursing programmes in Canada began in the mid-1970s and continue to this day. A 1976 resolution at the CNA 1976 Annual Meeting called for leadership in relation to doctoral preparation for Canadian nurses. In 1978 the Kellogg National Seminar on Doctoral Preparation for Canadian Nurses was held at the initiation of the CNA, in conjunction with the CNF and CAUSN, and funded by a grant from the W. K. Kellogg Foundation of Battle Creek, Michigan (Zilm et al., 1979). Participants at the seminar reached consensus that 'the greatest and most pressing priority is the initiation of a Ph.D. (Nursing) programme or programmes in Canada'. Since that time there have been four initiatives to establish Canadian PhD in nursing programmes.

In 1986 the University of Alberta's PhD in nursing programme proposal was approved by its Board of Governors and Universities Coordinating Council, 'subject to appropriate funding'. In the meantime three 'special case' PhD (Nursing) students were admitted for doctoral study in September 1988. Funding for the approved programme was eventually secured in 1990 and it began in January 1991, with a projected annual intake of four students and a total enrollment of up to 16 students (Alberta, 1991).

The conjoint PhD in nursing programme proposed by the University of Montréal and McGill University has been reviewed once by the Quebec Council of Universities and the Ministry of Higher Education and Sciences and has, at the time of writing, been sent back for a second review. The conjoint committees of the Quebec Council of Universities and the Conference of University Principals have acknowledged the necessity of a PhD in nursing. As McGill University has a clause in its regulations permitting *ad hoc* programmes three 'special case' students have undertaken studies towards a PhD in nursing. However this avenue is limited as there are no programme funds provided by the Ministry of Higher Education and Sciences.

The University of Toronto (UT) and University of British Columbia (UBC) have both been engaged in planning PhD programmes in nursing. It is anticipated that the UBC course will be operational in 1991 (Willman, 1991) and the UT one in 1992 (Pringle, 1991).

During the 15-year effort to establish doctoral programmes in nursing little attention has been given to post-doctoral preparation. Although a number of funding councils consider post-doctoral preparation to be necessary for the development of independent researchers it is likely to be some time before such education is the norm in Canadian nursing. Over the next decade attention must be given to the development of post-doctoral programmes and fellowships for nurses. In the latter respect the one exception is that, in 1990, the Alberta Foundation for Nursing Research established a post-doctorate funding category.

RESEARCH LITERATURE AND LIBRARIES

While some of the Canadian nursing research literature is available in both English and French much of it is available in only one of the two. English if the first language for approximately two-thirds of Canadian nurses and French is the first language of one-third, most of whom live in Quebec. Many Canadian nurses are bilingual but if literature is to be useful to *all* Canadian nurses, it must be available in both official languages.

Research literature

Canadian nurses have relied greatly on nursing research journals from other countries, especially the US and the UK, for research articles to read and for opportunities to publish. Since the early 1970s opportunities in Canada have increased but there is as yet only one peer-reviewed nursing research journal in Canada. The 'Canadian Journal of Nursing Research/ Revue canadienne de recherche en sciences infirmières', is the CAUSN's official journal, has a circulation of approximately 1000 and has been published by the McGill University School of Nursing since 1969. The 'Canadian Nurse/L'infirmière canadienne', the official journal of the CNA, publishes some research articles in both languages, providing abstracts in the other language. The newsletters or journals of some nursing specialty organizations and of provincial nursing associations, such as 'Nursing Québec', the official journal of the Order of Nurses of Quebec, also publish some research articles. Health-related periodicals, such as the 'Canadian Journal of Public Health' 'Santé mentale au Canada', and 'Revue de L'administration hospitalière et sociale', provide additional opportunities for Canadian nurse researchers to publish in their first language.

The proceedings of the National Nursing Research Conferences (NNRCs) that began in 1971 constitute the most comprehensive collection of research articles by Canadian nurses. Although in the earliest years these proceedings were published in both English and French the financial constraints in recent years have led conference organizers to publish articles in the language of presentation with an abstract in the other language (King et al., 1986). There have been changes in the content of Canadian nursing research, as reflected in the proceedings of NNRCs and International Nursing Research Conferences (Nursing Studies Research Unit, 1982; Stinson et al., 1986). The emphasis on nursing education and nursing administration at the first conference (King, 1971) changed to an emphasis on clinical practice (Allen and Thibaudeau, 1973), with a considerable increase in literature on the conceptualization of nursing and health (Godden & Cahoon, 1974; King et al., 1986; MacKay & Zilm, 1981). These proceedings also indicate an expansion of the methods used by Canadian nurse researchers, a greater use of nursing conceptual frameworks and an extended research locus, from hospitals to community health settings such as the home and the workplace.

Master's and doctoral theses constitute an important source of Canadian nursing research literature. Access to these is facilitated through 'Dissertation Abstracts International', the CNA's collection of theses and its bilingual index of nursing research by Canadian nurses (Canadian Nurses Association, 1987), an on-line computerized list of completed master's theses available through the University of Alberta Faculty of Nursing's CAMN system, and the extensive collection of nursing theses at the University of Montreal (all PhD theses in nursing done in the US since 1978 and all PhD theses done in the US dealing with nursing topics).

Libraries

The best nursing library in Canada is the CNA's Helen K. Mussallem Library, located at its headquarters in Ottawa. (Virginia Henderson [1984] has lamented the fact that the US has produced nothing comparable to the CNA, Royal College of Nursing or Japanese Nursing Organization libraries.) The CNA's holdings include hundreds of theses, research reports and proceedings of research conferences as well as an extensive archives collection. Another library of importance in Ottawa is the federally operated Health Science Resource Centre of the Canada Institute for Scientific and Technical Information (CISTI).

All Canadian schools of nursing have nursing libraries; however the better nursing research libraries can be found in the 11 universities offering graduate degree programmes in nursing. The libraries of some of the provincial nursing associations, notably the Alberta Association of Registered Nurses, systematically collect nursing theses and research reports completed by their members. The 84 teaching hospitals in Canada also maintain libraries that include some material on nursing research.

In Quebec there are three large French language libraries located at the University of Montreal (UM), University of Laval and the Order of Nurses of Quebec (ONQ). These holdings probably constitute the largest collection of French language nursing research literature in the world. Although the CNA's library has collected all the Canadian research publications available in French it does not have a comprehensive collection of French language unpublished documents and reports.

RESEARCH NETWORKS

As Canada is large in size (over 11 000 km from coast to coast) and has a relatively small population (under 27 million) communication has always been a challenge. With regard to nursing research networking has been facilitated by national and international conferences, universities, nursing and funding organizations and research committees.

Conferences

The NNRCs were at first planned on an *ad hoc* basis, sponsored by one or more universities and provincial nursing associations, and organized on the classical model of presentation and critique of scientific papers. Since the 1980s these have been open to any interested persons; thus networking is enhanced. The annual NNRCs are now sponsored by the CAUSN in cooperation with the faculty or school of nursing of the university that hosts the annual meeting of the Learned Societies. Nursing research development was enhanced by a series of 'Evaluation Seminars', initiated in 1970 at McMaster University and sponsored by the NHRDP. These seminars facilitated networking and helped nurses to design studies and prepare funding proposals. Provincial professional conferences focused on a variety of health-related topics, as such as care of the chronically ill, computers in health care and quality of care evaluation, and also provide research networking opportunities.

Canadian nurses have participated in international nursing research conferences and established networks through their attendance at the conferences of the Workgroup of European Nurse Researchers (WENR), the International Council of Nurses (ICN), Sigma Theta Tau International Honor Society and other national and international organizations. The first international nursing research conference was sponsored by the Department of Nursing Studies of Edinburgh University in 1981; the second was held in Edmonton in 1986, sponsored by the University of Alberta Faculty of Nursing in collaboration with the CNA, CAUSN, Alberta Association of Registered Nurses, University of Calgary, University of Lethbridge, WENR and American Nurses' Association (ANA). These International conferences have been of key importance in extending nursing research networks and stimulating the organization of new conferences on a wide variety of research topics.

Research organization and committees

A discussion on the merits of establishing a national organization of nurse researchers in Canada took place at the 1975 NNRC, based on a paper prepared by Stinson (1975). Debate on the topic continued for a number of years. Points of controversy included the purpose and financing of a national organization, the role of a new organization *vis à vis* the CNA, CAUSN and CNF (all of which have had roles in nursing research development) and the membership, structure and activities of such an organization. At the 1986 International Nursing Research Conference approximately 80 nurse researchers met informally and agreed to establish a national nursing research group. The bylaws of the Canadian Nursing Research Group (CNRG) were adopted the following year. The CNRG has recently become a CNA Interest Group and its major goals have been described as developing 'nurse researchers, nursing research, and a nursing research reality' (Giovannetti, 1991).

National, regional, provincial and local committees have been important in the development of research networks as early as the 1950s and 1960s. In addition to the series of CNA research committees since 1971 a number of organizations have brought nurse researchers together from across the country and within provinces or cities. For example the Quebec Region of the CAUSN began to assemble a repertory of ongoing nursing research by 1984. The CNF had also established a research grants committee by the mid-80s, providing a new structure for the networking process. Also at the national level the NHRDP's interdisciplinary research review committees continue to provide networking opportunities for nursing and other health-related disciplines.

At the local level a number of structures are in place that provide opportunities for nurse researchers to meet and develop their research skills. These structures include local nursing research interest groups, health agency research committees, nursing research units, joint appointments, inter-institutional collaborative projects, open lectures by nurse researchers and community-based nursing research seminars.

RESEARCH FUNDING

There has been a paucity of funding for nursing research in Canada. In 1986 the CNA's former Executive Director noted that while more than $30 billion were spent annually in providing health care in the country only one half to just over one million dollars were spent in support of nursing research (Canadian Nurse/L'infirmière canadienne, 1986). Little has changed since 1986 and funding is needed not only for the conduct of investigations but also for research training, clinical researchers in universities and health agencies, research development programmes, scientific travel, conferences, journals and the development of research units.

National level funding

As mentioned earlier the NHRDP has been the major supporter of nursing research at the national level through grants for projects, fellowships for students and support of conferences. Nurses have also been involved on NHRDP committees for many years. Although the MRC has awarded funding to a few nurses engaged in basic 'medical' research these projects cannot be classified as *nursing* research. The CNA and CAUSN voiced their concerns about the lack of support from the MRC and, in 1983, the MRC established an *ad hoc* committee on nursing research. The report of this group (Medical Research Council, 1985) contained a series of recommendations for the development of nursing research in Canada. To date although there has been some increased funding of a few nurse researchers there has been no fundamental support for nursing research development as envisioned by the *ad hoc* committee.

In 1986 the CNA's Executive Director was appointed as a member of the MRC for a two-year term and, during the past few years, some nurses have been included on MRC committees, such as the Clinical Trials Committee, a Studentship Committee and the joint NHRDP – MRC Development of Research in Nursing Committee (Medical Research Council, 1990). Recently a nurse administrator has been appointed as a member of Council.

The CNF has offered a modest number of scholarships (44 for a total of $147 000 in 1989–90 for baccalaureate, master's and PhD study) and several years ago the CNF initiated a small research grants programme (awarding $21 582 to six projects in 1990) for nursing research (Bisson, 1991). Health-related voluntary organizations, such as the Kidney Foundation of Canada and the National Cancer Institute (Canadian Nurses Association, 1985b), also provide some funding for nursing research training and projects, but these are of limited importance in the development of an infrastructure for nursing research.

Provincial level funding

At the provincial level nurse researchers have obtained limited amounts of funding from health research organizations, local foundations and provincial government agencies. For example in Ontario some nursing research has been funded and some nurses engaged in nursing research training have been supported by the Ministry of Health in Ontario. Similarly in Quebec university professors of nursing who work in research teams that include a number of graduate students are eligible for funding from the Formation des chercheurs et aide à la recherche (FCAR). This year the Fonds de la recherche en santé du Québec (FRSQ) is establishing a special competition for 'emerging teams' in nursing that will provide funding for staff and equipment. The Conseil québécois de la recherche sociale (CQRS), which focuses on social health and welfare, has in the past funded (to a maximum of $120 000 per grant) many nursing research projects. On occasion larger grants are awarded through a special competition when there are issues considered to be by government a priority. For example in Ontario in 1990 a proposal for a Quality of Nursing Worklife Research Unit submitted by the Faculty of Nursing, University of Toronto, and School of Nursing, McMaster University, received funding to the tune of $2 million funding over five years (Bethune, 1991). To our knowledge at the provincial and state level there is only one government world-wide that has established a structure and earmarked funds exclusively for nursing research: the Government of Alberta. The Alberta Foundation for Nursing Research (AFNR) was established in 1982 when that government allocated $1 million over a five-year period for this purpose, followed in 1988 by a minimum amount of $1.2 million for the subsequent five years. (It is that same government which earmarked funds to establish and maintain Canada's first PhD in nursing programme in 1990.)

Non-governmental sources of support at the provincial level include provincial nursing associations, private foundations and service organizations. Some nursing associations designate a small amount from operating funds to make research grants, scholarships or conference funds available while others have established foundations that make small research grants. Provincial counterparts to several national health foundations and agencies also provide similar funding. While the amounts are generally quite small (e.g. from $100 for a computer search to a few thousand dollars) there is a wide variety of such organizations that support nursing research to a limited extent.

There has been no published comprehensive review of the sources and extent of nursing research funding in Canada although unpublished, informal surveys and estimates have been produced at the national level and in some of the provinces. Periodically the CNA publishes a document on sources of funding for which nurses are eligible (Canadian Nurses Association, 1985b) and national overviews on funding have been published by Kerr (1986), Stinson (1977) and Wilmot (1986).

CANADIAN NURSING RESEARCH IN THE FUTURE

Nursing research development in Canada seems uncertain in the short term. However when viewed in the long-term there is reason to be optimistic. At the time of writing Canada is in an economic recession, federal and provincial governments are operating with deficit budgets and, despite cutbacks on research and other activities, the national debt remains high. The budgets of university nursing education programmes and nursing service departments are severely constrained, making new initiatives in nursing research unlikely.

The long-term view is a more positive one, especially when one considers the advances that have been made in the past 15 years. These accomplishments include the first government funded agency for nursing research, the establishment of a number of nursing research units, growth in the number of nurses with doctoral degrees, increased nursing involvement in funding council committees, the first PhD in nursing graduate from a Canadian university, the establishment of the first PhD in nursing programme with several more in the planning and approval stages, and the gradual but steady increase in the conduct of nursing research. What is remarkable is not the great development tasks yet remaining but the advances in Canadian nursing research that have been achieved in a relatively short period of time in difficult circumstances.

14

Planning for nursing

One major problem in attempting to plan for nursing in Canada is concerned with who should assume responsibility for the planning process. It is not clear what roles federal and provincial governments should play in planning for nursing, although they are ultimately responsible for generating the demand for nurses. Because educational programmes for nurses are controlled by Ministers of Education, rather than Health, it is also unclear what authority the educational system has for influencing the supply of nurses.

Accordingly a systematic, comprehensive programme for planning for nursing in Canada that would attempt to balance demand and supply of nurses has not been developed. Because there is no overall responsibility for planning by one agency imbalances in supply and demand for nurses (over- or undersupply) may produce a variety of somewhat impulsive responses and reactions from a number of different groups, including federal government, provincial governments, hospital associations, nursing associations, universities and colleges. Statistics Canada, a federally operated programme, keeps annual figures, widely available to those interested in planning, on supply and demand of all health professionals including nurses.

MEASUREMENT OF THE DEMAND FOR NURSING SERVICES

In 1990 the population of Canada was 26.6 million (World Almanac, 1991), an increase of over five million since 1972. Quebec and Ontario together account for more than half this number. The percentage of gross national product spent on all health expenditure in 1987 was 8.6, an increase of only 1% since 1976. In 1988 the breakdown of health expenditures by sector was as follows:

	$ million
All hospitals (acute and psychiatric)	12 470.0
Homes for special care (long-term care facilities)	4 117.7
Physician services	4 414.3
Dentist services	1 682.6
Other professional services (chiropracters, optometrists, Victorian Order of Nurses	467.2
Drugs and appliances	3 275.3
Other health care costs (public health)	3 660.6
Total	30 087.7

Source: Canadian Hospital Directory, 1988.

It may be noted that by far the largest proportion of health expenditure is on hospital services. The proportion of health expenditure on hospitals has remained relatively consistent: in 1972 it accounted for 3.28% of the gross national product and in 1982 3.49%.

The bed complement of public hospitals in Canada from 1973 to 1987 is shown in Table 14.1. It should be noted that there has been an increase in number of hospital beds, from 142 069 in 1973 to 156 132 in 1987. When numbers of beds are examined by type and size of hospital, as shown in Table 14.1, it can be seen that there has been a decrease in the number of beds in general, non-teaching hospitals; however there has been an increase in the public hospitals that now have beds allocated to long-term care patients. These figures suggest that some acute hospital beds have been recategorized as long-term care.

Although the number of hospitals beds has increased there has been little change in the bed:population ratio: for example the number of hospital beds per 1000 population in 1979 was 6.66 and in 1984 6.08. Bed occupancy rates in hospitals in Canada in 1987 averaged 83%, an increase from 79% in 1974; occupancy rates tend to be low in small hospitals and high in large hospitals. There are also some interprovincial differences in occupancy rates, the highest rates being in British Columbia, Quebec and Ontario and the lowest in the NorthWest Territories and Newfoundland.

In Canadian hospitals in 1987 total paid hours for all categories of staff per patient day was 15.14. Paid hours per patient day for nursing services in 1987 was 6.74, i.e. a little under 50% of the paid hours in hospitals. Again there were interprovincial differences, with larger, more populated provinces providing fewer paid nursing hours than smaller, isolated provinces. For example Quebec paid 6.51 and the North West Territories 8.48 nursing hours per patient day in 1987.

Since 1985 there has been growing concern that demand for registered nurses has exceeded supply. Meltz and Marzetti (1988) identified four

Table 14.1 Approved bed complement of operating public hospitals classified by type and size, Canada, 1973–1986/7

Public hospitals type and size	1973	1974	1975	1976	1977/8	1978/9	1979/80	1980/1	1981/2	1982/3[1]	1983/4	1986/7
Gen Non-Tch No LTU												
Beds												
1– 24	3 275	3 208	3 228	3 289	3 177	3 172	3 097	2 991	3 005	2 641	2 429	2 277
25– 49	6 176	6 219	5 943	5 544	5 287	5 102	4 923	4 885	4 788	4 594	4 295	3 989
50– 99	6 987	7 363	5 791	6 196	5 805	5 665	5 121	5 124	4 851	5 067	4 913	4 182
100–199	10 408	10 437	9 205	8 234	7 521	7 119	6 679	6 666	6 169	6 046	5 785	5 631
200–299	19 768	19 092	18 752	8 190	7 612	6 834	5 846	6 489	5 983	4 965	5 071	4 392
300+				11 833	10 343	10 327	8 554	7 620	8 688	8 595	7 259	6 068
Subtotal	46 614	46 319	42 919	43 286	39 745	38 219	34 220	33 775	33 484	31 908	29 752	26 539
Gen Non-Tch LTU												
Beds												
1– 49	3 544	3 680	3 867	995	1 567	1 567	1 859	1 937	1 938	2 439	2 765	2 856
50– 99				3 842	4 218	4 366	5 190	5 173	5 493	5 293	5 698	6 947
100–199	5 156	5 628	6 882	8 018	9 267	9 279	8 949	8 839	9 018	8 973	9 119	9 188
200–299	16 375	20 785	23 666	7 708	7 151	7 922	9 864	9 755	9 995	10 288	9 797	10 278
300+				20 768	23 185	25 143	24 947	27 094	28 811	28 289	30 838	34 614
Subtotal	25 075	30 093	34 415	41 331	45 301	48 277	50 809	52 798	55 255	55 282	58 217	63 883
Non-Tch Total	71 689	76 412	77 334	84 617	85 133	86 496	85 029	86 573	88 739	87 190	87 969	90 422
Tch. (Excl.)	(33,968) (12 608)	(35 035) (12 915)	(34 993) (13 081)	35 253	36 606	36 027	35 828	36 527	36 044	37 647	38 299	39 187
Gen. total:	118 265	124 362	125 408	119 870	121 739	122 523	120 857	123 100	124 783	124 837	126 268	129 609
Ped.	2 774	3 205	3 116	2 884	2 843	2 772	2 756	2 747	2 741	2 844	2 874	2 858
All Spec.	21 030	20 711	23 269	32 654	33 745	34 493	35 340	35 266	34 649	34 422	35 317	23 665
Pub grand total	142 069	148 278	151 793	155 408	158 327	159 788	158 953	161 113	162 173	162 103	164 459	156 132

Prior to 1976, this hospital size classification was not used.
[1] Preliminary figures.
[2] Prior to 1976 teaching hospitals were classified as full teaching (top number) and partial teaching (bottom number) hospitals.
Source: Statistics Canada.

factors underlying the increase in demand for RNs: 'an increase in the number of RNs per hospital bed (largely the result of substitution of RNs for RNAs, aides and orderlies); a shift from full-time to part-time work; some growth in non-hospital jobs for RNs; and an increase in the number of hospital beds'.

MEASUREMENT OF THE SUPPLY OF NURSING SERVICES

Figures are available on the number of registered nurses, nursing assistants and nursing orderlies by Canadian population. It may be seen from Table 14.2 that population per registered nurse has been decreasing. In 1976 there were 129 people for each registered nurse and in 1986 there were 108. As with previous figures on demand for nursing services it is clear from Table 14.2 that larger provinces such as Ontario have more registered nurses per population than smaller, more remote provinces or territories.

Similarly, as shown in Table 14.3, the supply of registered nursing assistants per population has been decreasing. In 1973 there were 362 Canadians for every registered nursing assistant but by 1986 there were only 309.

ATTEMPTS TO BALANCE SUPPLY AND DEMAND

In 1979 the Principal Nursing Officer for Canada, a special advisor on nursing matters to the Federal Minister of Health, examined the employment status for registered nurses in Canada (Flaherty, 1979) in an attempt to obtain the perceptions of a variety of representatives from nursing associations, governments and hospital associations about the needs for various types and levels of registered nurses and other nursing personnel. As Flaherty states:

> From time to time, since the beginning of this century, there have been periods of acute shortages and periods of significant surpluses of registered nurses in this country. These situations have been precipitated by a variety of factors – social, cultural, economic and situational (wars, depression, prosperity, fiscal constraints associated with government policies, *et al*) – that have made effective manpower planning for nurses difficult.

Flaherty was interested in obtaining information about the supply of nurses associated with filling vacancies and on communications between the employers of nurses and those previously responsible for educating nurses for practice. Survey results showed a number of regional differences in the balance of supply and demand for nurses. For example

Table 14.2 Population per nurse registered, by province of employment/residence, Canada, 1976/86

Province	1976	1977	1978	1979	1980	1981	1982	1983	1984	1985	1986
Newfoundland	176	163	159	180	181	161	135	148	148	131	117
Prince Edward Island	127	121	120	144	148	138	139	141	131	129	114
Nova Scotia	135	129	127	151	137	126	116	115	109	105	102
New Brunswick	135	127	130	136	130	130	122	115	111	116	103
Quebec	117	168	131	142	126	125	123	127	126	118	116
Ontario	102	102	100	102	101	101	101	99	100	99	98
Manitoba	132	128	126	133	130	135	130	126	122	121	116
Saskatchewan	132	130	133	140	141	128	130	129	121	121	116
Alberta	135	127	123	138	136	134	130	121	114	114	111
British Columbia	137	131	126	135	130	143	120	120	118	116	116
Yukon and Northern Territories	129	126	124	191	178	174	175	182	175	162	166
Total	129	125	117	124	119	119	115	114	113	110	108

Table 14.3 Population per licensed nursing assistant, by province of licensure, Canada, 1976–86

Province	1976	1977	1978	1979	1980	1981	1982	1983	1984	1985	1986
Newfoundland	344	336	328	320	313	286	294	238	244	236	232
Prince Edward Island	238	220	218	233	253	272	253	248	262	248	257
Nova Scotia	410	378	355	341	297	279	264	262	257	264	261
New Brunswick	343	338	320	325	321	309	320	311	322	317	324
Quebec	407	381	374	363	345	351	349	344	342	345	368
Ontario	260	254	265	254	256	256	258	257	263	267	269
Manitoba	302	288	266	260	270	308	283	272	281	258	255
Saskatchewan	388	380	379	390	3 043	386	416	411	434	398	397
Alberta	339	349	314	362	309	310	321	297	284	289	274
British Columbia	386	383	378	370	369	365	371	382	410	433	451
Yukon	317	400	328	283	299	337	377	388	418	398	395
Northwest Territories	407	359	366	396	450	431	471	398	329	424	485
Total	324	314	313	308	303	302	304	298	302	304	309

many provinces, such as Saskatchewan, Manitoba, Ontario and parts of the Maritimes, reported a surplus. British Columbia, specifically Vancouver, reported a shortage of nurses for critical care, obstetrics, gerontology, operating theatres and psychiatry.

The major scarcity of nurses, however, was found by Flaherty to be in the northern areas of Canada:

> The most difficult staffing problem, however, is in the one-person nursing station situations in the very small communities. The nurses in these stations must be experienced and be prepared to assume high levels of responsibility. They require experience in both active treatment and community health nursing as well as the personal strength and stamina to be on call virtually 24 hours a day, seven days a week. The rigours of isolation are extreme in these communities; hence, nurses at these stations must be personally stable, resourceful, mature and experienced. Such nurses are difficult to find and to recruit.

Similar problems of recruitment are also reported in northern Alberta, Manitoba, Ontario and Newfoundland. Nurses willing to work in isolated places are rare. The added responsibility of being the only health worker in a community without a doctor on call, and in some places without paved roads, is frightening to many nurses, who fear they do not have adequate skills to cope with potential emergencies. In some northern areas the nurse may be the only non-native in the community and be expected to play a major community leadership role that young nurses are not necessarily able to assume.

The importance of Flaherty's work, however, was that it clearly demonstrated the lack of systematic planning for a balance in the supply and distribution of nurses. The organizations surveyed, including provincial nursing associations, governments, hospital associations, educational institutions and individual health care facilities, showed that no specific type of organization was assuming responsibility for nursing planning and that there was little communication or coordination among the agencies involved.

Since 1985 there has been growing concern over increasing nurse vacancy and turnover rates. An unpublished CNA document (1989) lists 56 national or provincial studies and/or reports undertaken since 1985 to examine the issues surrounding the nursing shortage and other work-related issues. Many of the studies combined a market analysis of the labour situation with a survey that sought information regarding nurses' opinions, attitudes and feelings towards their work and work environment (Alberta Association of Registered Nurses, 1985; Carson *et al.*, 1987; Collinge, 1988; Meltz and Marzetti, 1988; Ministere de la Santé et des Services Scoiaux du Quebec, 1987; Nurses Association of New Brunswick

1988; Registered Nurses Association of British Columbia, 1987; Registered Nurses Association of Ontario, 1988;).

Generally they found that vacancies were more likely to be found in critical care, long-term care and psychiatric care areas. Reasons for vacancies ranged from nurses' general dissatisfaction with their work environment, due primarily to lack of control over conditions of work such as scheduling and decisions affecting their ability to carry out their work effectively, to the increase in clerical duties and part-time workers. Recommendations from the majority of reports addressed the need to improve in the following areas:

1. Work environment: increase of orientation programmes, scheduling patterns, staffing, including the appropriate mix of personnel, and organizational communication, including involvement of nurses in policy development within their institutions.
2. Compensation: adoption of premium pay scales, increase in the range between starting salary and maximum rate of the RN pay scale, and remuneration congruent with education and professional activities.

Other areas included increasing the scope and opportunities for career enhancement and advancement as well as determining ways to support nurses in the pursuit of advanced education. The Registered Nurses Association of Ontario (RNAO) (1988) emphasized that human resource planning for nursing should not be carried out in isolation. They recommended that 'the governing bodies of Ontario's self-regulating professions examine their proposal to establish an independent institute for Coordinated Health Manpower Planning'.

The responses of government to these reports have varied. Alberta and Ontario announced specific retention and recruitment programmes to which they allocated a significant amount of money. In both instances a senior nurse consultant was hired to advise the Ministry of Health on human resources issues. In Ontario a $5 million innovation fund was established to encourage hospitals to solve staff and scheduling issues and universities to set up continuing education programmes.

Alberta and Ontario also decreed that nurses be involved in key hospital decision making committees. The Minister of Health in Ontario announced amendments to the Public Hospitals' Act, which governs hospitals, to allow nurses an active voice in administrative, financial, operational and planning decisions in their hospitals. Under the new regulations Ontario hospitals are required to amend their bylaws to allow both staff and management nurse representation on various hospital committees. Each institution is also required to set up a fiscal advisory committee that includes staff and management nursing representatives. Only hospitals that have complied with the changes are eligible to access monies from the innovation fund. A nursing human resources databank was also established.

To date the majority of provinces have responded to the conclusions of the studies by setting up nursing advisory committees on nursing human resources. To ensure that some measure of coordination occurs a federal/provincial committee on nursing human resources planning also meets, at a minimum on a yearly basis.

PROGRAMMES TO INFLUENCE THE SUPPLY AND DISTRIBUTION OF NURSES – THE ROLE OF STRATEGIC PLANNING

Although, in general, attempts specifically to balance the supply and demand for nurses have only now been coordinated there have been a number of attempts to influence the direction of Canadian nursing through strategic planning processes. The most important of these programmes are outlined below.

A blueprint for nursing

Since 1967 the Council of the College of Nurses of Ontario has attempted to plan systematically for the future by holding regular 'brainstorming' sessions to discuss potential changes in Canada's health care system and the implications for nurses. Aware that today's decisions may shape the future of nursing, the College of Nurses of Ontario in 1980 commissioned a study of the future of nursing in the year 2000 (Lemieux-Charles, 1980). Terms of reference for the survey included consideration of the future delivery of health care and where and how it will be given and by whom, identification of the kinds of nurse who will be needed and consideration of the future of nursing for the next 10–20 years.

This innovative study was based on the premise that the future is not entirely unforeseeable, inevitable or unpredictable and that a range of alternative futures can be identified. Not only do informed choices increase the likelihood of achieving the desired future but also influence can be exercised to affect the likelihood of that future being achieved (Lemieux-Charles, 1980).

To identify the changes foreseen in nursing over the next 20 years a panel of nursing experts comprising registered nurses (RNs) and registered nursing assistants (RNAs) resident in Ontario was selected. The panel, consisting of 175 RNs and 38 RNAs chosen for their expertise, were sent open-ended questionnaires and asked to identify five major changes that they expected to occur in nursing by the year 2000. Through processes of content analysis and refinement of statements 48 changes were identified, which included changes in educational requirements to practice, in specialization, in educational programmes and in nursing management. The panel were then asked to evaluate the likelihood of each of the 48 changes taking place, given three possible future conditions that had been described in a survey conducted by Ottawa-Carleton District Health Council in 1979 (Lemieux-Charles, 1980).

1. Future I features rapid economic growth, regionalized government and increased awareness of health care services by the consumer.
2. Future II features slow economic growth with cutbacks in the health care sector.
3. Future III features a health system with continued growth but little change from the present structure and composition.

The experts were asked to complete the questionnaire twice, the second time after receiving feedback on the group's initial response.

A survey of a random sample of the membership of the College of Nurses of Ontario assessed the perceptions of the desirability of the predicted changes in nursing. Over 1000 nurses completed this assessment and their perceptions of the changes were compared with those of the panel of experts. Although there were some differences in the perceived desirability of certain changes in nursing between experts and College members, and between RNs and RNAs, there were many similarities. The changes in nursing considered desirable by all participants in all three future conditions were that there would be:

1. More course time in nursing education programmes for clinical practice;
2. More nurses voluntarily taking continuing education courses;
3. Certification of entry to clinical nursing specialities;
4. Restriction of the practice of nursing to registered personnel;
5. A view of nursing as a long-term career commitment;
6. Greater specialization, especially in mental health, stress-related illnesses and gerontological nursing;
7. Requirement of increased technical skills as medical technology becomes more complex;
8. A patient advocate function;
9. More political action by nurses.

The study was restricted to Ontario and the results were relatively complex in that there was no agreement about where nursing might be in the year 2000, but the blueprint has been extremely important in stimulating discussion across Canada.

Canadian Nurses Association (CNA) initiatives

The objectives of the CNA include not only functioning as a voice on behalf of Canadian nurses but also developing strategies that will guide the future development of nursing practice, education, administration and research. In all these areas the Association has taken a pro-active approach, involving and informing its membership of all planning activities. To this end the CNA has developed a series of five-year plans for research, nursing administration and entry to practice.

Plan for nursing practice

The overall goal of the plan for development of nursing research in Canada, set up in 1984, is to establish a scientific foundation for the practice of nursing. The plan, revised in 1990 (Statistics Canada, 1990), outlines detailed objectives for nursing research in Canada as well as specific strategies to be taken by the CNA each year to achieve these goals. The main objectives are to develop nurse researchers, nursing research and nursing research reality.

Plan for nursing administration

A national plan for nursing administration in Canada began following the report of Leatt (1981) on educational opportunities for nursing administrators. A position paper on the role of nursing administrators and standards for nursing administration was subsequently developed by the CNA in 1983. As Besel, president of the CNA at that time, said (Besel, 1985):

> Our profession urgently needs politically and economically astute leaders who have a solid background in management, a broad philosophical perspective on health services and a clear vision of the type of health care system we ultimately want to see in place.

The main goal in developing the national plan for nursing administration in Canada was to outline objectives and strategies necessary to create an environment that facilitates the provision of high quality nursing care to Canadians (Canadian Nurses Association, 1985). After being revised the plan was presented for approval at the Boards in the autumn of 1990. Similar to the plan for nursing research the one for nursing administration outlines particular steps to be taken by the CNA during specified time periods. The main objectives are:

1. To promote implementation of the CNA 'Position Paper on the Role of Nurse Administrators and Standards for Nursing Administration' (1983, revised 1988):
   (a) to increase nurse administrators' awareness of the position paper;
   (b) to encourage use of the position paper in health care agencies;

2. To enhance educational opportunities available for nursing administrators:
   (a) to promote increased accessibility of degree-granting educational opportunities in nursing administration;
   (b) to facilitate professional development opportunities for nursing administrators;
3. To enhance leadership in nursing administration:
   (a) to enhance visibility of current leaders in nursing administration;
   (b) to support nurses with leadership potential for nursing administration;
   (c) to foster increased communication among nursing administrators;
   (d) to promote opportunities for leadership development;
4. To promote the development of research in nursing administration:
   (a) to promote a supportive climate in which research into nursing administration can be conducted;
   (b) to identify financial support available for research in nursing administration;
5. To increase funding to support improved preparation of nursing administrators:
   (a) to increase sources of financial assistance for improved education of nursing administrators;
   (b) to increase financial resources for educational programmes in nursing administration;
   (c) to communicate information on educational funding sources for nursing administrators;
   (d) to seek funding to support opportunities for nursing administrators (actual and potential) to increase knowledge and skills in relation to policy and programme development in government.

In 1987 the Boards of Directors of the Canadian Hospital Association, Canadian Public Health Association, Canadian College of Health Service Executives and the Canadian Association of University Schools of Nursing and the CNA approved a joint statement on nursing that states that there is a need to strengthen nursing administration through improved educational preparation. The associations have established a joint working group that has developed strategies and actions to meet the objectives. They have also co-sponsored two national conferences on nursing administration.

A Plan for entry to practice

In 1982 the CNA's Board moved that by the year 2000 the minimal educational requirement for entry into the practice of nursing should be a baccalaureate degree in nursing. This decision was based on discussions from 1980 and a background paper that had outlined the historical development of nursing and made some projections about the future health care needs of Canadians (Canadian Nurses Association, 1982). In April 1984 the CNA issued the first 'Entry to Practice Newsletter', which has been used as a vehicle for the exchange of information about provincial and territorial association positions on entry to practice (Canadian Nurses Association, 1984). In February 1984 the CNA's Board accepted a national plan for the implementation of its position on entry to practice. The plan outlined specific objectives for the CNA in attempting to achieve that goal by the year 2000 and ways in which the Association would work with the provincial associations to help them interpret the CNA's position.

In a latter (June 1984) issue of the newsletter the Association clarified differences between its position and that of the American Nurses' Association. Whereas the American Nurses' Association identifies two categories of nursing practice (professional requiring a baccalaureate degree in nursing and technical requiring an associate degree in nursing) the CNA aims to recognize one category of nursing practice, that is professional, for which a baccalaureate degree in nursing will be required.

The 'Entry to Practice Newsletter', issued quarterly, has provided invaluable service to the provinces, clarifying issues such as the effect of the proposed change on costs of nursing education, quality of care, teacher education and nursing supply and demand. Considerable activity has been stimulated at the provincial association level, such as the formation of task forces to examine issues at local levels.

The CNA National Plan for Entry to Practice has been revised annually since 1984. The 1989 plan has the following outcome orientated objectives:

1. There is broad support among nurses for changes in educational preparation for the future.
2. The number of nurse educators is sufficient to meet the increase in size and number of baccalaureate programmes.
3. The number of baccalaureate programmes and their size will produce sufficient graduates.
4. Students are attracted to baccalaureate programmes in order to produce the required numbers of graduates.
5. The future educational requirement is understood and accepted by non-nursing health care colleagues.
6. The public understands the role of the nurse and supports changes in educational preparation.
7. Changes in the educational preparation of nurses are supported by governments.

8. Plans for an increased proportion of baccalaureate-prepared nurses are made by:
   (a) employers in all sectors;
   (b) licensing bodies;
   (c) nurses;
   (d) non-nursing health care workers.
9. Research in nursing education and administration of nursing education addresses issues in the transition to baccalaureate education and in improvements of baccalaureate education.

CONCLUSIONS

Attempts to plan for an adequate supply of nurses in Canada have been made by several different groups including governments, hospital associations and nursing associations. Statistics Canada makes available information on supply and demand for all health professionals, including nurses. From the reports available, perceptions from the field have generally suggested that, at least since 1985, there has not been a shortage of nurses in specialized areas of hospitals, such as critical care units, that tend to have a higher turnover than other units. More attention has been paid to the work environment and strategies to improve conditions of work. In addition there appears to have been a chronic shortage of nurses prepared to work in the northern, isolated areas of Canada where there are few medical back-ups or support systems. The working conditions in the north and the stamina required of nurses working in the isolated nursing stations do not appear to have changed since the settling of Canada in the 1600s.

Although issues of supply and demand for nurses seem to be balanced in the marketplace rather than by an overall scheme, strategic planning for nursing in Canada has been a major focus of activities since 1980. The CNA has provided the leadership for the systematic development of plans for the future of Canadian nursing. These plans emphasize improving the quality of nursing rather than increasing the quantity of services. Quality of nursing will be achieved in the future through upgrading the requirements for entry to practice, improving nursing administration and carrying out more nursing practice.

Part Four

The United States

15
Historical evolution of the health care and nursing systems

The history of health and nursing systems in the US has been, as Anderson (1984) had said, 'a growth enterprise for a hundred years'. Health and nursing services began to expand about 1875 but have grown more in the past 20 years than in the entire history of the US. The development of health and nursing services can, for convenience, be grouped into seven periods. As Figure 15.1 shows each period can be succinctly described in terms of major developments, trends and issues associated with the period.

Years	Major developments, trends and issues
Before 1865	Primitive status of health and nursing systems.
1865–1900	Rise of formal training. First stirrings towards professionalism. Establishment of first training school for nurses.
1900–1930	Rapid growth in number of hospitals, physicians and trained nurses. Impact of First World War. Concern with quality of nursing education.
1930–1950	Great Depression. Second World War. Entry of federal government into support of nursing education, health care research and health facilities. Beginning of rapid growth in nursing and concern with nursing shortage.
1950–1965	Expansion of federal role in health care and training of health care personnel. Significant advances in treatment of disease. Intensification of concern about nursing shortage.
1965–1980	Entry of federal government into a national health insurance programme. Rapid expansion of federally supported health programmes as part of the 'Great Society'. Inflation in medical care costs. Continued concern about nursing shortage.
1980–	Growth of corporate medicine. Concern with containing health care costs. Cutbacks in public funding of care. Nursing shortage appeared to be surplus at beginning of decade but a shortage once again at the end as enrolments to nursing schools declined. By 1988 enrolments began to rise.

Figure 15.1 Major periods in the development of health and nursing systems in the US.

PRIOR TO 1865

The spirit of 'rugged individualism' that had pervaded the establishment of the US as a nation and the expansion of its frontier had filtered into the area of health care. Hospitals, caring largely for the sick poor or transients, were in hideous condition and being 'dirty, unventilated and contaminated by infections, actually facilitated the spread of disease' (Kalish and Kalish, 1978). The professional status of physicians was quite low, improvement being blocked by 'popular resistance, internal division and an inhospitable economic environment' (Starr, 1982). Professional nursing did not exist and there were no training schools. The only disciplined nursing services were provided by religious sisters in nursing orders.

Much health care during this period was on a do-it-yourself basis. 'Care of the sick was part of the domestic economy as each wife assumed responsibility'. Buchan's 'Domestic Medicine', originally published in Edinburgh in 1769, was 'an attempt to render the Medical art more generally useful, by showing people what is in their own power both with respect to the Prevention and Cure of Disease'. Although the nation's health was not of governmental concern the federal government did establish the Marine Hospital Service in 1798 to provide direct medical care for sick and disabled seamen. European nations had already seen the wisdom of providing health care to a group of such vital importance to a nation's economy. This federal programme operated until the early 1980s when it was abolished in the move to privatize health functions.

In the mid-1860s a most traumatic event in US history occurred – the Civil War. It is an interesting historical phenomenon that important advances in health care often occur as a consequence of war. Florence Nightingale had earned her reputation during the Crimean War and the British National Health Service had its origins in the Second World War (Watkin, 1978). While, as Roberts points out, no nurse in the Civil War had emerged with such prestige as had Miss Nightingale in the Crimean, 'many splendid women served as nurses during the Civil War' (Roberts, 1954). One was Dorothea Dix, appointed by the Union Secretary of War to be superintendent of women nurses. Louisa May Alcott, author of the novel 'Little Women', also worked as a nurse. These and others, after the war's end, helped to establish nursing as a profession through the creation of formal training programmes.

The Civil War also stimulated growth of hospitals. The Union Army had built a huge hospital system of over 130 000 beds by 1865. Standards were much higher in these hospitals than in the charity wards of the typical voluntary hospitals of the time.

1865–1900

Remarkable improvements took place in health care and nursing during this period. Hospitals as settings for health care made great progress with the understanding of the principle of antisepsis, which, along with anaesthesia, resulted in an improved rate of successful surgical operations. Improvements were made in pharmaceuticals and diagnostic tools such as X-rays, discovered by Wilhelm Roentgen in 1895. As a result of these and other advances, as well as increased urbanization, the number of general hospitals grew from fewer than 100 in 1875 to more than 4000 in 1900.

Another development in the health care infrastructure was the creation of the first effective state Board of Health in Massachusetts, earlier ones in Louisiana (1855) and New York City (1867) being essentially inoperative. Health boards took increasingly active roles in promoting sanitary conditions of food and water as the links between poor hygiene and certain illnesses and epidemics grew stronger. Louis Pasteur's elucidation of the germ theory of diseases and Robert Koch's isolation of the tuberculosis bacillus gave doctors a rational basis for techniques in controlling the spread of communicable diseases in what became a main function of public health departments. Establishment of the American Public Health Association in 1872 gave public health workers a mechanism to develop professional standards through exchange of scientific, medical and managerial information.

Advances in the professionalization of nursing were much in evidence at this time. Agitation for improvement of the practice and education of nurses began in earnest. Susan Dimock, who, at the age of 22, had received a medical degree in Zurich, returned to the New England Hospital for Women and Children to help establish in 1872 the first general training school for nurses, based on some of the principles of Florence Nightingale. The first US nursing school to be completely modelled on Miss Nightingale's school was the New York Training School at Bellevue Hospital, opened in May 1873. Several weeks later the Connecticut Training School for Nurses opened, as did the third American school of nursing based on the Nightingale system, the Boston Training School for Nurses at Massachusetts General Hospital (Kalish and Kalish, 1978).

By 1900 there were over 400 training schools for nurses, a remarkable growth in the 28 years since the opening of the first school. By the turn of the century an estimated 640 fully trained nurses were in practice (Tibbitts and Levine, 1953). Professionalism continued to grow with the founding of the two major nursing associations, today known as the American Nurses' Association and the National League for Nursing. (Roberts, 1954).

1900–1930

In the aftermath of another war, the Spanish–American War of 1898, Dr Walter Reed and co-workers, in studies on yellow fever and malaria conducted in Cuba, proved that these diseases were transmitted by mosquitoes, a discovery of major public health consequence because the southern US periodically experienced horrific death rates from these diseases. Such research was part of a number of studies on the aetiology of disease that eventually led to marked improvements after public health services began campaigns of quarantine, isolation, vaccination and health education in personal hygiene. Also consequent to the Spanish–American War military medical and nursing services were improved. The Army Nurse Corps was established in 1901, followed by the Navy Nurse Corps in 1908. The importance of these organizations was that for the first time in US history nursing services composed entirely of graduates of formal training schools were established.

Landmark studies

A major event affecting health care was the establishment in 1904 of a Council on Medical Education by the doctor's professional organization, the American Medical Association, to improve the quality of medical education by setting academic standards. It had been only in 1893 that the first medical school, at Johns Hopkins University, had required all entering students to have baccalaureate degrees. The Council invited the Carnegie Foundation for the Advancement of Teaching to evaluate the 160 medical schools then in existence. The study, conducted by Abraham Flexner and published in 1910, is considered a landmark in medical education (Flexner, 1910). Known as the Flexner Report it recommended that the majority of medical schools, primarily the proprietary medical colleges, be closed and that the curriculum for preparation of doctors be substantially upgraded (Roberts, 1954). By 1915 the number of medical schools had declined to fewer than 100, most of which had become associated with institutions of higher learning. Watched over by physicians' organizations the number of doctors remained relatively fixed until the 1960s when national concern about a doctor shortage led to federal government intervention to increase the supply of doctors.

With substantial growth in the number of nursing schools and graduates similar concern was raised about the quality of nurses and nursing education. By 1930 there were nearly 1800 schools of nursing with enrolments of 100 000 students. Between 1913 and 1917 more than 500 new schools were opened. Over 200 000 graduates of formal nurse training programmes were in practice by 1930.

One major step towards improvement of nursing education and practice was the adoption by state governments of nurse practice acts. Beginning in 1903 in North Carolina and ten years later extending to 38 other states, laws were passed setting standards – at first quite minimal – for school curricula and the registration of graduates (Roberts, 1954). Registration laws today have become more strict, more demanding and more uniform from state to state.

Towards collegiate education

Early nursing schools had been located in hospitals. The beginnings of collegiate education for nurses came in 1909 when, subsumed under the College of Medicine, a nurse training school was established at the University of Minnesota. By 1930 over 30 colleges and universities were conducting nursing courses that offered bachelor's degrees in nursing.

A report similar to the Flexner Report on Medical Education resulted in improved quality of nursing education. In 1919, with support from the Rockefeller Foundation, a Committee for the Study of Nursing Education was appointed. Although its original purpose had been to examine the education of public health nurses, more highly specialized and trained professionals, the study was broadened to nursing education in general. The report of the Committee in 1923, authored by Josephine Goldmark, found many deficiencies among schools (Committee for the Study of Nursing Education, 1923). Although it did not advise removing the training of nurses from hospitals to colleges or universities the Report did recommend that nursing leaders be trained at higher education institutions. One year after release of the Goldmark Report Yale University opened the first independently operated nursing schools to offer a collegiate degree, but it was not until the 1960s that collegiate education for nurses expanded significantly.

Another result of the Goldmark Report was the creation in 1926 of a Committee on the Grading of Nursing Schools. The Committee had three objectives:

1. To study nursing supply and demand;
2. To conduct an analysis of nursing activities in hospitals;
3. To prepare a grading of schools of nursing.

The first study, completed in 1928 under the direction of Mary Burgess, concluded that there were too many poorly trained nurses (Burgess, 1928). The implication was that there really was a shortage of nurses from a qualititative standpoint. Although it did not have an immediate impact on nursing education or nursing service, the study did have a major long-range impact because it focused on the need to improve nursing quality, an issue of continuing importance. The Burgess study laid the foundation for future studies of nursing supply and demand.

The other two projects of the Committee on the Grading of Nursing Schools – job analysis and grading of schools – were completed in the 1930s. Like the supply and demand study these studies are still influencing nursing. They concerned issues that are always important – the performance of nurses in hospitals and the degree to which schools of nursing maintain desirable standards.

Trends in the health services system

As to developments in the health system in general and the role of government during this period several major trends can be discerned. First during this time the personal health services system that exists in the US today settled firmly into place. It is a system conducted largely in the private sector on a fee-for-service basis. Advocacy of national health insurance also began during this period, but no such programme has yet materialized. This advocacy originated outside government and, as in other countries, was related to the labour movement, of which one organization, the American Association for Labor Legislation, published a draft of health insurance legislation in 1915. Like its European antecedents it limited coverage to workers in the lower wage brackets and their families. Benefits included payment for the services of doctors and nurses, sick pay and maternity benefits. Agitation for health insurance proposals continued for several years, finally being laid to rest because of lack of strong governmental support as well as opposition from employers and, surprisingly, a major workers' union, the American Federation of Labor. Even more surprising was the initial support by the American Medical Association, always a staunch opponent of national health insurance.

Although compulsory national health insurance was defeated voluntary health insurance began with the creation of Blue Cross in 1929 to provide school teachers in Dallas, Texas, with 21 days of hospital care a year for $6 per subscriber. Prior to Blue Cross private health insurance generally took the form of an agency agreeing to provide health services for a flat fee per subscriber (capitation), similar to today's health maintenance organizations.

An expanding government role

The role of government in health continued to expand, in part again related to war (the First World War). Public health agencies broadened their responsibilities by strengthening the visiting nurse programme and establishing clinics to try to control venereal diseases and prevent infant mortality and heart disease. In 1902 nurses began working in New York City schools, marking the start of the school health programme. Gradually the focus of public health programmes expanded from concern with community sanitation and containing the spread of communicable disease but also with illness prevention and health promotion among individuals. The expanded approach to public health led to establishment in 1912 of the US Public Health Service, which acquired the Marine Hospital Service and is today the federal government's major health agency, with responsibilities that range from service to research. Adoption of the Pure Food and Drug Act in 1905 marked the beginning of the regulation of drugs, medical devices and foods by the federal government in response to a public outcry over unhygienic and hazardous conditions in their preparation.

The World Wars

One immediate health consequence of the First World War was the passage of the War Risk Insurance Act of 1917, which provided treatment in hospitals for injuries received in military service and vocational rehabilitation for the service disabled. A Veterans Bureau, created in 1921, the antecedent of which was the veterans benefits introduced in England in the 16th century, was expanded into the Veterans Administration in 1930 (since 1987 the Department of Veterans Affairs) and is today the largest single hospital and medical care system in the US providing free services. But perhaps the clearest example of the expanded role of government in health was the creation in 1930 of the National Institute of Health from the Hygienic Laboratory to conduct research on medical problems other than infectious disease.

1930–1950

This was a period full of dramatic events, beginning with the Great Depression, the impact of which was felt throughout the 1930s, and ending with the Second World War. In this period health care entered the age of antibiotics, with the demonstration that penicillin, first developed by Alexander Fleming in 1929, had curative properties for a number of illnesses. The technological revolution in diagnosis and treatment of diseases began in this period, with advances in instrumentation, surgical procedures and drugs, at least partly resulting from the treatment and rehabilitation of war casualties.

In nursing the period began with issuance of two more reports by the Committee on the Grading of Nursing Schools. One report, 'Nursing

Schools – Today and Tomorrow', issued in 1934, had provided a basis for accreditation of schools of nursing and its recommendations were effected in 1952 under the management of the National League for Nursing (Committee on the Grading of Nursing Schools, 1934). The other report, 'An Activity Analysis of Nursing', provided the first systematic classification of nursing activities in hospitals, although its major focus was on assessing curricula and not on improving nursing management. This study initiated a productive period of research in the late 1930s and 1940s into how most efficiently to organize and deliver hospital nursing services (National League for Nursing Education, 1937). Methodology was developed that laid the groundwork for present day research on patient classification and nursing workload measurement.

Nurse training Acts

Training of nurses received a major boost from the Second World War. Congress passed the Nurse Training Act of 1943, administered by the US Public Health Service, which made nurses the first professional health occupation whose training was subsidized by the federal government. Federal programmes to combat the ravages of depression of the 1930s, such as the Federal Emergency Relief Administration and the Social Security Act of 1935, had provided modest funding to the states for nursing services and the training of public health nurses. The Nurse Training Act 'laid the groundwork for what would become the largest experiment in federally subsidized education in the history of the United States up to that time' (Kalish and Kalish, 1982). The Act set up a Cadet Nurse Corps organized on a quasi-military basis that provided cadets with full support for training. By the time the programme was terminated in 1948 the federal government had spent over $160 million on it and 125 000 people had graduated as nurses. Not until 1964 would the federal government again establish a programme to support the basic training of nurses.

Although the Cadet Nurse Corps was disbanded after the war ended the US Public Health Service retained the organizational unit established to administer the Nurse Training Act. First called the Division of Nursing Education the unit became the Division of Nursing Resources in 1949 with, as its primary mission, assistance to states experiencing nurse shortages. These shortages were the consequences of termination of the nurse training subsidies and the attrition that occurred as nurses left the profession in large numbers when the war ended. The US began a period of about 30 years when the shortage issue was a dominant theme in nursing.

Entry of the federal government into the support of nurse training was only one expansionary trend of the federal role in health during this period. In the midst of the economic depression a compulsory health insurance programme had been considered as part of the Social Security Act of 1935, but it was deleted under pressure from the American Medical Association and other groups. Major benefits of the Act were provisions for old-age pensions, unemployment insurance and financial grants to states for maternal and infant care, rehabilitation of crippled children and general public health. National health insurance came up for consideration in the 1940s but was again defeated when vociferous opponents such as the American Medical Association raised the alarm of 'socialized medicine'.

Enlarged public health services

Over time the Public Health Service had been substantially enlarged as new functions were added and in 1939 it was moved from the Treasury Department to the newly created Federal Security Agency (which also administered the Social Security Act). The Cadet Nurse Corps had been a major foray into the education of nurses but the government's primary role remained the provision and management of funds; actual training was conducted by schools in the private, state or local government sectors. In 1937 the National Cancer Institute was created under the aegis of the Public Health Service's National Institutes of Health and for the first time financial grants were authorized to researchers outside the federal government. The research grants programme, which began with barely $2 million, had grown to $9 billion by 1992, the funds supporting the extramural programmes of nearly a dozen institutes. A third major scheme with considerable impact on the health system was the Hospital Survey and Construction Act of 1946, the Hill–Burton programme, which provided grants to states and individual organizations to construct hospitals and long-term care and ambulatory facilities. Nearly $4 billion has been spent under this programme by the federal government and nearly $10 billion by state and local governments in matching funds.

This period, therefore, is one in which there were substantial increases in the size and scope of the nursing and health care systems and in the governmental role in health. From 1930 to 1950 national health expenditure rose from $3.6 billion to $12.5 billion, its share of the gross national product rising from 3.5% to 4.4%. Perhaps most striking of the statistics is the doubling of expenditure on health from public funds from 13.6% to 27.2% of the total expenditures. Also with the repeated rejection of compulsory health insurance voluntary health insurance, a rarity in earlier times, began to expand. By 1950 nearly 10% of all personal health care expenditure was paid by private health insurance.

1950–1965

Although the number of employed registered nurses had reached 300 000 by the beginning of this period there was widespread agreement that a severe shortage of nurses existed. With rapid expansion in the number of hospital beds and other health care facilities, and increased utilization of all health resources, calls for nurses rose sharply. The large number of nurses who had left employment since the Second World War, as well as higher accreditation standards for nursing schools, had had its effect. Discontinuance of the use of student nurses to provide patient care other than that necessary to obtain adequate clinical experience also contributed to the shortage. Health care, aided by significant advances in medical service as well as by increased use of, especially, private insurance plans, also stimulated the demand for nurses.

The early 1950s' agitation to re-institute a federally supported programme for basic nurse training was unsuccessful. The 1950s were a time when the federal role, under President Dwight Eisenhower, was non-interventionist. The Division of Nursing of the US Public Health Service spent much time trying to figure out how best to relieve the shortage. It provided technical assistance to states in surveying their nursing needs and resources. It also conducted landmark studies on patient classification, staffing, job satisfaction and turnover. Methodology was developed in these and other areas that applied techniques of industrial engineering, operations research and the social sciences (Abdellah and Levine, 1986). Considerable progress was made in establishing databases on nursing supply and developing methodology for forecasting needs (Marshall and Moses, 1965). Even though federal funds were not provided for basic training the Eisenhower years were not without some activity. Two important programmes geared to promoting qualitative rather than quantitative improvement were begun. In 1955 the Nursing Research Grants Program was launched, providing funds for nursing-orientated research in universities and health facilities. Beginning in 1955 with an annual budget of a $625 thousand dollars, the programme had by 1990 reached a peak of nearly $300 million.

In 1956 an educational support programme for registered nurses was adopted to provide funds, mostly at the master's degree level, for training in supervision, administration and teaching. The traineeship programme was intended to respond to the need for nurses with advanced academic preparation. A 1958 conference evaluated the initial years of this scheme and concluded that, because there was a severe shortage of nurses in leadership positions, the federal government should expand its programme of support for at least five years (United States Department of Health, Education and Welfare, 1964).

Studies on personnel shortage

From 1950 to 1965 a number of federally supported commissions and conferences studied the increasing shortage of health personnel. In 1952 the Report of the President's Commission on the Health Needs of the Nation reported severe shortages of doctors, dentists and nurses and recommended federal aid to health profession schools (United States President's Commission on the Health Needs of the Nation, 1952). Federal support for training doctors and other health professionals began in 1963. The Report of the Surgeon General's Consultant Group on Nursing in 1963 ended the series of studies on health profession shortages and led to passage of the Nurse Training Act of 1964, a major programme of federal support of nursing education at all levels that continues to the present day (United States Surgeon General's Consultant Group on Nursing, 1963).

In response to the nursing shortage, schools preparing registered nurses expanded their enrolments significantly. These increased from 98 000 in 1950 to 136 000 in 1965 (United States Public Health Service, 1969). During this period a new type of programme, the Associate Degree Program, to prepare registered nurses began. In 1952 an experiment was set up to determine whether RNs could be prepared to provide many services in entry level positions in hospitals by a two-year programme that would be associated with community (two-year) colleges. This two-year programme became so successful that it now prepares more RNs than either the baccalaureate or hospital-based diploma programmes. The other licensed category of nurse, the practical nurse, with vocational training of one year, also grew substantially in number. In 1965 there were 25 000 licensed practical nurse graduates compared to fewer than 3000 in 1950. The extensive growth of associate degree and licensed practical nurses led to concern about appropriate education for entry level positions. With three educational routes to becoming a registered nurse, (the two-year associate degree, three-year diploma and four-year baccalaureate degree) there was much concern about which was the most appropriate education. Another question concerned where the practical nurse fitted in. In 1965 the American Nurses' Association issued a controversial 'position paper' that declared that the education of all those licensed to practise nursing should occur in an institution of higher education. Moreover, minimum preparation for entry level professional practice should be a baccalaureate degree while minimum preparation for technical practice should be an associate degree (American Nurses' Association, 1965). This meant that diploma and practical programmes would be eliminated and associate degree graduates would have lesser status. These goals have not yet been attained.

Cabinet status for health agency

One significant governmental action at this time was the raising to cabinet status of the Federal Security Agency, renamed the Department of Health, Education and Welfare. The relatively passive Eisenhower years ended in 1961 with the inauguration of John Kennedy. Although he had spoken of 'getting the country moving again' only the groundwork for his health programme had been laid by the time of his assassination in 1963. The Community Mental Health Center programme was his administration's only significant achievement in the health area. President Lyndon Johnson then began an unprecedented period of federal health legislation, which, together with other social programmes, became known as the 'Great Society'. During Johnson's administration Congress had adopted two significant pieces of legislation with major impact on nursing, the already mentioned Nurse Training Act of 1964 and the Medicare and Medicaid programmes in 1965. The Medicare programme was the first, and to this day only, programme of compulsory health insurance and is limited to the aged, the disabled and those with end-stage renal disease. The other scheme, Medicaid, provides assistance to the states for medical care of the poor.

1965–1980

This was undoubtedly the most eventful period in health care in the history of the US. As mentioned above the Medicare and Medicaid programmes were adopted in 1965. In 1966, the first year of Medicare operation, total payments were $1 billion, mostly for hospital insurance. By 1984 payments totalled $63 billion: $43.3 billion for hospital insurance and $19.7 billion for supplementary medical insurance (Gornick et al., 1985). The federal government, under the renewed and expanded Nurse Training Act of 1964, has spent over $2 billion on nursing education and related schemes over the 30 years of the programme.

Federal legislation stemming from the 'Great Society' aftermath affected every area of health care. Figure 15.2 shows by title some of the major health legislation adopted during this period. National expenditure on health increased from $42 billion in 1965 to $247 billion in 1980. Of these amounts federal expenditure rose from $5.5 billion to $71 billion, primarily because of the Medicare and Medicaid programmes. The proportion of health dollars of the gross national product rose from 6.1% to 9.4%. State and local expenditures rose from $5.5 billion to $34.3 billion.

Year	Legislation
1965	Health insurance for the aged and grants to states for medical assistance – Medicare and Medicaid programmes. Heart disease, cancer and stroke programme for research training and dissemination of knowledge.
1966	Comprehensive health planning programme to promote health planning and improve public health services. Clean water act to combat water pollution.
1967	Air Quality Act to combat air pollution.
1968	Health Manpower Act continued and expanded training support for nurses and other health professions.
1970	Comprehensive Drug Abuse and Prevention Act. Occupational Safety and Health Act. Alcohol Abuse and Alcoholism Prevention Act.
1971	National Cancer Act expanded efforts against cancer.
1972	Consumer Product Safety Act. Noise Control Act. Extended Medicare to disabled and end-stage renal disease patients. Established professional service review organizations.
1973	Health Maintenance Organization Act.
1974	National Planning and Resource Development Act.
1979	Nurse Training Amendments of 1979 – continued support of nurse training at reduced level.
1980	Prospective Payment System adopted, based on Diagnosis Related Groups for reimbursement under Medicare.
1983	Health Care Quality Improvement Act – to monitor performance of physicians and other health care providers.
1988	Nursing Shortage Reduction and Educational Extension Act – continues support for nurse training.
1989	Physician Payment Reform through prospective reimbursement.
1990	Disadvantaged Minority Health Improvement Act.

Figure 15.2 Selected health legislation adopted by the US federal government, 1965–1990.

Rising health costs

As health expenditure soared and hospital costs rose at a rate of 15% each year during the 1970s alarm arose over whether the health care system was going out of financial control. Although the increases were generally attributable to growth of the Medicare and Medicaid programmes, new technology and increased utilization of health services, ways in which health expenditure was financed were also major causes of the growth. By 1980 over 70% of all personal health care expenditure was financed by third parties, not directly by the consumer: 30% by private health insurance and 40% by government. Payment for insured health care was on a retrospective basis, for costs incurred, with no incentive to hold down costs; instead providers benefited from higher costs.

Attempts to hold down costs directly continued through the 1970s. In 1971 the Nixon administration imposed a limit on annual increases in doctors' fees and hospital charges, a freeze that lasted several years. President Carter, in the late 1970s, attempted to have legislation adopted to contain annual increases in hospital charges but was blocked by Congress and opposition of the American Hospital Association. Some states, however, adopted their own programmes of hospital cost-containment through rate setting. Indirect mechanisms to contain health care costs included planning legislation, health maintenance organizations (HMOs) and professional services review organizations (PSROs). Also great emphasis was placed on improving the efficiency and effectiveness of the health system and health care providers.

Although there were discussions on national compulsory health insurance, concern over rising costs prevented adoption of any such programme during this period because, purportedly, it would have drastically increased utilization of health services and driven up health care costs even more. Attempts to put the brakes on 'overutilization' took the form of increased cost-sharing by the insured through higher deductibles and co-payments. Also the concept of competition among providers and insurers took hold. As more for-profit organizations entered the health care industry the market concept became a reality. Lastly, health promotion gained added importance as a way both to contain costs and improve quality of care.

Nursing also underwent significant changes. The growth in number of students and nurses was phenomenal. In schools preparing RNs enrolment reached an all-time high of 250 000 in 1975. By 1980 the number of employed RNs was estimated at 1.3 million. Another significant occurrence was the realization of important qualitative changes. Financed largely by the federal government more nurses sought graduate degrees. Several programmes offering doctoral degrees in nursing were established. New and expanded roles were developed, such as the nurse practitioner and clinical nurse specialist. Primarily as a result of federal support there was great expansion of nursing research, including research on health care costs/benefits that examined the administration of nursing services and nursing productivity and quality (United States Public Health Service, 1979).

This period is, therefore, one of great expansion in health care services, providers and costs. Towards the end of the period two major organizational changes were made in the Department of Health, Education and Welfare. It was renamed the Department of Health and Human Services and the Health Care Financing Administration was created within the department to deal with problems of costs of quality care. Ronald Reagan's administration sought restraints on the health care system, particularly on the governmental role.

1980–1990

Although health care expenditure continued to grow (inflation and increases in intensity of care were big factors), reaching over $500 billion by the decade's end, attempts to limit the federal government's role by elimination and reduction of health programmes characterized the Reagan administration's policies. Although reductions were made support continued through 1991 due to the action of Congress. The federal role in supporting health planning was greatly diminished and only a few states maintain planning programmes. Support for health profession education programmes was reduced. A major piece of health legislation was aimed at controlling the costs of hospitalized Medicare patients through the mechanism of diagnosis related groups (DRGs; Chapter 2), which went into effect on a 'phased in' basis in 1983 (Levine and Abdellah, 1984). With incentives to hold down costs of care per patient there was considerable activity during the 1980s to promote cost-effectiveness.

However, entrepreneurship still dominated the health care industry. Health economists and industrial engineers became leading 'experts' in improving management of the health care system. The concept of 'managed care' emerged, in which insurers for health care exerted greater control over care of its beneficiaries. Health maintenance organizations (HMOs) became models of managed care. Nursing journals began to devote considerable space to subjects such as costs of nursing services, productivity and efficient management of the nursing service. A new journal entitled 'Nursing Economics' appeared; in the not-too-distant past the humanitarian ideal of nursing would have been considered incompatible with what Thomas Carlyle called the 'dismal science' – economics.

The issue of a quantitative nursing shortage disappeared in the early 1980s. The shortage was addressed in qualitative rather than quantitative terms. A major study of nursing, issued in 1983 by the National Academy of Sciences, reinforced the need for quality improvements (National Academy of Sciences, 1983). Advanced education for leadership was promoted, rather than entry level education. Although enrolments in basic training programmes dropped below the peak year of one-quarter million in 1976 they rose again in 1983 and, despite the mood of restraint, the registered nurse supply, the number of nurses actively engaged in nursing, grew to an all-time high of about 1.6 million in 1988 (United States Department of Health and Human Services, 1990). The percentage of gross national product devoted to health care is at an all-time high of over 11%, although the growth may be slowing. By the end of 1989, however, the nurse shortage reappeared, attributed to an increase in demand caused by advances in health care technology and increased use of services. Also, beginning in 1984, enrolments in nursing schools began to decline, although by the end of the decade enrolments again began to increase.

This historical overview has presented only the highlights of what is a lengthy, rich and complex development of health care in the US. Ensuing chapters dealing with specific aspects of the nursing system will provide additional historical detail. In closing some pertinent data will be presented on three important areas: the organization of the federal government's leading health agency, the Department of Health and Human Services, the federal budget for health and a statistical profile of health in the US.

DEPARTMENT OF HEALTH AND HUMAN SERVICES

Of the 14 departments of the federal government the Department of Health and Human Services has the major responsibility in the area of health. The Public Health Service is among its varied and important functions and includes health research (National Institutes of Health), support to health professions' training and health maintenance organizations, protection against pharmaceutical and medical hazards (Food and Drug Administration), control of communicable diseases (Centers for Disease Control) and provision of health services to American Indians and Alaskan Natives. The Division of Nursing, responsible for administering the research and training support progammes in nursing, is located in the Public Health Service. The Department of Health and Human Services includes the Health Care Financing Administration, which administers the Medicare and Medicaid programmes.

Some health functions are given to other agencies of the federal government. The Occupational Safety and Health Administration in the Department of Labour regulates employee safety and health. The Environmental Protection Agency, independent of cabinet departments, regulates quality of air and water as well as waste disposal, pesticide use and noise pollution. The Department of Veterans Affairs, also an independent agency, operates a major programme of health care for veterans in 175 hospitals located in every state in the continental US. The Defense Department, with the largest budget in the federal government, operates an extensive programme of health care for armed forces members, both on active duty and retired, and their dependents.

THE FEDERAL BUDGET

The federal budget for the year beginning October 1st 1991 is more than one trillion dollars, an amount impossible to conceive. Because health activities are scattered throughout many departments and agencies it is difficult to obtain an accurate account of the amount budgeted by each for health. We do know that total federal spending is estimated to be $150 billion on health – 15% of the budget.

Table 15.1 Appropriation for selected programmes of the the US Public Health Service for fiscal year ending 1991 (in millions of dollars)

Health care delivery	874
Nursing research	40
Nurse training	60
Indian health	1 100
Centers for disease control	1 010
National institutes of health	7 987
Alcohol, drug abuse and mental health	2 829
Other	1 159
Total	15 059

Table 15.1 shows the Public Health Service budget that was enacted for the fiscal year ending September 30th 1991. The total, $15 billion, is slightly below that of the previous year because of actions taken to reduce the federal deficit resulting from the Gramm-Rudman-Hollings bill. The Health Care Financing Administration, the agency that administers the Medicare and Medicaid programmes, had a 1991 appropriation of $85.9 billion.

SOME HEALTH STATISTICS

Although direct governmental intervention in health is considered to be minimal in the US, there is obviously a substantial infusion of public funds into the system. Together the federal, state and local governments are the source of 40% of health expenditure money. Because of this large public investment there has been considerable debate over what has been accomplished. After all the US spends over 11% of its gross national product on health, a percentage nearly twice as high as that of the UK with its nearly total publicly supported and operated health system. Tables 15.2 and 15.3 give an overview of some important health indicators. With these data and with the historical development presented earlier as background we can now move into a detailed examination of the US nursing system.

Figure 15.2 The US: a statistical profile

Population: 248.7 million
Population density: 69 per square mile
Population per square mile urban: 79.2
Median age: 32.3 years
Percentage of population under 5 years: 7.6
Percentage of population 65 years and over: 12.5
Percentage of population who are black: 12.3
Number of foreign born: 14 million
Average number of people per household: 2.7
Median family income: $30 853
Percentage of population living in poverty: 13.5
Percentage of population who are literate: 99.0

Note: Most data are for 1988. Total population is for 1990.
Source: US Bureau of the Census (1990), *Statistical Abstract of the United States, 1990*. Washington, DC: GPO.

Table 15.3 The US: a health profile

Life expectancy at birth: 74.9 years
Death rate: 541.7 deaths per 100 000 population
Infant mortality rate: 10.0 deaths per 1000 births: White 8.9, Black 18.0
Fertility: 65.4 live births per 1000 women 15–44 years old
Death rates: heart disease 175.0 deaths per 100 000 population; cancer 133.2 deaths per 100 000; motor vehicle accident 19.8 deaths per 100 000; maternal mortality 7 deaths per 100 000
Acquired immunodeficiency syndrome (AIDS) cases: 100 000
Percentage of population rating their health excellent: 40.3
Percentage of population seeing physician in past year: 76.6
Physician visits per person: 2.7 per annum
Dental visits per person: 2.0 per annum
Days of care in short-stay hospitals: 622.7 per 1000
Average length of stay in short-stay hospitals: 6.7 days
Surgical procedures per 1000 population: 76.4
Number of short stay hospitals: 60 35
Number of nursing homes with 25 or more beds: 16 033
Hospital care *per capita* expenditure: $745
Nursing home care *per capita* expenditure: $158
Percentage of population not covered by health insurance: 13.0

Note: Data for various years, 1986–1988.
Source: Department of Health and Human Services (1990), *Health United States, 1989*. Washington, DC: GPO.

16

Nursing Education

HISTORICAL EVOLUTION

The previous chapter presented the historical evolution of nursing education in the US within the larger context of the nursing and health care systems. Figure 16.1 presents highlights in the history of nursing education. In brief nursing education evolved from the model developed by Florence Nightingale based on her experiences in military hospitals during wartime. Hospital-based and heavily work-orientated this apprenticeship model dominated education of nurses until the years following the Second World War, when the shift towards colleges and universities gained momentum. The Goldmark report in 1923 (Committee for the Study of Nursing Education, 1923) began a continuing debate about the appropriate entry level for nursing, with consensus forming around two – professional and associate – both requiring college or university preparation.

Nursing education has matured considerably in the US since its beginnings in 1873. The curriculum has been enlarged to accommodate increased scientific and health knowledge, students are more thoroughly grounded in theory, psychosocial aspects are emphasized, as is the wellness model, and services to patients are no longer provided by students – clinical experiences have become truly educational experiences. Postgraduate education has a high priority, with many nurses enrolled in programme leading to master's and doctoral degrees.

Professional associations and state and federal governments have played important roles in the quantitative and qualitative growth of nursing education. As a result of frequent examination by professional organizations of practice, education and other activities, the curricula in schools has been upgraded through the years and higher accreditation standards set. All state governments have adopted licensing laws for nurses as well as standards for approving the operation of schools. While the federal government's primary role has been as financier of nursing education it has also promoted nursing education research and practice through grants to universities and other agencies and by conducting studies of the education system.

Year	Event
1873	First trained nurse in America, Linda Richards, graduates from New England Hospital for Women and Children in Boston.
1873	Three schools of nursing, based on the Nightingale system are opened: Bellevue Hospital Training, New York City; Connecticut Training School, New Haven Hospital; Boston Training School for Nurses, Massachusetts General Hospital.
1894	Birth of first national nursing organization, the American Society of Superintendents of Training Schools of Nursing. Became the National League for Nursing Education in 1912 and National League for Nursing in 1952.
1896	Nurses' Associated Alumnae of the United States and Canada organized. In 1908 Canadian alumnae withdrew to later form the Canadian Nurses' Association. Remaining group became the American Nurses' Association in 1911.
1899	First graduate course for nurses, in hospital economy, at Teachers College, New York City.
1900	American Journal of Nursing began publication.
1903	First nurse registration legislation in North Carolina. Registration soon spread to other states. State approval of nurse training schools accompanied nurse registration legislation.
1917	*Standard Curriculum for Schools of Nursing*, published by National League of Nursing Education. Set forth the three year course for hospital schools of nursing.
1923	Publication of report *Nursing and Nursing Education in the United States* by the Committee for the Study of Nursing Education. This was a landmark report on nursing education, based on study by Josephine Goldmark, which criticized the apprenticeship system of education in nursing schools and emphasized the importance of university based programs for the education of nurse leaders.
1924	Yale School of Nursing, the first collegiate school of nursing to be established as an independent university department. After a few years, offered a Master of Nursing degree in a 2½ year course open to holders of baccalaureate degrees.
1925	Committee on the Grading of Schools of Nursing established. Committee issues three classic reports, including *Nurses, Patients, Pockets (1928)*, which investigated the supply of and demand for nursing services.
1927	Publication of *A Curriculum for Schools of Nursing* by NLNE further raised the standards of schools of nursing contained in the earlier *A Standard Curriculum for Schools of Nurses*. In 1937 another revision by NLNE was issued, entitled *Curriculum Guide for Schools of Nursing*.
1935	Social Security Act authorized funds for scholarship stipends for public health nurses.
1941	Federal Government appropriated $1.8 million for nurse training, for refresher training and for schools of nursing to increase enrolments.
1943	*Nurse Training Act* established US Cadet Nurse Corps.
1944	Beginning of the State Board Test Pool Examination for licensing graduates of nursing schools.
1948	Report by Esther Lucille Brown, *Nursing for the Future* recommended that nursing education be conducted in institutions of higher education.

Year	Event
1949	Division of Nursing resources (now the Division of Nursing) established in the US Public Health Service. Has served as main agency of Federal Government administering support programmes for nursing education and research.
1950	The National Committee for the Improvement of Nursing Services, established to implement the Brown Report conducted an evaluation of schools of nursing, published in *Nursing Schools at Mid–Century*.
1952	Beginning of the nursing school accreditation programme administered by the NLN. Development of two-year associate degree programme to prepare RNs began.
1956	Federal Nurse Traineeship programme commenced providing support for registered nurses for training in administration, supervision and teaching. Programme later incorporated into Nurse Training Act of 1964.
1963	Report of the Surgeon General's Consultant Group on Nursing, *Toward Quality in Nursing*, which recommended substantial Federal aid to nursing education to eliminate the nursing shortage.
1964	Nurse Training Act adopted providing federal funding support for basic and graduate nursing education.
1965	The American Nurses' Association issues a *Position Paper* recommending two levels of nursing, *professional* with baccalaureate degree entry level education and *technical* being the associate degree.
1967	National Commission for the study of Nursing Education created by the NLN and ANA. Recommended qualitative changes in nursing in its final report, *An Abstract for Action (1970)*.
1983	Report of the Institute of Medicine's Committee on Nursing and Nursing Education, *Nursing Policies and Private Actions*. Recommended further qualitative changes in nursing education.
1985	The NLN supports ANA in the recommendation for two categories of nursing, professional and associate.
1988	The Nursing Shortage Reduction and Education Extension Act of 1988 continued Federal Government support of nursing education. This followed the issuance of the report by the US Department of Health and Human Service's Secretary's Commission on Nursing.

Figure 16.1 Major Milestones in the Development of Nursing education in the United States.

BASIC EDUCATION FOR NURSES

The two categories of licensed nurses are registered nurses (RNs) and practical nurses (LPNs). Currently education for licensure as a registered nurse is offered in three types of programme, all requiring high school certificates for entry.

Associate programme

Newest of the three programmes, initiated in 1952, the associate programme is usually located in a two-year community college course and confers an associate degree (AD). It includes academic and clinical training.

Diploma programme

Oldest of the three programmes, diploma study is located in hospitals. A diploma is offered after three years' training. Academic courses are usually provided by educational institutions or two- or four-year college courses.

Baccalaureate programme

Begun in the 1920s this four-year programme in colleges and universities leads to a bachelor's degree in nursing. The usual pattern is a two-year nursing major after two years of course work in the sciences and liberal arts.

Other programmes

In addition there are a few programmes that offer master's or doctoral degrees as basic education for entry into practice. However these are extremely rare and will probably not become more numerous in the future.

Numbers in basic education programmes

In 1989 there were nearly 1500 programmes preparing students to become registered nurses. Of these 50% were associate programmes, 33% were baccalaureate programmes and 12% were diploma programmes. All 50 states have nursing programmes. Heavily populated states such as California, Pennsylvania and New York have nearly 100 programmes each. But, whereas most of California's courses are for either associate or baccalaureate degrees, over one third of Pennsylvania's programmes are for diplomas. Western states, in which governmentally supported institutions of higher education predominate, have been especially hospitable to college-based courses.

About 70% of all basic nursing education programmes are accredited by the National League for Nursing (1990b). All must be approved by state boards of nursing to remain in operation. State standards, which must be met to operate a school, still may not be sufficient to meet accreditation by the National League for Nursing, the main reasons being that the majority of non-accredited programmes are associate, the programmes relatively new and the length of schooling brief.

Admissions, graduation and enrolments

Table 16.1 contains data on the number of basic registered nurse programmes and their admissions, enrolments and graduations since 1950. The data show a generally consistent growth in the number of students entering training and graduating from 1950 to 1984, with the largest growth occurring before 1975, a significant decline up to 1988 and a rise again from 1988–9. There are striking differences among the three types of programmes. Admissions to associate degree two-year courses have grown steadily from 1950 to 1884, at the same time that hospital-based diploma three-year programmes have declined by nearly 90%. More than half the total admissions are now to associate programmes. Baccalaureate programmes also grew substantially – nearly eight-fold since 1950. However even though total admissions, graduations and enrolments grew substantially until 1984, mainly because of growth in associate programmes, even these programmes declined after 1984. Graduations from baccalaureate courses declined from 1984 to 1988, a source of concern to those educational planners who favour the baccalaureate as the route of entry to professional nursing.

The decline in admissions to basic registered nurse programmes in the mid-1980s has been attributed to several factors. One is the decline in the pool of potential entrants due to the fall in the number of 18-year-olds. Also other professions – for example medicine, computer sciences and management – are now more accessible.

Practical nursing

The education of practical nurses shows a growth pattern similar to that of registered nurses. Today there are over 1300 training programmes for practical nurses; in 1950 there were fewer than 300. More than half these programmes are currently in trade, technical or vocational education schools and the remainder in a variety of agencies, including hospitals and secondary schools. Courses vary in length and average between nine months and one year.

Enrolments in practical nurse education programmes followed the same pattern as RN programmes declining in the mid-1980s from a peak over 57,000 in 1982 and then rising in 1988, reaching nearly 47,000 in 1989. The decline is possibly related to the move to only two entry levels, professional and associate.

Characteristics of nursing students

Growth of the associate programme has resulted in significant changes in the characteristics of nursing students in registered nurse programmes. There are now more men and ethnic minorities among nursing students in registered nurse programmes (each group comprises less than 10% of

Table 16.1 Number of nursing education programmes preparing RNs, and their admissions, enrolments and graduations by type of programme, US, 1950–89

Year	All programmes	Associate	Diploma	Baccalaureate
Number of programmes				
1950	1 314	–	1 119	195
1955	1 161	34	981	146
1960	1 137	57	908	172
1965	1 182	172	813	197
1970	1 340	437	636	267
1975	1 362	608	428	326
1980	1 385	697	311	377
1984	1 477	777	273	427
1988	1 442	792	171	479
1989	1 457	812	157	488
Admissions				
1950	45 542*	–	37 140	5 402
1955	46 498	629	38 884	6 985
1960	49 166	1 598	40 013	7 555
1965	57 180	6 144	39 236	11 800
1970	74 596	25 142	30 514	18 942
1975	109 020	49 368	24 696	34 956
1980	110 201	56 899	17 494	35 808
1984	118 224	63 776	14 875	39 573
1988	103 025	63 973	10 010	29 042
1989	108 580	68,634	10 088	29 858
Enrolments				
1950	97,903*	–	89 420	8 483
1955	107 572	1 507	91 076	14 989
1960	118 849	3 254	94 812	20 783
1965	134 733	11 513	92 911	30 309
1970	162 924	43 855	70 412	48 657
1975	248 171	88 121	60 213	99 837
1980	230 966	94 060	41 048	95 858
1984	237 232	104 968	37 256	95 008
1988	184 924	95 986	18 860	70 078
1989	201 458	106 175	20 418	74 865
Graduations				
1950	29 016*	298	26 720	1 998
1955	28 729	199	25 862	2 704
1960	30 113	789	25 188	4 136
1965	34 497	2 510	26 611	5 376
1970	43 103	11 403	22 551	9 069
1975	73 915	32 183	21 562	20 170
1980	75 523	36 034	14 495	24 994
1984	80 132	44 394	12 200	23 718
1988	61 660	37 837	4 826	18 997
1989	66 088	42 318	5 199	18 571

For data on programmes the year refers to 15 October of each year. For all other data the year refers to the beginning of the academic year 1 August through 31 July.

* 1952 data. Source: National League for Nursing.

total enrolment) and the average age of students has risen, although the majority are under 20 years of age on entry to the courses. National League for Nursing (1990a). Among practical nursing students there is a higher proportion of minorities than among registered nurse students.

POST-RN BACCALAUREATE AND HIGHER DEGREE PROGRAMMES

The number of nurses pursuing advanced degrees has increased substantially, especially since 1965 and with greater availability of financial support through the Federal Nurse Training Act. In addition the profession has promoted the need for advanced preparation for leadership positions in research, administration and clinical practice. The role of nurses has expanded substantially in recent years and new roles have been created in response to technological and sociological developments in health care. The complexities of the modern health care system require much higher levels of knowledge and skill that must be acquired to practise good, quality nursing.

Table 16.2 shows the trend in the number of graduates from post-RN education programmes. Although the course is not strictly a postgraduate level programme in the true graduate educational sense there has been a sharp increase in the number of baccalaureate degrees awarded to registered nurses who had for the most part received their nursing training through diploma or associate programmes. The impact of the profession's attempt to establish the baccalaureate degree as the entry level requirement for *professional* nursing undoubtedly accounts for this trend.

Annual graduations from master's degree courses have doubled since 1974 to nearly 6000 in 1988, about three-quarters of whom are in clinical practice. Graduations from doctoral programmes in nursing reached 324 in 1988. However these are not the only advanced degrees awarded to nurses, since many nurses obtain master's and doctoral degrees in fields other than nursing education, for example in biological, sociological and management sciences. Awarding of the doctoral degree, doctor of nursing science, by nursing education programmes is of recent origin. Today many nurses still obtain non-nursing doctorates.

FACULTY STAFF MEMBERS

There are nearly 30 000 faculty staff members in all nursing programmes in the US: about 24 000 in programmes preparing registered nurses and 5000 in practical nursing programmes (National League for Nursing 1990a). Most are registered nurses and nearly three-quarters are employed full time by their educational institutions. Full-time faculty members, especially in baccalaureate programmes, are very well prepared educationally. In all programmes nearly all have at least baccalau-

Table 16.2 Number of graduates from post-RN baccalaureate, master's and doctoral programmes located in nursing education programmes, 1975–88

Year[1]	Baccalaureate (for those with RN qualifications)	Master's	Doctorates
1974	3 791	2 694	74
1975	4 759	3 437	62
1976	5 455	3 830	59
1977	6 146	4 271	53
1978	6 414	4 621	101
1979	7 318	4 778	125
1980	8 238	5 026	121
1981	9 171	5 085	137
1982	8 893	5 085	139
1983	10 085	4 669[2]	183
1987	11 168	5 933	284
1988	11 546	5 777	324

[1] Academic year beginning 1 October of the year stated.
[2] Excludes eight programmes which did not prepare data.

Source: National League for Nursing.

reate degrees, over 70% have master's degrees and over 10% have doctorates. In accredited baccalaureate programmes one third have doctoral degrees. Administrators of nursing education programmes are especially well prepared. In baccalaureate educational programmes, more than three-quarters of administrators have earned doctoral degrees. Educational preparation of faculty members has greatly improved in recent years, with emphasis on continuing education as a means of keeping pace with change and new developments. In 1964 20% of faculty staff did not even have baccalaureate degrees.

While the number of students per faculty member varies from programme to programme, the average is approximately 32 students in classroom settings and nine in clinical settings for registered nurse programmes. Of the three types diploma programmes have the fewest students per staff member in both classroom and clinical settings. Full-time faculty members in diploma programmes average around 47 hours of classroom teaching and 13.5 hours of clinical teaching per week, more teaching time than those in other programmes.

FINANCING OF NURSING EDUCATION

Government investment in higher education in the US is considerable. It is estimated that over $30 billion was spent on higher education by federal and state governments in 1988, three-quarters of this by state governments. Prior to the Second World War nursing education had been entirely financed by the private sector. The wartime US Cadet Nurse Corps marked the entry of the federal government, under pressure of large numbers of casualties, into financing nursing education. State and local governments also expanded their financial support of nursing education about the same time as they lost nurses to the military. The growth of associate programmes since 1952, mostly state and local governmentally supported, increased public involvement in financing nursing education. Current baccalaureate programmes are about equally divided between receiving private and public support. Diploma programmes, dwindling in numbers, have mostly been financed by the private sector.

With the passage of the 1964 Nurse Training Act the Federal government began financially supporting nursing education. It has provided over $2 billion from 1964 to 1990 that has been roughly equally divided between institutional support and support to students. Institutional support has included grants for construction of schools (no longer available), to defray costs of special projects, to improve teaching programmes and to encourage schools to expand enrolments (called capitation grants and also no longer available). The Medicare programme also reimburses hospitals for nursing education. Schools are awarded funds, in addition, for nurse training at the master's and doctoral level, for nurse practitioner training and for traineeships in administration, supervision and teaching. Fellowships have also been available to pursue research at doctoral and postdoctoral levels. Students at undergraduate levels have been awarded loans and scholarships but this support has been more available to students in financial need and has been curtailed in recent years.

The majority of students enrolled in nursings schools receive some type of public financial support, either directly through loans or scholarships or indirectly through lowered tuition and other fees in publicly run schools. Private schools preparing registered nurses are more costly than public schools, the average annual tuition fee in 1988 being nearly $5000 in private schools and $1400 in public schools. Over and above tuition and other fees students must pay for books, housing, transportation and other personal expenses, which may amount to several thousand dollars per year in total expenses. This does not include potential earnings foregone while pursuing an education, making the preparation to become a registered nurse in the US a costly endeavour indeed.

LICENSURE OF NURSES

Because state governments have established their own mechanisms for regulating health occupations students, in addition to successfully completing the course of study, must also meet certain requirements, including physical, mental and character standards and proficiency in the English language, and pass a written licensing examination. In April 1989 nearly 90% of US educated candidates who took the National Council Licensure Examination for Registered Nurses passed on their first attempt. Only about half the foreign educated nurse graduates passed the exam the first time. Fewer than half the US graduates who took the examination more than once passed and only 22% of foreign nurse graduates who repeated the exam passed.

Practical nurses (in some states called vocational nurses) must also take licensure examinations as well as meeting educational, age, character and English proficiency standards. In 1983 51 074 graduates of practical nursing programmes took the examination for the first time and nearly 90% passed. Among candidates who were re-examined only 40.5% passed. Foreign nurse graduates fared considerably worse than US graduates on both first-time and repeat bases.

SOME CURRENT ISSUES IN NURSING EDUCATION

Current issues in nursing education in the US centre around controversy, change and collaboration. Controversy underlies the question of an appropriate educational route to being a registered nurse; change is evident in the slowing of growth of educational programmes and numbers of students; collaboration refers to a revival of closer relationships between nursing education and service. An additional issue is the decline of federal financial support for nursing education. These issues will be discussed briefly to conclude this chapter.

Education for entry into practice

As already described nurses can become registered nurses through one of three educational routes: associate, diploma or baccalaureate. Licensed practical nurses are trained in more homogeneous education programmes. No definitive data exist about relationships between the three educational pathways to the registered nurse title and the proficiency of graduates. This does not mean that no differences exist but more likely reflects absence of methodology to make a proper assessment.

A key difference is that the baccalaureate degree is essential for career mobility to higher level positions as administrators, managers, educators and researchers. The educational credentials for these positions are the master's degree or, increasingly, the doctorate. The nursing profession – the American Nurses' Association in 1965 and the National League for

Nursing in 1985 – had called for two levels of licensure: professional and associate. The baccalaureate degree would be the entry into the professional category and the associate degree, the entry into the associate (formerly technical level) level, thereby eliminating both the diploma and practical programmes. Implementation of such a system requires action by 50 state boards of nursing, a formidable task that will take many years, given the differences in financial status and educational levels among the states.

Growth in education programmes

Basic educational programmes appear to have reached the limits of their growth, at least for the present. Several factors account for this. All higher education programmes in the US are faced with falling enrolments because of the combination of a decline of college-aged people, steep rises in tuition costs and competition from careers not requiring years of higher education. In addition nursing is faced with other negative factors, such as the rise in opportunities for women in other professions, including medicine, where the percentage in some classes has lately risen to one third. Compounding this dilemma is the recent decline in federal support for nursing education. Financially disadvantaged students find it increasingly difficult to undertake an educational programme that costs thousands of dollars. The question, too, is being raised as to whether the return on such an investment is as high in nursing as in other fields. Although salaries have continued to rise many nurses feel that increases have not been commensurate with accompanying responsibilities.

While growth in basic education has ceased postgraduate preparation is expanding, although more slowly than a few years ago. Full-time enrolments (5,860) in master's degree programmes in 1989 have actually declined below the peak of 7300 in 1980, but part-time enrolments have more than doubled since 1980, to nearly 17 000. Enrolments in doctoral programmes located in nursing education schools reached a peak of 2309 in 1988 but nearly 60% of these are part time. Federal government support for postgraduate nursing education, a significant factor in enrolment increases since 1965, has thus far not been reduced as much as support for basic education.

COLLABORATION BETWEEN EDUCATION AND SERVICE

Nursing education in the US began as hospital-based training in which student service to patients was the major part of the educational experience. Directors of nursing often did double duty as directors of nursing education. Beginning in the 1950s nursing education moved away from hospital control and apprentice-type training to college-based programmes in which classroom teaching was emphasized. But, in recent years, hospital nursing administrators have voiced some dissatisfaction about college-based, particularly associate, programmes for turning out nurses lacking in clinical skills and unprepared for the realities of hospital work. They have also claimed that nurse educators are too far removed from the actual clinical setting to provide proper instruction. Nurse educators have countered with arguments that nursing administrators do not provide the challenging assignments in work settings that would build on the type of education received by associate and, particularly, baccalaureate graduates.

To bridge the gap between practical service and academic education nursing leaders have in recent years proposed numerous collaborative approaches. These include lengthening the time devoted to clinical experiences of students, joint nursing service and education planning to facilitate the new graduates' entry into practice, providing faculty staff with opportunities to maintain their clinical practice skills and providing joint nursing service/nurse faculty appointments. Federal grants had been available to fund cooperative arrangements between educational institutions and hospitals for the years 1977 and 1980 but were eliminated in 1981. With the current move to limit the federal budget there is little likelihood that funding to promote collaborative arrangements will be available again soon.

THE GOVERNMENTAL ROLE

All levels of government have played an important role in funding nursing education during the past 25 years. Financial support – to institutions and students – has been the major way in which the federal government has had impact on nursing education since control over education policies, processes and content has traditionally rested with state and local govenments and the private sector. The philosophy of the Reagan administration was that the federal government should not even have a role in funding nursing education.

What impact reduced federal funding will have on enrolment in nursing schools is conjectural. Although data are very sketchy it can be estimated that at the peak of federal appropriations the majority of both basic and postgraduate students received some form of federal aid (Kalish and Kalish 1982). But for many students this assistance had to be supplemented with other sources, including personal finances. As for the educational institutions themselves federal support has been an important factor in providing resources for expansion and improvement. Undoubtedly the next 20 years will see in the nursing field a different pattern but one that is not yet discernible.

17

The practice of nursing

The total population of nursing personnel is about four million, including approximately two million registered nurses (RNs), over 800 000 licensed practical nurses (LPNs) and about one million nursing aides and attendants, trained on the job and unlicensed (United States Department of Health and Human Services, 1990). The number of employed RNs and LPNs was about 2.3 million in 1988. They are the nation's licensed and trained nurse supply, defined as the entire group of nurses working in nursing or seeking work (a small fraction of the total). The population of nurses includes all those who were ever licensed, whether or not presently employed.

At the turn of this century, a little more than 25 years after the first school of nursing was established, there was still only a handful of trained nurses. Since then growth of the nurse supply has been phenomenal. Table 17.1 below shows that the growth in number of RNs has been especially high since 1950. Moreover settings within which nurses work have expanded into many new areas as a result of new technology, better education and increased public demand for services. In the early days almost all nurses worked in hospitals. Although the majority of both RNs and LPNs still do so, there are now large numbers employed in the new settings. The role of nurses in these settings is described below.

PREVENTIVE CARE AND PRIMARY CARE

Public health nurses, numerically small compared to the number of nurses in hospitals, serve the important functions of illness prevention and health promotion. Recent concern with wellness has focused increased attention on these nurses, among the most highly trained of all nurses. Several categories of agencies are involved in preventive health care. Known as community health agencies they include clinics run by school health programmes, employee health units in federal and non-federal government agencies and home care programmes operated by visiting nurse associations (Anderson, 1984). Of the estimated 16 000 community health agencies the majority are governmentally operated by local health departments and boards of education. More than half the community health nurses work in health programmes in schools and colleges. There are about 3000 community health agencies in local health departments and about 2000 occupational health units in business and industry.

Nurses who work in community health agencies are primarily concerned with providing services to groups rather than individuals, unlike nurses employed in acute and long-term care settings. Their major focus is on promoting healthier life-styles, identifying individuals and groups with abnormal risks of contracting certain illnesses, facilitating entry into and promoting effective utilization of the health care system and providing skilled nursing services in non-institutional settings.

ACUTE CARE

The approximately 6000 acute care and short-stay hospitals in the US are, for the most part, the most numerous of all types. They contain nearly 1.2 million beds which have an occupancy rate of 65%. During a year there are over 30 million admissions to these hospitals, which have a higher volume of nursing services than do other health care settings because of a higher ratio of nursing staff to patients. For each 100 average daily patients there are approximately 120 full-time equivalent staff nurses, half of whom are RNs and the remainder practical nurses and aides.

The governmental role in acute care settings is less than in preventive care, the majority of hospitals being controlled by non-governmental agencies:

Voluntary	55%
State and local government	26%
For-profit organizations	14%
Federal government	5%

Only one-third of acute care hospitals are governmentally controlled. The for-profit sector, although presently only 14%, is growing. Many belong to multi-hospital organizations such as the Hospital Corporation of America and Humana.

Nursing practice in acute care settings is now considerably more technically demanding than ever before. Also in these settings the average patient, who is older than in the past, requires a higher intensity of nursing services each day because lengths of stay have been shortened by cost containment policies. In addition, since more complex procedures are being performed in these settings and cost-containment measures discourage hospitalization of less acutely ill patients nursing services are further intensified. Tertiary hospitals, which provide highly technical services such as cardiovascular surgery and care of low birth-weight infants, have great need for specialized and competent nursing services.

The practice of nursing in acute care settings also encompasses critical care nursing. Critical care is defined as multidisciplinary care for patients who have sustained or are at risk of acute life-threatening single or multiple organ system failures secondary to disease or injury. Critical care may occur in emergency rooms of hospitals, operating rooms and intensive care units as well as at the scene of an accident in which severe injury has occurred. Registered nurses play a key role in critical care because they provide continuity of care to patients whose conditions necessitate sustained observation and therapy.

LONG-TERM CARE

Because patients in long-term care have chronic illnesses and problems not amenable to short-term treatment the primary objective of long-term care is to restore or maintain the patient's capabilities to function rather than to provide a cure. Patients requiring long-term care include physically handicapped children at one end of the age spectrum and, at the other, elderly people requiring assistance with their infirmities and basic activities of daily living. Nursing care of long-term care patients occurs in a variety of settings. Non-institutional settings include patients' homes, day care and residential centres, clinics and physicians' offices. Institutional settings include chronic and psychiatric hospitals, nursing homes and hospices. Nursing homes are the most numerous, there being an estimated 16 000 with 25 or more beds, caring for about 1.6 million patients. Three-quarters of a million nursing personnel, the majority of whom are nursing aides, are employed to care for these patients. Only about one in ten nursing home personnel is a registered nurse and many nursing homes offer only minimally skilled nursing services, the primary mission being provision of supportive and personal care services.

Psychiatric and mental health care have both long-term and acute care components. Some psychiatric disorders are treated in acute care settings and many acute care hospitals have psychiatric wings and special treatment centres for alcoholics and drug abusers. With the movement towards de-institutionalizing psychiatric patients, psychiatric hospitals are becoming short-term care facilities. Of nearly 600 psychiatric hospitals over one-third are now short term.

The government's role in long-term care is greatest for institutionalized psychiatric patients. Of about 391 long-term psychiatric hospitals state and local governments operate 226 and the federal government 18. In contrast state and local governments operate less than 20% of the short-term psychiatric hospitals and the federal government none. The majority of short-term psychiatric hospitals are controlled by private, for-profit companies. As the for-profit sector takes over control of nursing homes governmental and non-profit agencies' control diminishes. This is also true among for-profit home care agencies providing nursing services to patients at home, of which there are thousands. While entrepreneurship dominates the long-term care sector more than it does preventive and acute care it is certainly growing in the latter area.

Perhaps as much, if not more, than in the acute care area the role of the registered nurse in long-term care is rapidly increasing in response to both an increased elderly population and increased federal financing of long-term care services through Medicare and Medicaid. Nurses, moreover, are performing more highly skilled and technical services in long-term settings whereas in previous years the main function of registered nurses in nursing homes was to supervise aides. As prospective payment systems are leading to earlier discharge from acute care hospitals patients are increasingly being admitted to nursing homes or to home care programmes for continued care of a highly skilled nature. Also long-term care patients, formerly consigned to receiving supportive services only, now receive nursing intervention aimed at restoring functional capabilities.

THE REGISTERED NURSE SUPPLY

The latest data on the RN supply is available from the US Public Health Services' Division of Nursing, which conducts periodic sample surveys of RNs, the most recent of which was in November 1988 (United States Public Health Service, 1988). That sample consisted of 33 000 RNs selected from the licensing lists of the 50 states and the District of Columbia. After correction for duplicate registration – one nurse holding registration in more than one state – the data were projected to determine state and national totals.

Table 17.1 shows that the number of employed RNs in 1988 was 1.6 million, i.e. 662 nurses per 100 000 population. In addition there were, in 1988, about 400 000 RNs not actively employed in nursing. Therefore about 20% of the total RN population was not employed in nursing. This proportion has declined since 1980 when it was estimated to be 24.4%. Moreover those not employed in nursing in 1988 were older that those in 1980. Nearly 45% of the not employed were 55 years of age or older in 1988, compared to 35% in 1980. It appears that the not employed group contains a higher proportion of the truly retired. In years past the proportion of the total RN population not employed in nursing was much higher and the average age was considerably lower; it consisted largely of young, married nurses who had left employment, perhaps temporarily, to raise families. In 1949, for example, 40% of the total RN population was not employed in nursing, of whom only 10% were aged 55 or older.

Table 17.1 Number of employed RNs and number per 100 000 population, US, 1900–88

Year	Number of employed RNs	Number of RNs per 100 000 population
1900	11 804[1]	16
1910	50 476	55
1920	103 879	98
1930	214 292	175
1940	284 159	216
1950	374 584	249
1960	504 000	281
1970	722 000	355
1977	1 055 000	472
1980	1 273 000	562
1984	1 486 000	628
1988	1 627 035	662

[1] Includes students and nurses. Latter estimated to be 640.

Source: National Sample Survey of Registered Nurses, September 1977 and March 1988.

EMPLOYMENT SETTINGS

Table 17.2 shows the distribution of RNs according to major health care settings in 1988 and changes since 1977, the year of the first RN sample survey. Data show clearly that hospitals, meaning mostly acute care hospitals, employ the majority of RNs, the percentage having increased substantially since 1977.

Table 17.2 Number and percentage of RNs employed, by field of employment, US, 1977 and 1988

Field of employment	1977 n	1977 %	1988 n	1988 %
Hospital	601 011	64.4	1 104 978	67.9
Nursing home	79 647	8.1	107 805	6.6
Nursing education	37 826	3.9	30 005	1.8
Community/public health	77 139	7.9	110 886	6.8
Student health	41 365	4.2	47 792	2.9
Occupational health	24 317	2.5	21 857	1.3
Ambulatory care setting	69 263	7.1	125 813	7.7
Private duty and other self-employed	28 563	3.4	33 191	2.0
Other	18 856	1.5	43 321	2.7
Unknown	247	0.0	1 387	0.1
Total employed nurses	978 234	100.0	1 627 035	100.0

Source: National Sample Survey of Registered Nurses, September 1977 and November 1988.

Although the federal government's cost-containment effort in hospitals, the prospective payment system for Medicare patients based on Diagnostic Related Groupings (DRGs), came in effect in late 1983, its impact on RN employment in hospitals is not discernible in these data. Currently patient numbers in acute care hospitals are dropping as a result of a reduction in the length of stay, which could slow the growth rate of RN numbers. However these short-stay hospitals are reporting shortages of RNs because of increasing demand for RN services. While most RN employment settings have grown rapidly since 1977 a few show little growth. Nursing education is a notable example, reflecting the levelling off of student enrolment.

FULL-TIME NURSING

For all RNs the full-time working percentage has dropped slightly since 1977, from 68% to 67.6%. The extent to which nurses work less than full time must be considered in assessing a nation's nursing resources. Because hours of employment vary from one country to another international comparisons should be based on the full-time equivalency of nurses. In the UK, for example, a smaller proportion of the nurse supply works part time than in the US.

THE LICENSED PRACTICAL NURSE SUPPLY

The only data on the practical nurse supply come from the November 1983 national sample survey of licensed practical or vocational nurses (LPNs), the first such survey for LPNs, which has not been updated in recent years. Conducted by the same method as the sample survey of RNs the sample was drawn from lists maintained by state nursing boards that were checked to eliminate (a very small number) duplication of nurses who held licenses to practise in more than one state. Presently an estimated 400 000 practical nurses are actively employed. Like RNs LPNs are employed more in hospitals than in any other setting. The second largest setting by far, is nursing homes. More LPNs work in nursing homes than do RNs. About equal numbers of RNs and LPNs work in private duty.

THE HIERARCHY OF NURSING

The settings distribution of nurses represents the horizontal specialization in the practice of nursing. In addition there is a distribution according to managerial and administrative level as well as clinical expertise and specialty, which is called the vertical or hierarchical specialization.

As seen in Table 17.3 two-thirds of all RNs are classified as staff nurses, at the base of the organizational pyramid in nursing. Practically all LPNs are classified as staff nurses although a few do rise to managerial positions. In hospitals, the most bureaucratic of nursing settings, there is a hierarchy that extends from staff nurse to head nurse (in charge of a single nursing unit that usually contains between 16 and 40 beds, depending on the medical category of the patients in the unit) to the supervisor (in charge of several nursing units) to the top administrator – variously called director of nursing, nursing administrator or vice president for nursing. Community health agencies, particularly large ones, also have many organizational layers extending from staff nurse to agency director. Increasingly managerial positions require advanced educational preparation.

Table 17.3 Number of employed RNs, by position title, US, March 1988

Title	Employed n	%
Administration	98 382	6.0
Certified nurse anesthetist	16 831	1.0
Clinical nurse specialist	28 975	1.8
Consultant	17 625	1.1
Head nurse or assistant	85 911	5.3
Instructor	62 558	3.9
Nurse clinician	17 628	1.1
Nurse practitioner/midwife	23 535	1.5
Private duty nurse	19 988	1.2
Researcher	4 783	0.3
Staff nurse	1 087 878	66.9
Supervisor or assistant	91 538	5.6
Other	71 403	4.3
Total	1 627 035	100.0

Source: National Sample Survey of Registered Nurses, March 1988.

NURSE PRACTITIONERS

In addition to managerial titles, there are a number of non-managerial nursing positions that require advanced education. Although numerically a small (but growing) group nurse practitioners (NPs) have received considerable attention in recent years. Substantial federal support has been provided for the education of practitioners, beginning with the Nurse Training Act of 1975. The initial impetus for such support was the view that nurse practitioners could extend the services of physicians who, at that time, were thought to be in short supply.

Nurse practitioners have completed a formal programme of study as preparation for an expanded role in delivery of primary health care in a variety of health care settings – hospitals, public health agencies, health maintenance organizations and physicians' offices. Increasingly, educational programmes for NPs offer master's degrees, although certificate programmes still exist. Functions of NPs include health assessment, health promotion and disease prevention, physical examination and management of certain self-limiting acute and chronic health problems.

Nurse practitioners tend to specialize. While some practise in general primary care others specialize in pediatrics, family health and care of the elderly. Although not strictly classified as a nurse practitioner there is usually included with this group the long-established speciality of nurse-midwife. Perhaps even more than a nurse practitioner the nurse-midwife is perceived as an extension to the role of the physician. Midwives function most actively in rural areas and inner cities where physician services are least available. Studies of cost-effectiveness of nurse practitioners and midwives show that they compare favourably with physicians. This holds true for nurse anaesthetists, another extension role. With the emerging surplus of physicians demand for extension roles may subside. In 1988 63 000 RNs had formal nurse practitioner/nurse-midwifery training. Most were employed in nursing. Less than 30% were employed in hospitals, the majority working in ambulatory or community health settings.

CLINICAL NURSE SPECIALISTS AND CLINICIANS

Since 1977 the number of RNs with these titles has grown from approximately 17 000 to over 45 000. These RNs are considered to be experts in specialized fields of clinical practice. Some have advanced academic degrees, although many earn these titles through years of practical experience. The functions of RN clinical specialists/clinicians include the provision of care to patients in secondary and tertiary care settings, the management of complex clinical situations and service as consultants or mentors to less experienced nurses and students. Although not directly analogous clinical specialists play a role in nursing similar to that of MD specialists in medical care. The latter outnumber primary care physicians, a situation considered to be undesirable by critics of the American health care system. In nursing clinical experts form a very small minority.

NURSES EMPLOYED BY THE FEDERAL GOVERNMENT

The federal government employs a substantial number of nurses. In addition to approximately 13 000 RNs in the military nurse corps nearly

40 000 civilian RNs are employed by various departments and agencies. The majority of civilian RNs are found in the Department of Veterans Affairs, the largest single health care system in the nation. Federal nurses also perform a variety of other functions, including serving in employee health units of departments and agencies and on Indian reservations, conducting nursing research and providing consultation on research, education and nursing management.

In addition to RNs the federal government also employs practical nurses and aides, mainly for hospital work. The total number of federal nursing personnel of all types is around 100 000, about 6% of the total nursing supply in the US. State and local governments employ an estimated 300 000 nursing personnel, about 18% of the total. About 75% of all nursing personnel in the US work in the private health sector.

FACTORS INFLUENCING NURSING PRACTICE

The practice of nursing in the US is subject to a number of factors that undoubtedly affect the way nursing services are provided. A few of the major ones will be discussed briefly.

Expansion of the nursing role

Beginning in the late 1960s the practice of nursing was expanded into new areas and functions (Levine, 1985). A major reason for this was the doctor shortage and attempts to alleviate it by giving nurses functions formerly in the domain of medicine. Nurse practitioners (NPs) began working as 'physician extenders' and their federal training support was largely based on the belief that they would be available for primary care in underserved areas. Because of current projections that there will be a significant surplus of physicians in the future, concern is now expressed about the effect of the surplus on demand for NPs. Efforts are underway to justify the role of the NP in nursing rather than medical terms.

Cost-containment

Cost-containment measures, such as the prospective payment system based on DRGs, are believed to have an effect on the demand for RNs (Levine and Abdellah, 1984). To cut costs hospitals could replace RNs with lower paid practical nurses and aides. Because hospital population is dropping patients now admitted are more acutely ill, and shorter lengths of stay mean an intensification of services. Moreover the technological complexity of health care is increasing, requiring greater nursing input. A strong focus on the promotion of wellness will actually increase demand for nurses who can play an important role in this area.

Slowdown of RN growth

The large increases in RN supply of the 1960s and 1970s appear to have ended, at least for now. Table 17.4 shows that, whereas the average annual increase in the nurse:population ratio reached its highest level (6%), between 1977 and 1980, it declined to 2.9% between 1980 and 1984 and to 1.4% between 1984 and 1988. We are witnessing a slowdown in the large increase in demand for nurses that followed the adoption in 1965 of the Medicare and Medicaid programmes. Recently reported shortages of nurses are most likely to be due to increases in demand that have exceeded increase in nurse supply. There is also considerable evidence that *qualitative* shortages continue to exist and, in fact, may have worsened as the complexity of nursing practice has increased.

Table 17.4 Ratio of employed RNs per 100 000 population and average annual percentage increase, US, 1950–88

Year	Ratio per 100 000 population	Average annual percentage increase from previous period
1950	249	–
1962	298	1.7
1966	313	1.3
1972	380	3.6
1977	472	4.8
1980	562	6.0
1984	628	2.9
1988	662	1.4

Source: National Sample Survey of Registered Nurses, September 1977 and March 1988.

Role of federal government

The federal government role in nursing practice is less than that in nursing education. The private sector dominates provision of health care. The federal government employs less than 5% of the total nurse supply for its own health care systems. The only other influence of the federal government on nursing practice is through its research and consultative programme, not a minor influence, but with cutbacks in federal spending on domestic programmes the nursing research and consultative aspect is in danger of diminishing.

18

The nurse at work

Nursing in the US has undergone remarkable changes in recent years. This chapter will discuss various aspects of nursing within the context of the changes that have occurred in the following areas:

1. Settings in which nurses work;
2. Nursing roles;
3. Characteristics of the working nurse;
4. Pay and benefits for nursing;
5. Politicization of nursing.

SETTINGS IN WHICH NURSES WORK

Acute care hospitals are the dominant setting in which nurses in the US – nearly 70% of registered nurses (RNs) and 60% of licensed practical nurses (LPNs) – work. An additional 7% of RNs and 22% of LPNs work in nursing homes. Almost all nursing aides work in hospitals or nursing homes. Thus the large majority of nurses work in institutional settings. Notwithstanding recent discussion of how nursing must move away from the sickness-orientated medical model towards the wellness model, nursing care in the US is still practised within a framework that emphasizes care of the sick.

Some new settings have appeared in recent years but employ only a small, but increasing, number of nurses. The health maintenance organization (HMO), employing less than 1% of RNs and offering comprehensive medical services on a pre-paid basis, is not actually a new setting because it provides services in traditional hospitals and ambulatory care facilities; however it provides for closer management of the care patients receive. Thus HMOs and related organizations, such as Independent practice organizations (IPOs), have become known as 'managed care settings'. Several years ago there was much excitement about independent *nursing* practice organizations, such clinics or offices being run by nurse practitioners, but these settings have not proliferated, understandably, as they are not welcomed by most physicians.

Recently there has been much talk about recurrence of a nursing shor-

Table 18.1 Percentage increase in the number of RNs employed in major settings, 1977–88

Employment field	Percentage increase
All fields	66.3
Hospitals	83.6
Nursing homes	35.3
Community/public health	43.8
Nursing education	−20.7
Ambulatory care settings	81.6

Source: National Sample Survey of Registered Nurses, September 1977 and March 1988.

tage, particularly in the hospital setting. As Table 18.1 shows the growth in hospital employment of RNs from 1977 to 1988 has been greater than in any other field, although percentagewise ambulatory care settings have grown nearly as much. The estimated number of full-time equivalent RNs per 100 average daily patients in non-federal short-term hospitals in 1988 has increased more than four-fold since 1950, when it was 23. In 1984 the impact of the prospective payment system based on Diagnosis Related Groups (DRGs) for hospital care began to be felt. For several years thereafter hospitals engaged in cost-cutting, reducing nursing staff and 'eliminating' shortages. In 1986, however, shortages began to reappear, perhaps related to such factors as an increasing demand for nurses due to increasing utilization of health services, especially by those with more intense needs for nursing services. Another possible factor is a recent decline in the number of LPNs working in hospitals.

Some hospitals have utilized RNs and LPNs interchangeably for many of the more basic and routine nursing tasks. When shortages of RNs were most severe LPNs, who were more plentiful, were hired as RN substitutes. In the early 1980s when RNs became more available the substitution was reversed – RNs for LPNs – and was considered a cost-efficient measure because RNs had greater skills and knowledge. Also for recently qualified staff, wages for RNs were not that much higher than for LPNs.

NURSING ROLES

Although there has not been much change in the distribution of nurses according to major practice settings – except to further emphasize institutional settings – there have been significant changes in the roles of RNs within these settings. In short-term hospitals there is much evidence that patients are more acutely ill than in the past. Reduced lengths of stay, partly a consequence of the prospective payment system, have increased and complicated patient requirements for nursing care. New technology and medical procedures have intensified demands for nursing care and increased the skill and knowledge levels required for proper care. Specialized hospital units, such as critical care, coronary care, intensive care, neonatal intensive care, neurological intensive care and rehabilitation, are proliferating. These units require technical and clinical knowledge in depth, including the ability to precisely monitor and assess patients' conditions and take appropriate action. The acutely ill patient with highly complex requirements is now the typical patient in American hospitals, a situation greatly changed from just a few years ago.

Not only are more nurses working in acute care settings but also larger numbers are working in positions of direct care to patients. As Table 18.2 shows the largest increase in the percentage of RNs employed in nursing was in positions providing direct care to patients, such as clinical nursing specialist, nurse clinician, nurse practitioner and general duty/staff nurse. The number of managerial positions, such as supervisor and head nurse, has grown at a slower rate, although top positions as administrators doubled from 1977 to 1988.

Table 18.2 Distribution of employed RNs, by type of primary position held, September 1977 and March 1988

Type of position	September 1977	March 1988	Percentage increase 1977–88
Administrator	47 563	98 382	106.8
Consultant	4 639	17 625	279.9
Supervisor or assistant	66 883	91 538	36.9
Instructor	48 369	62 558	29.3
Head nurse or assistant	84 770	85 911	1.4
General duty/staff nurse	622 170	1 087 878	74.9
Nurse clinician	7 045	17 628	150.2
Nurse practitioner/midwife	9 634	23 535	144.3
Clinical nursing specialist	8 065	28 975	259.3
Nurse anesthetist	13 046	16 831	29.0
Private duty nurse	28 563	19 988	−30.0
Other	37 486	76 185	103.2
Total	978 233	1 627 035	66.3

Source: National Sample Survey of Registered Nurses, September 1977 and March 1988.

The availability of more care to hospital patients has been accompanied by an increase in hospitals of an organizational pattern for nursing that brings nursing care closer to the patient. In the organizational form known as primary nursing, an RN assumes responsibility for all nursing care provided to a group of designated patients throughout their hospitalization. Over one-quarter of acute care hospitals now have this form of organization, the purpose of which is to provide more holistic and integrated care while giving more decision making autonomy to the RN. Older forms of organization, however, still dominate hospital nursing and include team nursing, in which care is provided by a team of nursing personnel directed by a registered nurse (25% of hospitals), and functional nursing, in which personnel perform certain specialized tasks, such as giving medication and taking temperatures (9%). A study of hospitals reputed to give patients a higher quality of nursing care revealed that primary nursing was the dominant organizational pattern.

As Table 18.2 (above) makes clear the trend in nursing roles is towards increasing those roles that require considerable advanced educational preparation and provide RNs with the most autonomy in practice. These include consultants, nurse practitioners, clinical nurse specialists and nurse clinicians, all relatively new practice roles. Evolution of these expanded roles has been due in no small part to the financial support of the federal government which, since the mid-1960s, has provided grants for training nurse practitioners and others in roles requiring advanced preparation. About $150 million has been spent by the federal government for nurse practitioner training alone since support began in 1976.

Nurse practitioners have completed formal educational programmes that prepare them for expanded roles in primary health care in a variety of settings. These education programmes range from a nine-month certificate programme to full-time graduate study of one to two years in a university. Their functions include health assessment, physical examination, treatment of acute self-limiting illnesses as well as longer-term illnesses, health promotion and illness prevention activities, instruction, counselling and coordination of services. Practitioners often specialize in areas such as child health care and care of the elderly.

Clinical nurse specialists and clinicians are experts in a specialized clinical field of nursing. Although clinical specialists are often educationally prepared at the master's degree level the majority have entered the role by on-the-job experience. Clinical specialists are employed in all health care settings. Among the fastest growing of all nursing roles (Table 18.2 above), clinical nurses are developing some of the most innovative nursing practices incorporating functions based on both illness and wellness models.

Although these newly developed roles, blending aspects of both sickness and wellness models and moving nurses towards more autonomous practice, have received considerable media attention, numerically they form only a small proportion of the RN workforce. Together nurse practitioners, clinical nurse specialists and clinicians total 70 000. Although services are still mainly organized and delivered as in the past, the number and proportion of RNs in these specialized categories have significantly increased since 1977 when they numbered 25 000 and 2.6% respectively.

CHARACTERISTICS OF THE WORKING NURSE

The typical registered nurse in the US is a married, white female in her late thirties. Although these characteristics have been dominant among working RNs for the past 30 years there are several small changes that are quite significant (Table 18.3). The proportion of male nurses has increased, as has the proportion of nurses from minority groups (black, Hispanic, Asian and American Indian). In addition the proportion of employed RNs with children at home has increased, reflecting the trend towards families with two wage earners.

Table 18.3 Statistical profile of employed RNs, US, September 1977 to March 1988

Characteristic	1977	1980	1984	1988
Median age	37.7	36.3	37.5	36.6
Percentage male	2.1	3.0	3.3	3.3
Percentage minority group	7.5	8.3	9.4	9.1
Percentage married	68.9	68.1	68.7	69.5
Percentage married with children at home	43.8	46.3	47.7	48.3

Source: National Sample Survey of Registered Nurses, September 1977, November 1980, 1984 and March 1988.

Although the increase in the proportion of male RNs may not seem large, particularly in light of recent efforts to bring more men into nursing, the growth in numbers from 1977 to 1988 is sizeable. In 1977 there were about 21 000 men employed as RNs; in 1988 there were 58 242. The increase in percentage of RNs who are members of minority groups is quite significant. Thirty years ago, when hospital-based diploma programmes dominated nursing education, non-white students were rare. The growth of associate degree and baccalaureate programmes has opened the doors to both minorities and men. In 1988 nearly 10% of all RNs employed in nursing were from a racial/ethnic minority group.

The characteristics of LPNs provide an interesting contrast to those of RNs. While age, marital status and percentage of males among employed LPNs are similar to those of RNs, the proportion of LPNs from racial/ethnic minority groups was higher: 13.8% in 1983.

Educational preparation

An important characteristic of RNs is their educational preparation. Table

18.4 shows a substantial increase in the academic credentials of RNs. In 1977 nearly two-thirds of employed RNs had diplomas in nursing as their highest preparation. Eleven years later this group had declined to 36.5%. In 1977 4.4% of employed RNs held master's or doctoral degrees; in 1988 this proportion was 6.4%. These are remarkable changes, considering that in 1952 the highest credential for 91.8% of employed RNs was a diploma in nursing and only 1.0% held master's or doctoral degrees. Clearly the federal government has played an important role in this rise in educational level through support of graduate education since 1956. Moreover professional associations for many years have promoted the baccalaureate degree preparation as the entry level and established advanced academic degrees as credentials for leadership positions.

Table 18.4 Percentage of employed RNs according to highest educational preparation, September 1977 to March 1988

Highest educational preparation	1977	1980	1984	1988
Diploma	63.4	50.9	41.8	36.5
Associate degree	13.5	20.0	25.1	28.0
Baccalaureate	18.5	23.2	26.6	28.7
Master's or doctorate	4.4	5.3	6.1	6.4
Unknown	0.2	0.6	0.4	0.4
Total	100.0	100.0	100.0	100.0

Source: National Sample Survey of Registered Nurses, September 1977, November 1980, 1984 and March 1988.

Academic preparation of registered nurses varies considerably according to role. As would be expected nurse educators have the highest academic credentials, followed by clinical nurse specialists, researchers, consultants and nurse practitioners. The vast majority of these nurses have at least a baccalaureate degree and more than one-third have graduate degrees. Interestingly supervisors, mainly employed in hospitals and nursing homes, have among the lowest level of academic credentials, with nearly half having the diploma as their highest attainment. Many supervisors attain their positions through on-the-job experience, which is considered more valuable than academic knowledge. Although only about one in five nursing administrators holds an advanced academic degree the number is growing rapidly as the role has been broadened to include more involvement in institutional planning and policy making. Then, too, as health care institutions have become more complex, administrative decision making has become more demanding. Thus, even though the majority of top and middle level nursing executives do not now hold graduate degrees, there is undoubtedly a trend in that direction.

In discussing the population of RNs earlier it was pointed out that, in addition to RNs employed in nursing, there is a substantial number of RNs who are not employed at all. In 1988 it was estimated that there were about 291 000 RNs in this category. In addition about 114 000 RNs were employed in occupations other than nursing.

For many years the unemployed group, thought to consist of nurses who had left the workforce temporarily, were considered a resource for the nursing supply. Only a small proportion were considered permanently lost to the field. Today this idea is not believed to be true. For one thing unemployed nurses form a considerably smaller proportion, about 15%, of the RN population than in the past. In 1951 40% of the RN population was not employed in nursing. With the many programmes and facilities to help working mothers today, as well as the pressure for married women to continue as wage earners, there is greater opportunity for married nurses with small children to remain in the workforce. Thus the median age of RNs not employed in nursing is 51 years, compared to 36.6 for employed RNs. About 5% of employed RNs are 60 years of age and over compared to 33% of RNs not employed in nursing.

A higher proportion of LPNs are not employed in nursing: 31%, as compared to 2% of RNs. The median age of these LPNs is 41.3 years, considerably less than that of RNs not employed in nursing. One factor may be lesser opportunity for career advancement among LPNs.

PAY AND BENEFITS FOR NURSING

According to the 1988 Sample Survey average annual earnings of RNs working full time were $28 383. This is an increase of 119% since 1977, when average annual earnings were $12 948. This may seem a significant rise in 11 years but it was also a period of high inflation. Adjusted for inflation the rise was about 20%, barely keeping up with increases in the cost of living.

As Table 18.5 shows earnings vary among types of position and employment setting. Administrators of nursing education programmes are the highest paid of all, other than nurse anesthetists who are considered closer to the medical profession than to nursing. Nursing administrators in hospitals are also relatively highly paid but, compared to non-nursing administrators in similarly sized organizations with comparable responsibilities, they are woefully underpaid. There is a substantial number of hospital administrators and deans of medical schools who earn well over $100 000.

In general percentage increases in earnings were similar for all positions. As a group earnings rose a little more for nurses in hospitals than for other nursing positions. Except for nurse clinicians all positions rose in percentage terms more than the national average salary. The highest percentage increase was for nurse anesthetists.

Unlike most other professions there is not a large difference in the average earnings of newly qualified nurses and those in higher level positions that carry greater responsibility and require more education and experience. Administrative personnel in hospitals now earn about 32% more than staff nurses, a smaller spread than in 1977 (43%). The difference between a dean or director of a nursing education programme and an instructor was only 35% in 1988, actually less than in 1977. Research-

Table 18.5 Estimated average annual salaries of RNs employed full-time in selected nursing positions, September 1977 and March 1988

Nursing position	September 1977	November 1988	Percentage increase
All full-time RNs	$12 984	$28 383	$118.6
Hospital			
Administrator	17 532	39 905	127.6
Supervisor	14 196	31 207	119.8
Clinical nursing specialist	14 472	32 062	121.5
Nurse clinician	14 400	31 003	115.3
Head nurse	13 464	31 475	133.8
Staff nurse	12 252	27 196	122.0
Nurse anesthetist	19 896	47 556	139.0
Nursing home			
Administrator	14 064	27 601	96.3
Staff nurse	10 572	22 381	111.7
Nursing Education			
Administrator	19 716	41 050	108.2
Instructor	13 752	30 335	120.6
Public health			
Administrator	14 664	32 108	119.0
Supervisor	14 064	27 362	94.6
Staff nurse	12 096	23 635	95.4
Student health			
Staff nurse	11 244	22 460	99.8
Occupational health			
Staff nurse	13 368	27 389	104.9
Physicians' office			
Staff nurse	9 720	21 528	121.5
Nurse practitioner/midwife	14 220	31 807	123.7

Source: National Sample Survey of Registered Nurses, September 1977 and March 1988.

ers, many of whom have advanced degrees, earned only a little more than staff nurses in hospitals.

Differences in average annual earnings, according to highest level of educational preparation, are also not especially significant. As would be expected nurses with doctorates have the highest earnings – $43 092 – whereas nurses whose highest educational preparation is associate degree earn the lowest salaries – $26 532.

Moreover there is not a large difference in earnings between RNs, in positions such as staff nurse in hospitals, nursing homes or doctors' offices, and LPNs. In 1983 an LPN staff nurse in a hospital earned $15 083, in a nursing home $13 449 and in a doctor's office $12 801. At the other end of the scale the difference between physicians' and nurses' incomes is enormous. Physicians earn on average over $100 000, about four times the average nurse's salary. Comparisons of nurses' earnings with those of other professions – social workers, teachers and health professionals such as physical therapists – also show nursing at a disadvantage.

Earnings of nurses have not improved substantially, nor have other aspects of working conditions. Hours of full-time work average about 40, shift rotation is required in acute care hospitals and fringe benefits, e.g. vacation time, sick leave, education support and retirement benefit, are modest. Compared to 20 years ago when the average salary was about 20% of what it is today, and fringe benefits were virtually non-existent, there have been some improvements. However, except in certain employment areas, such as government, most nurses today do not have the benefits of a true career system with proper career ladders and incentives for long tenure.

Economists explain that nursing wages and benefits have been constrained by agreements among employers of nurses to pay the same salaries rather than pay competitively. That nursing is mostly a woman's profession is also advanced as an explanation of disadvantaged pay and benefits because women professionals do not exert the political clout seen in male dominated professions, doctors being a notable example. Then, too, collective bargaining for improved pay and benefits in nursing is a recent phenomenon. Although the major professional association, the American Nurses' Association (ANA), has had since 1897 an economic and general welfare programme concerned with working conditions for nurses, it was not until 1966 that the ANA House of Delegates adopted the first national minimum salary goal of $6500; the average annual salary was then $4700. In the mid-1970s, after collective bargaining in non-profit hospitals was permitted, the ANA became the collective bargaining agent for RNs. Nearly 150 000 RNs now work under contracts negotiated by state constituents of the ANA.

Opposition to the collective bargaining activities of the ANA has arisen from a number of sources. Some nurses and employers of nurses believe that the primary mission of the ANA is to be a professional organization rather than a trade union (even though professional issues are often intertwined with economic ones). The ANA is also challenged by trade unions, such as the American Federation of Teachers and the Federation of Nurses and Health Professionals, who also believe that a professional association should not function as a trade union.

The injection of economic issues into nursing in a major way is new. Past sentiment was that the introduction of 'mercenary' issues would detract from the altruism and dedication of the nursing profession. With the increase of entrepreneurship in the health care industry, however, nursing cannot afford to isolate itself from the economics of health care. For example an important economic issue today is how to determine accurately nursing costs in the delivery of care. These costs are usually lumped with other costs, which, in hospitals, have been rising faster than nursing costs, and nursing is often unfairly blamed for cost inflation. There is a lack of valid measures for nursing costs, and the lack of a valid measure of income generated by nurses hides the fact that nursing is indeed cost-effective, generating more income than it costs.

Job satisfaction within nursing

Although job satisfaction is a popular topic most such studies have been very localized, making it difficult to draw generalizations for states or the country as a whole. In the late 1950s Levine and Wright, in a nationwide sample of hospitals, found high rates of turnover among all categories of RNs and an association of job dissatisfaction with the high rates. Among the causes of dissatisfaction were low status, low pay, lack of career incentives and fragmentation of work. In the late 1960s and 1970s, when the nursing shortage was supposedly at its peak, job dissatisfaction appeared, from the many articles in journals, to be quite high. A widely used term was 'burnout', denoting the point reached in a nurse's working life when she had to leave nursing because she had reached 'the end of her tether'. Causes of burnout included overwork, coupled with underutilization of nursing skills and knowledge, this coming at a time when the intensity of services in hospitals was markedly increasing. Restraints on the authority of nurses – continuation of the role of 'handmaiden' to the physician –, at the same time education of nurses was expanding, also contributed.

United States Department of Health and Human Services (1986) suggests that job satisfaction may be higher than during the 1970s and that turnover rates may be lower. This could be attributed to improvement in salaries and fringe benefits, which, however modest, do represent a positive change, unlike the years prior to 1965 when salaries remained absolutely flat. Also the nurse supply has increased and more nursing care is available per patient, reducing the shortage and decreasing work pressure. However the shortage is again on the increase because the greater intensity of nursing care required by patient work pressures undoubtedly increases the need for nurses. Finally the 1980s were characterized as a period of complacency, in contrast to the turmoil of the 1960s and 1970s, and that may be another explanation of increased job satisfaction. Like the previous explanations it is not supported by facts.

LICENSURE

Licensure of nurses is administered by governmental organizations called boards of nursing, maintained by each state and the District of Columbia, Guam and the Virgin Islands. Mechanisms for regulating various health occupations were established by state governments, and qualifications of applicants for RN and practical nurse licensure are specified by nurse practice acts and generally relate to the applicant's age, educational attainments, character and English language competency. Graduates must pass a written examination – the National Council Licensure Examination for Registered Nurses (NCLEX-RN) or the NCLEX-LPN – to become licensed. About 90% of US graduates pass these examinations the first time, while only about one-third of foreign nurse graduates do. Success rates are lower for those who retake the tests.

Although each state board operates autonomously there are procedures that permit a nurse with a licence in one state to obtain a licence in another by endorsement rather than examination by the other state. Licences must be reviewed periodically by filing a renewal application and paying an appropriate fee. Renewal periods vary, with a few states having annual or triennial periods but the majority having biennial periods.

Nurse practice acts vary in requirements and definitions of scope of nursing practice. A few states, for example, require that nurses take continuing education courses as a condition of licence renewal. As to scope of practice some states define the nursing role more broadly than others by having statutory or regulatory references to advanced nursing practice of the kind engaged in by nurse practitioners.

Nearly 100 000 foreign-graduated nurses are licensed by various state boards. About 20% are from the UK and Canada. The Commission on Graduates of Foreign Nursing Schools (CGFNS) administers a testing and evaluation programme for graduates of foreign nursing schools to determine the probability of their passing the examination for RN licensure.

Passing the examination, which includes an English proficiency requirement, provides the foreign graduate with a certificate that enables them to take the licensing examination. Foreign nurse graduates seeking to enter the US for temporary employment must have the CGFNS certificate, as must foreign nurse graduates seeking to enter permanent employment; additionally they must have a labour certificate issued from the US Department of Labour in order to obtain an immigrant occupational preference visa.

There are 47 state boards that administer both RN and LPN licensure, six that administer RN licensure and seven that grant only practical nurse licensure. Sixty agencies belong to the National Council of State Boards of Nursing. The Council serves as coordinating body on matters of common interest and provides services and consultation to the state boards on all issues relating to entry into practice.

PROFESSIONAL ORGANIZATIONS

There are several large professional associations for nurses. The American Nurses' Association (ANA) is for RNs and has about 190 000 members, less than 10% of the total RN population. The ANA is a federation of constituent state associations that have representation in its House of Delegates, the governing body. The scope and concerns of the ANA include nursing education, practice, research, services, economic and general welfare and human rights. Thirteen councils provide forums for nurses on such specialized topics as clinical nurse specialists, computer applications in nursing, cultural diversity in nursing practice and nurse researchers. An important activity is labour relations, including collective bargaining to determine pay and benefits.

In addition there are several important organizations adjunct to the ANA, including the American Nurses' Foundation, which provides funds for nursing research and conducts its own research in areas such as health policy. The Nurses' Coalition for Action in Politics, the ANA's political action arm, endorses candidates for national office and provides financial support to their campaigns. The American Academy of Nursing (AAN) is concerned with advancing new concepts in nursing and health care and identifying and proposing solutions to major problems in nursing and health care. The AAN is an organization of Fellows selected by the membership committee and voted upon by the entire membership. Membership is composed of nurses who have made significant contributions to nursing administration, practice or research. The purpose of the Academy is to keep the profession at the forefront of issues in health and nursing and to address new concepts, ideas and solutions. Another important organization is the Association of Nurse Executives, which includes nurses in managerial and administrative positions. This organization is part of the American Hospital Association.

The National Federation of Licensed Practical Nurses is the LPN counterpart of the ANA. It consists of 34 constituent state associations and is governed by a House of Delegates. Major functions include establishment of education programmes for members, liaison with other nursing and health organizations and an economic and general welfare programme.

Another major organization, the National League for Nursing, is composed of agency membership – schools of nursing, health agencies – and nurses, other health care professionals and consumers. It maintains a number of important educational and consultative services such as accrediting nursing education programmes at all levels, administering a testing programme for educational courses and health institutions and providing continuing education workshops and institutes. The American Association of Colleges of Nursing is an organization of schools of nursing in colleges and universities offering degrees in nursing. The National Council of State Boards of Nursing administers the licensing examinations for nurses.

The National Student Nurses' Association has constituent organizations in all states and territories and the District of Columbia. It is concerned with promoting undergraduate nursing education and advancing the interests of students, career planning and aiding transition to active nursing. Other organizations, such as the American Association of Critical Care Nurses, are of recent origin, reflecting the trend towards greater specialization and the highly pluralistic nature of American society.

THE POLITICS OF NURSING: NURSING INFLUENCE ON NURSING AND HEALTH POLICIES

The power of nurses to influence health policies and, to a lesser extent, nursing salaries has been quite limited. Lack of political clout has been attributed to several factors. Because it is overwhelmingly (97%) a women's organization it has suffered from the undervalued role of women throughout history. Most of the power in the health care industry has been wielded by doctors and by hospital and other health care administrators, all predominantly male. With increasing entrepreneurship in the health care industry business and financial managers, also mostly men, are assuming the power positions. The view of nurses is not as leaders but as followers and the result is inadequate economic reward and little authority and autonomy, but, at the same time they bear the responsibility for doing whatever necessary things are in danger of not being done at all.

However the power of nurses to influence policies is greater today than ever before. In general nursing's influence has increased at several levels: in matters pertaining to nursing as a profession, in administration and management of health agencies and in policy making at the national, state and local levels.

Nursing as a profession

Internal matters relating to education, licensure and nursing research have always largely been in the hands of the profession. Schools and licensure boards have always been run by nurses and educational policies regarding curriculum, accreditation and credentialling have been determined by professional associations such as the National League for Nursing and the American Nurses' Association. The practice of nursing, including such important areas as pay and benefits and, increasingly in recent years, defining nursing roles, establishing standards of care and determining certification for specialty areas have also fallen within nurses' purview. Future strength of professional associations in these areas is difficult to assess in view of the financial difficulties of the traditional major nursing organizations, loss of membership and increasing competition from other newly created nursing associations.

Although the work of nurses within health agencies, particularly hospitals, has been largely controlled by physicians, there has been a tendency in recent years towards increased autonomy. Expanded roles, such as clinical nurse specialists, clinicians and nurse practitioners, are examples, the most extreme being the independent nurse practitioner, whose role is almost totally autonomous. Moreover recently developed concepts such as nursing assessment, nursing diagnosis and the nursing process have enlarged the influence of nursing on patient care. However these expanded roles are relatively few in number and the move towards placing health care on a more business-like basis could counteract the trend towards greater autonomy by promoting task orientation in patient care.

Administration and management of health agencies

Although hospital and other health agency administrators have been non-nurses and men the administration and management of nursing departments have always been controlled by nurses. Since these departments are usually the single largest cost centres they have had some degree of influence – at least in the domain of nursing – by virtue of the power of money. The current concern with the 'profitability' of nursing has undoubtedly increased this influence. In some health agencies nursing administrators have been elevated to positions of influence over the entire operation of the agency. As vice-presidents in charge of nursing they may serve as policy makers for the whole hospital. Another example is the nurse director of a home health care agency that provides a broad range of health care services – physiotherapy, speech therapy and social work – in addition to nursing services.

National, state and local government health policies

Governmental health programmes are dominated by the federal government, in terms of both financing and conduct of programmes. The federal government's role has undergone a major expansion since the mid-1960s and, although federal support of nursing research and education predates that period, nursing influence on federal policies is most clearly seen in the past 25 years. Although the most significant nursing input would be as a member of a federal legislative body – the House of Representatives or Senate – nurses have only rarely served on these bodies, as have other women. Fewer than 5% of the US Congress and 15% of state legislators are women. Only a handful of state governors or city mayors – the chief executive officers – are women and, of course, a woman has never served as president or vice-president of the US. Only 20% of high level posts in the federal government, and an even lower proportion at the state and local government level, are held by women. A notable example of a nurse holding a high level executive position in the federal health establishment is the former administrator of the Health Care Financing Administration, Dr Carolyn K. Davis. Another is Dr Faye G. Abdellah, former Deputy Surgeon General of the US Public Health Service.

Although the overall influence of nurses on federal health policy in general may not be great, nursing's influence on federal policies on nursing education and research has been substantial. The Nurse Training Act of 1964 established an advisory body to help formulate policy, the National Advisory Council on Nurse Training, which consists mainly of nurses from various fields outside the federal government. The Division of Nursing, the agency within the federal government that administers the Nurse Training Act, is headed by a nurse and consists of professionals who are mostly nurses. The recently established Center for Nursing Research in the National Institute of Health, which administers the federal programme of support for nursing research, also consists mostly of nurses, as does the review panel that judges the merits of grant applications for nursing research projects.

The Nurse Training Act has had important influences on areas of great concern to nurses: the nursing shortage, quality of nursing care and expansion of the role of nurses. Since the early 1970s various administrations have attempted to reduce funding for the programme or, in the case of the Reagan administration, eliminate it entirely. Opposition to funding stems from the claim that the shortage no longer exists and, currently, that federal spending on social programmes must be curtailed. The nursing profession has been able, through its lobbying efforts in Congress, to keep the programme alive, albeit with reduced funding levels. However future survival of the programme is in doubt.

Nevertheless, despite reverses, the influence of the nursing profession on health policies in general is, although not substantial, probably greater than ever before. And the influence on nursing policies and practices, although seemingly waning after a period of growth, is still felt. Predictions for the future cannot be made with any degree of certainty because of the many changes taking place in the health care industry.

19

Nursing research

Nursing research in the US includes both research conducted by nurses and research on nursing care. Research conducted by nurses includes scientific enquiry into causes, diagnoses and prevention of diseases, promotion of health in the processes of human growth and development and the impact on health of environmental hazards. Research on nursing care is concerned with understanding the nursing care of individuals and groups and the biological, physiological, social, behavioural and environmental mechanisms that influence health and disease and are relevant to that care.

Nursing research has come a long way since it began over 60 years ago as time studies of nursing activities in hospitals and surveys of schools of nursing. Today the focus is on nursing care research – or clinical nursing research as it is sometimes labelled – and on the theoretical and conceptual underpinnings of such research on the impact of nursing care interventions. Currently an estimated $40 million is being spent annually on nursing research, provided primarily by the federal government and by professional associations, foundations, hospitals and health agencies. Compared to the size of the profession it is not really a very large amount of money. About $8 billion is spent on medical research.

DEVELOPMENT OF NURSING RESEARCH

Until 1950 the major thrust of nursing research was on practical, management improvement type studies. One of the earliest recorded studies was a survey of hospitals on the work of nurses that revealed some of the problems in carrying out the sometimes confusing and conflicting physicians' orders. As a result of the 1923 Goldmark report (Committee for the Study of Nursing Education 1923) various evaluative studies were conducted in nursing schools. Perhaps the most elaborate of the early studies was reported by the then National League for Nursing Education (now NLN) in 1937 (National League for Nursing Education, 1937). Entitled 'A Study of the Nursing Service in Fifty Selected Hospitals', it gathered data on the distribution of time spent with patients in hospitals in New York City by graduate and student nurses and other personnel. This study initiated a long series of time studies, which, with the introduction of industrial engineering and operations research techniques, have become increasingly sophisticated. Today these management engineering studies have assumed considerable importance as hospitals and other health agencies attempt to increase cost-effectiveness in response to constraints on health care costs.

The creation of the Division of Nursing Resources in the federal government in 1949 provided a great stimulus to nursing research. Begun as a means to assist states in coping with nursing shortages after the Second World War, the Division initiated state nursing surveys of needs and resources – systematic approaches to assembling facts on a state's nursing manpower situation and developing plans to meet documented deficiencies. The Division conducted or financed major studies on more specific studies of nursing manpower issues, on developing methodologies for surveys of nurse staffing, turnover, job satisfaction and quality of performance, as well as on the relationship between nursing care and patient welfare. Under the leadership of Margaret Arnstein, the Division's first chief, a design was developed in the early 1950s for an experimental study in which contrasting patterns of nursing care could be tested in terms of various outcome measures, in essence a clinical trial model that, through the years, has influenced the design of numerous research studies in nursing care.

An important milestone was the appearance in 1952 of 'Nursing Research' the first journal devoted solely to nursing research and aimed at communicating results of nursing studies and research methodology. In 1953 Leo Simmons and Virginia Henderson of the National Committee for the Improvement of Nursing Services conducted a survey and assessment of nursing research that produced a typology of nursing research that is still useful. In 1954 the American Nurses' Association established a Committee on Research and Studies to plan and promote studies relating to the mission of the association. Today the Association's organization includes a Cabinet on Nursing Research as well as a Council of Nurse Researchers and Center for Research. The ANA also supports the American Nurses' Foundation, which provides small grants to nurse researchers. The National League for Nursing maintains an active research programme through its Division of Public Policy and Research.

A major step in the advancement of nursing research in the US was the creation of a Research Grants and Fellowships Program in the Division of Nursing Resources in 1955 to stimulate and provide financial support and training for researchers. Funded for approximately one-half million dollars for research project grants and $125 000 for research training grants the programme averaged, at its inception, less than $5 million per year in grants. In fiscal year 1985/86, as a result of a recommendation from the Institute of Medicine (National Academy of Sciences) study that the 'federal government should establish an organizational entity to place nursing research in the mainstream of scientific investigation', and because 'an adequately funded focal point is needed at the national level to foster research', approximately $10 million was made available. In that year the research component was moved from the Division of Nursing to the National Institutes of Health (NIH), the major federal health research organization. Called the Center for Nursing Research and located within a complete research milieu, funding is now more generous than previous nursing research budgets of the federal government. The Center becomes an Institute in 1993.

Another milestone was the publication in 1965 of the first textbook on nursing research, 'Better Patient Care Through Nursing Research', by Faye Abdellah and Eugene Levine. This was followed by the publication of a variety of textbooks and other materials relating to nursing research. Many schools of nursing now offer courses in nursing research, both at undergraduate and graduate levels. Another barometer of increased emphasis on research is the growth in the number of nurses with doctoral degrees, many of whom have participated in research for their doctoral dissertations. An estimated 5000 registered nurses have earned doctoral degrees and 5000 registered nurses designated nursing research as their field of employment in the March 1988 Sample Survey.

THE CURRENT STATUS OF NURSING RESEARCH

The current status of nursing research shows a 'great leap forward' over the past 30 years. More nurses are trained in research methodology, more nurses are employed full time in research, more money is being allocated and many more projects that can be labelled nursing research are being conducted. Considerable credit for this progress can be given to the federal government, through its funding of research by people outside government as well as within its own agencies. Although no definitive data are available on the total amount of money spent yearly on nursing research the federal government's Center for Nursing Research spent about $40 million in the most recent fiscal year (1992).

In addition the Division of Nursing, another Public Health Service (PHS) agency, conducts research, mainly manpower studies, with its own staff as well as through outside agencies. The National Institutes of Health conducts categorical medical research in many disease areas, generally within a multidisciplinary framework. Other PHS agencies, e.g. the National Institute of Mental Health and the Agency for Health Care Policy and Research (AHCPR), to a small extent also support nursing research, as do other organizations outside the PHS, such as the

Health Care Financing Administration, which supports research related to the administration of the Medicare and Medicaid programmes.

Other possible supporters of nursing research are state and local governments, professional associations and private foundations that award grants to researchers on a competitive basis, e.g. the Kellogg Foundation in Battle Creek, Michigan, and the Robert Wood Johnson Foundation in Princeton, New Jersey. In addition hospitals and community health agencies conduct nursing studies, although these are usually management engineering type studies concerned with improving organization. Finally, in fulfilment of academic requirements, students on master's and doctoral programmes conduct studies in nursing, many of which are of high quality and published in nursing literature.

NATIONAL CENTER FOR NURSING RESEARCH

Authorized by Congress in 1985 and established at the National Institutes of Health in 1986, the National Center for Nursing Research (NCNR) is now responsible for research project and training grants formerly administered by the Division of Nursing. Focus of the project grants is research on nursing interventions, procedures and delivery methods in the areas of patient care, promotion of health, prevention of disease and mitigation of the effects of acute and chronic illnesses and disabilities. As part of the National Institutes of Health, which focuses on clinical research, the projects of the Center for Nursing Research are intended to complement other biomedical research programmes primarily concerned with the causes and treatment of disease.

The process of applying for a research grant from the Center for Nursing Research has been carefully developed. A proposal is reviewed competitively for scientific merit in relation to other proposals and, if approved with a high enough score, is funded. About 20% of all new research proposals are funded each year. The average grant is somewhat less than $100 000 per year and three years is the usual maximum period for an award. However an investigator, after completion of work described in a proposal, can submit an application for renewal of the grant. Private foundations award grants for nursing research by a procedure similar to that of the federal government, except that the length and content of the proposal may be more modest and funding is generally lower – $50 000 to $100 000 for the entire project.

To encourage development of research capabilities among nurses the Center for Nursing Research maintains several programmes of financial support for students and new researchers. National Research Service Awards are training grants that offer support for individual fellowships and institutional grants to undertake post-doctoral training that emphasizes research. From 1979 until July 1st 1986, when a moratorium was placed on the programme, 16 schools of nursing had received funding from Nursing Research Emphasis Grants, the purpose of which was to stimulate research in areas that emphasize special health needs and advance the research efforts and resources of faculty staff in nursing schools offering doctoral programmes. The First Independent Research Support and Transition (First) Awards are intended to underwrite the first independent investigative efforts of an individual and to help effect a transition towards traditional types of National Institutes of Health research project grants.

Analysis of nursing research grants

It is revealing to analyse nursing research grants supported by the federal government through the National Center for Nursing Research. Data are available for grant applications for the fiscal year 1988. As Table 19.1 shows the majority were for research projects. The remaining applications were primarily for training in research. Seventeen, for example, were for schools of nursing to expand the research emphasis of doctoral programmes.

Table 19.1 Distribution of FY 1988 National Center for Nursing Research Applications, by type

Type of award	Number	Percentage
Research Project	148	41
Predoctoral Individual National Research Service	111	31
First Independent Research Support	27	7
Small Business Innovation Research	21	6
Academic Research Enhancement	17	5
Postdoctoral Individual National Research Service	14	4
Individual National Research Service	9	2
All others	15	4
Total	362	100

Source: National Institute of Health. Report of the 1989 NIH Task Force on Nursing Research. Bethesda, MD: NIH.

Although the subjects of applications for nursing research projects are wide-ranging, they tend to cluster in certain areas. Of the many ways of classifying nursing research a useful one for federally funded projects is according to five areas.

1. Fundamental nursing projects

Sometimes called basic research these studies seek to identify, describe and explain phenomena related to human systems and functioning. They are designed to provide new knowledge and develop, test and expand theories and models. Examples of such studies from the list of federally supported nursing projects include:

> The Adolescent and Her Child: A Longitudinal View; One-Parent Families: Women Transcending Options; Nasal Cannula and Transtracheal Delivery of Oxygen; Longitudinal Study of Touch and Taste Acuity in Diabetes; and Type A Behaviour: An Epidemiological Study of Twin Families.

2. *Nursing practice projects*

Sometimes called applied research these focus on the impact of nursing interventions or changes in the organization and delivery of nursing care to recipients of care. Included are outcome studies that assess the effectiveness of procedures, techniques and methods. A research model for these studies is the clinical trial of medical and nursing interventions. Examples of supported studies are:

> Nursing Factors in Pregnancy Health Behaviour and Outcomes; Behavioural Therapy for Urinary Incontinence in Females; A Study of Early Management of Breast Feeding; Influencing Adherence and Life Adjustment Post-Infarction; and Expanding Nursing's Role in Weight Control Counselling.

3. *Profession of nursing projects*

These studies focus on social and economic problems of the nurse and nursing as a profession, the 'image' of nursing and the status and prestige of nurses *vis-à-vis* other health occupations. Examples of such studies are:

> Role Conflict in the Nursing Profession; and Conceptualization of Nursing During Various Epochs.

4. *Nursing services administration research projects*

This category includes studies on increasing cost-effectiveness of the organization and delivery of nursing services, the role of the computer in nursing, quality of care, nurse staffing, satisfaction, turnover and the economics of nursing. Examples are:

> NURSE: A Nurse Staffing Requirements System; Technological Innovation for Home Care Nursing; Commitment, Satisfaction, Performance of Hospital Nurses; Design of a Tool to Evaluate Nurse Staffing System; Computer-Based Consultant for Nursing Care Standards.

5. *Nursing education*

These studies deal with the educational preparation of nurses, ways of improving educational resources, curricula, faculty staff and performance on licensing examinations, the optimal education system for preparing nurses for entry level positions and continuing and advanced preparation of graduates. Only one project was included in this category on the October 1985 list.

QUALITY INDICATIONS OF NURSING DOCTORAL PROGRAMMES

Most nursing doctoral programmes supported by the federal government falls into the areas of fundamental research and nursing practice. This reflects the emphasis of the federally supported programme to expand the scientific basis of nursing and to test and evaluate nursing interventions in a clinical setting. Among the clinical areas a very large number of projects are found in nursing in maternal and child health, although care of the elderly, cardiovascular disease and AIDS are receiving increasing attention.

DISSEMINATION OF NURSING RESEARCH FINDINGS

With the growth in nursing research activities in the US there has been a substantial increase in the volume of research information. One dissemination source is the periodical journal. Since 'Nursing Research' first appeared other journals have been initiated that provide vehicles for reporting study results, e.g. *Western Journal of Nursing Research, Image* and the Annual Review of *Nursing Research. Nursing Abstracts* provides brief summaries of research articles in journals and indexes such as the *International Nursing Index* and *Index Medicus*, a means of locating published research studies.

The National Library of Medicine, which publishes 'Index Medicus', is the largest health library in the world (and is located at the National Institutes of Health, Bethesda, Maryland). It collects and organizes biomedical information, for the use of researchers and others, from more than six million references to journal articles and books published after 1965 in the health sciences. It maintains the Medical Literature Analyses and Retrieval System (MEDLARS), a computerized literature search system available through a nationwide network of centres at 2000 universities, hospitals, government agencies and commercial organizations. Among the many databases computerized and accessed on-line in the MEDLARS network is Medline, which contains references to biomedical journal articles published in the current and previous three years.

A compendium of current year research projects supported by the

National Institutes of Health is available in the Research Grants Index published by the Institutes. The federal government makes available the complete reports of the research it funds through the National Technical Information Services. An important way of disseminating research findings is research conferences, bringing together both researchers and utilizers of research for presentations and critiques of findings; the Library is the repository of the published proceedings.

CURRENT RESEARCH EMPHASIS AND PRIORITIES

In the past, operating as an organizational unit of the Division of Nursing of the Public Health Service, the Nursing Research Grants and Fellowships Program, while emphasizing clinically-orientated research, did fund a few projects in nursing administration and education. These projects might now be excluded from support by the National Center for Nursing Research because the following research areas are excluded from National Institutes of Health grant allocation: historical, educational, health care delivery, philosophical, human resource and health policy. Because National Institute of health-supported research is supposed to adhere as closely as possible to the rules of experimental design it could be difficult to fund some otherwise meritorious research. Many, perhaps the majority of, nursing problems are not amenable to the experimental approach or even to the so-called quasi-experimental approach and, in fact, would be diminished by such approaches.

To focus the available funding the NCNR has identified research priorities. Current priorities include:

1. Low birth-weight: mothers and infants;
2. HIV infection: prevention and care;
3. Long-term care of the elderly;
4. Symptom management;
5. Information systems;
6. Health promotion;
7. Technology dependency across the lifespan;
8. Nursing shortage.

Many of the changes that have occurred in nursing research in the past 30 years have resulted from technological advances. These have outpaced the solutions to the sociological and psychological problems related to health, such as personal relationships, life-styles adverse to health, sociopsychological aspects of ageing and substance abuse (to name but a few). Areas seen as having high priority for future nursing research are:

1. Studies in preventive health care to determine how best to change an individual's behaviour and attitudes;

2. Determination of ways to decrease the negative impact of health problems on coping abilities, productivity and life satisfaction of individuals and families;
3. Research on long-term care of the elderly, mentally retarded and developmentally disabled, with emphasis on the design of assessment tools that will take into account the functional status, limited patient outcome goals and complex treatment processes characteristic of long-term care;
4. Studies of life-threatening situations, anxiety, pain and stress; research on ways to ensure that care needs of vulnerable groups are met with appropriate strategies;
5. Determination of phenomena that negatively influence the recovery process and that may be alleviated by nursing practice, such as anorexia, sleep deprivation and deficiencies in nutrition;
6. Research to enhance the care of patients who are culturally different from the majority and patients with special problems – teenagers, prisoners and the mentally ill – and those whose health needs are underserved, such as the poor and those living in rural areas.

Another important area is the determination of nursing cost-effectiveness, a high priority in view of diminishing money for health care. At an April 1986 conference on nursing productivity a research agenda was developed that included the following high priority research topics (US Department of Health and Human Services):

1. Research on differences in costs, health status and satisfaction with care among patients who have experienced different types of delivery systems;
2. Determination of how positive outcomes of preventive health can be measured;
3. Study of the effect of greater nursing involvement in health care on costs of nursing service and savings in total health care costs;
4. Study of the effect of varying levels of nursing skill mix (RNs, LPNs and aides as well as RNs prepared in different types of educational programmes) on patient outcomes;
5. Investigation of characteristics of centres of excellence in nursing to determine factors contributing to high productivity;
6. Study of possible iatrogenic effects of nursing care;
7. Using meta-analysis to examine existing databases to shed light on the cost-effectiveness of nursing interventions;
8. Research on the impact of incentives on the quality and quantity of nursing services produced;
9. Determination of the management model that optimizes clinical decision making to achieve planned or desired outcomes;

10. Research to identify, measure and weigh contextual factors for the practice of nursing.

It appears that a fundamental need identified for nursing research in future is methodology: the development of measures to assess *outcomes* of nursing interventions. Essentially the question to be asked is, 'What difference does provision of nursing care make – in terms of costs, health status of recipients of care, including functional capabilities, mental status and prognosis and satisfaction?' The need for such measures was recognized at the very beginning of nursing research as the key to the success of patient care research, when studies of 'patient welfare' attempted to develop indicators of quality of care. Although some progress in this measurement area has been made much remains to be done, particularly in view of the increased complexity of nursing and health care services and growing concern with optimizing resources consumed in the provision of these services.

20
Planning for nursing

What is health planning? It is an orderly and measured process of:

1. Defining the extent and characteristics of community health problems and identifying unmet needs;
2. Assessing available and potential resources;
3. Establishing priority goals by matching needs and resources and considering alternatives and their consequences;
4. Formulating the necessary administrative action to achieve programme goals;
5. Relating results to goals by continuing evaluative studies.

More specifically planning for nursing is a process in which overall or particular nursing needs are identified and resources examined. First the nature and scope of needs and resources are defined, related to their influencing factors and considered as a whole. Then the means available for meeting needs and augmenting resources are interposed and courses of action are developed to achieve the goals.

Planning is an important element in the success of any enterprise. In the US the importance of planning for nursing, recognized for a long time, has had some notable beneficial results.

THE HISTORY OF HEALTH PLANNING

Although government, both national and local, in the US play a lesser role in the provision of *direct* health care than it does in the UK or Canada, in some areas, such as licensing of health professionals and monitoring of quality of care, it is more active. In health planning the government exerts a strong influence, especially in planning for nursing where, at the national level, it has had a long history, especially in the areas of education, distribution and research.

Federal government involvement in health planning was initiated by the Hospital Survey and Construction Act of 1946, the Hill–Burton programme, which provided grant assistance to states for developing plans for hospital facilities based on need. An important step forward in planning was the Comprehensive Health Planning Act of 1966 that authorized grants to states to undertake comprehensive health planning in health care services and manpower. State and regional agencies were created by law for coordinating and developing plans. The most far-reaching federal programme, authorized by the National Health Planning Resources Development Act of 1974, created state- and area-wide health planning agencies, to perform the function of the Hill–Burton Act programmes in facility planning, and the Comprehensive Health Planning Organizations in services and manpower planning. In addition to state agencies, health systems agencies created within the states were charged with developing health system plans. In recent years this federal health planning programme has first been greatly reduced and then practically eliminated.

Planning for nursing has evolved outside these three major federal planning programmes. Of all categories of health profession nursing has undoubtedly had the most extensive and richest history in planning for needs and resources.

THE HISTORY OF NURSING PLANNING

The first important planning study in nursing was the Report of the Committee for the Study of Nursing Education (Committee for the Study of Nursing Education 1923), known as the Goldmark Report. Focusing on nursing education the Committee made a number of recommendations for improving the quality of education to adequately prepare nursing practitioners and leaders of the future. Following the Goldmark Report the Committee on the Grading of Nursing Schools, 1934 was established, which in 1926 undertook a survey of the nation's schools of nursing in order to grade them according to quality. In addition the Committee initiated a study of the supply of and demand for graduate nurses. Findings of this study, published in 1928, indicated that there was an increasing oversupply of graduate nurses. However, there were significant qualitative deficiencies in services because of inadequate training of nurses. The Committee's report on nursing education, published in 1934, contained a number of recommendations for addressing these inadequacies (Committee on the Grading of Nursing Schools, 1934).

The federal government's involvement in nursing planning began after the Second World War. By then the US Cadet Nurse Corps, a wartime programme for support for nursing education, was terminated. As a consequence a large number of nurses left active practice, which led to a severe shortage of hospital nurses throughout the country. The Division of Nursing Resources set about assisting the states and local areas to survey their nursing needs and resources and developing plans for meeting those needs. The Division issued a manual, 'Measuring Nursing

Resources' (Division of Nursing Resources 1949), to guide state groups in conducting these planning studies. The manual explained how to obtain data on the nursing population from state licensing boards. In the late 1940s a programme known as the Inventory of Registered Nurses was begun by the American Nurses' Association; it encouraged state boards of nursing to incorporate a uniform set of questions (on age, sex, marital status, field of practice, etc.) into the licensing application. The manual also described how to obtain data on the supply of nurses from the major employers – hospitals, community health agencies and physicians' offices – using existing data and survey questionnaires. Finally the manual explained how to assess demand for nurses, using an essentially 'professional judgement' approach in which a panel of experts determined optimum or desirable nurse staffing patterns in each major field of nursing. The methodology provided current as well as future estimates for both supply and demand, by projecting future changes in the organization and delivery of nursing services.

Although simplistic by today's standards the methodology in the 1949 manual provided a practical approach to assessing the extent of nursing shortage in a state and providing a statistical basis for developing long-range plans for nursing education and services. The momentum for conducting state nursing planning studies increased during the 1950s as the nursing shortage persisted. Also the Division of Nursing Resources provided technical assistance to states conducting studies, and consultants from the Division served as project directors to numerous surveys carried out by state committees composed of nursing education and service leaders, non-nursing professionals and lay persons. Funding for the committees came mostly from non-governmental sources, the major contributors being state nurses' associations, state leagues for nursing and state hospital associations. Early state nursing surveys cost on average $19 000.

In 1956 a new edition of the planning manual was issued, entitled 'Design for State-wide Nursing Surveys'. By that time most of the states had conducted initial nursing planning surveys and some were involved in re-surveys. The revised manual, while essentially describing the same approach to assessing supply and demand as the earlier one, promoted studies that would yield more extensive information on the nursing population than would simple head counts. These included studies of utilization of nursing personnel, patients' needs for services, job satisfaction, turnover and costs of nursing education. In addition, during the 1950s, the staff of the Division of Nursing Resources were engaged in developing a variety of methodologies for evaluating the quantity and quality of nursing resources. These were published as separate manuals and supplemented the state survey manual.

Among the many manuals and study guides published by the Division during the 1950s were:

How to Study Nursing Activities in a Patient Unit; How to Study Supervisor Activities in a Hospital Nursing Service; How to Study Nursing Service of an Outpatient Department; Patients and Personnel Speak – A Method of Studying Patient Care in Hospitals; New Ways to Measure Personnel Turnover in Hospitals; and Elements of Progressive Patient Care.

A DATA BASE FOR PLANNING

Beginning in the early 1950s the Division of Nursing Resources began to establish databases for use in state and national planning for nurses. In 1953 the Division issued the first of a series of source books (Table 20.1) on nursing statistics that contained compilations of data on nursing supply, demand, education and services pertinent to nursing planning and evaluation. Compared to the first 'Source Book' the 1981 book was an expansion in both the depth and breadth of coverage (215 pages versus 88).

Table 20.1 Data and their sources for nursing supply model

Data element	Sources
Current supply and population of nurses	Sample Surveys, RN and LPN
Mortality rates	Life tables for white females, by the National Center for Health Statistics
Net loss rates	Annual licensure statistics of American Nurses' Association. Sample Surveys, RNs and LPNs. Inventories of RNs and LPNs.
New licences	Annual licensure data of ANA
Activity rates	Sample Surveys, Inventories of RNs and LPNs
Graduates of schools nursing	Analysis of trends based on Annual Surveys of National League for Nursing

To obtain an understanding of nursing supply and demand the Division launched a number of statistical surveys in such areas as nurse staffing in hospitals, inactive and part-time nursing, patient and personnel satisfaction with nursing care, patients' requirements for nursing services and costs in nursing education. Professional associations also participated in important statistical surveys. Beginning in 1949 and concluding in 1977 the American Nurses' Association (ANA) conducted seven inventories of registered nurses (RNs) and two of licensed practical nurses (LPNs). These comprehensive studies were conducted through the mechanism of periodic licence renewal by state boards of nursing. The application form used in the renewal process contained a standard set of statistical questions to be answered by the nurse applicant. In a few states special surveys were required.

Data from each state were centrally tabulated and reports prepared by the ANA. As the costs of the inventories increased federal money was made available, beginning in the 1960s and 1970s, from the US Public Health Service Division of Nursing, formerly the Division of Nursing Resources. In 1977 the Division supported a sample survey of RNs, collecting a somewhat expanded version of the inventory data on a small sample of RNs. This survey was repeated in 1980, 1984 and 1988 and the latest in 1992. A survey of similar content was conducted for LPNs in 1983.

The ANA also gathers data on licensure of nurses and on salaries and fringe benefits. It periodically publishes these data in 'Facts About Nursing', which, like the 'Source Book', contains statistics on the characteristics of nurse supply, education and staffing in institutions. The National League for Nursing (NLN) conducts surveys of all nursing schools and publishes these annually in 'State Approved Schools of Nursing – RN' and 'State Approved Schools of Nursing – LPN'. The League also conducts a periodic census of nursing faculty members and, until recently, maintained a continuing survey of newly licensed nurses. Compilations of NLN survey and trend data are published in its annuals 'NLN Nursing Data Review' and 'Nursing Student Census'. The American Association Colleges of Nursing conducts an annual survey of faculty salaries in colleges. The American Hospital Association annually surveys hospitals for data on nursing and other hospital personnel.

Although the nursing database can be criticized for incompleteness in some areas and lack of timeliness in others the efforts of the federal government, in conjunction with the professional associations, have produced a rich statistical resource for planning, evaluation and research. An important mechanism in achieving this cooperative and coordinated effort has been the Interagency Conference on Nursing Statistics. This organization was begun in 1953 by members of the Division of Nursing Resources, ANA and NLN to discuss ways of estimating the registered nurse supply and to promote much-needed studies of supply and distribution. Meeting annually the members of the organization now also include the American Hospital Association, American Association of Colleges of Nursing, National Council of State Boards of Nursing and National Center for Health Statistics (of the Public Health Service). Although it is an informal organization the Interagency Conference has accomplished much in developing data-gathering methodology, refining the statistical analysis of data, promoting joint data collection among members and stimulating necessary surveys and analyses. The Conference has supported workshops such as one on nursing data gaps and needs (September 1985), which identified important areas in planning and evaluation where new data are needed. Considering the vast effort expended to develop a comprehensive database for planning the additional data needs underscore how complex planning for nursing has become.

In 1972 another state survey manual, 'Planning for Nursing Needs and Resources' was issued, which reflected the growing sophistication of the surveys and their comprehensive orientation towards planning over statistical surveys. In the 1970s state studies on needs and resources became more sophisticated and costly (the Illinois survey cost $100 000). In the late 1970s a project funded by the Division of Nursing and conducted by the Western Interstate Commission on Higher Education (WICHE) moved the state planning study effort to an even higher level by incorporating in its 1978 planning manual, 'Nursing Resources and Requirements: A Guide for State-Level Planning', concepts from systems analysis and econometrics.

Recent state surveys, considerably fewer than in the 1950s and early 1960s, reflect the greater depth in the methodological approach of the WICHE 1978 guide. They also reflect the impact of the 1974 planning legislation by occasional sponsorship by or involvement of a state or local planning agency although, for the most part, these agencies have not attempted to develop plans for nursing or any other health profession. Another recent trend is to approach health manpower planning on a multidisciplinary basis. This makes considerable sense, particularly in view of overlapping roles and the need to determine the most cost-effective way of providing health services. Finally, in view of the costliness of doing a comprehensive nurse planning study, a regional approach encompassing several states is being more frequently used. The study of the Mid-Atlantic Regional Nurses Association in the late 1980s, which includes four states and the District of Columbia, is an example.

PLANNING AT THE NATIONAL LEVEL

State planning studies for nursing – which were often joint efforts of the federal government and state and local organizations – is one approach to nursing planning. On another level the federal government has for many years engaged in nursing studies for national planning purposes, primarily to evaluate legislative programmes that assist nursing and to determine future federal legislative policies. In 1948 a report to the President entitled the 'Nation's Health' (the Ewing Report) recommended increased numbers of health professionals, a goal of one RN or LPN to 280 people, and federal aid to nursing schools and nursing students. Another presidential report in 1952, 'Building America's Health', also recommended aid to health professions schools and students.

Legislation in 1956 provided funds for graduate training for nurses in teaching administration and supervision and authorized a national conference in 1958 to evaluate this training programme and recommend future legislative action. This requirement of an evaluation of nursing training legislation and planning recommendations for the future set the pattern for all subsequent legislation to support nursing training. The data and analysis requirement of the planning and evaluation reports was a major source of financial support and stimulus for the many studies undertaken in recent years by the Division of Nursing, including the major efforts by the Western Interstate Commission on Higher Education (WICHE) and others to develop methodologies for determining nursing supply and requirements.

A landmark in federal nursing studies was the work of the Consultant Group on Nursing, appointed in 1961 to advise the Surgeon General on future nursing needs and to identify the appropriate role of the federal government in assuring adequate nursing services for the nation. The Consultant Group's report, 'Towards Quality in Nursing', issued in 1963 (United States Surgeon General's Consultant Group on Nursing, 1963), claimed that a severe quantitative shortage of nurses existed, but of equal importance was the fact of serious qualitative deficiencies. Using projection methodology similar to that of state nursing surveys the Consultant Group projected an optimum need for 850 000 RNs by 1970 and a feasible goal of 680 000 RNs. Since the number of employed RNs in 1962 was 550 000 even the feasible goal represented a formidable accomplishment. Substantial improvements in the baccalaureate and post-baccalaureate preparation of nurses were also recommended.

A direct result of the Consultant Group report was the Nurse Training Act of 1964 that initiated a significant programme of federal support for nursing education, which continues in a considerably reduced form. Approximately $2 billion has been appropriated by the federal government for nurse training through a series of legislative actions that continue support for nursing education. In order that Congress obtain information on the status of nursing needs and resources at the time the legislation came up for renewal, it required a report on progress made under the legislation (Table 20.2 below). Preparation of the reports has been, basically, the responsibility of the Division of Nursing and has entailed the collection and analysis of large amounts of data, including projections of nursing supply and requirements. The need for data for these reports has been the basis for many studies conducted by the Division of Nursing during the past 20 years, including the sample surveys of RNs and LPNs.

280 *Planning for nursing*

The mammoth planning study conducted by the Western Interstate Commission on Higher Education included numerous methodological studies to develop modelling and projection techniques for nursing supply and requirement. Table 20.2 contains a list of Reports to Congress since adoption of the Nurse Training Act of 1964 and briefly describes

Table 20.2 Reports to Congress under the nurse training acts, 1968–90

Year and title	Major findings
Nurse Training Act of 1964: Program Review. US/DHEW, Pub. no. 1740, December 1967	Since NTA of 1964 demands for nurses increased significantly due to Medicare and Medicaid programmes of 1965. Also Comprehensive Health Planning Act of 1966 placed new emphasis on national planning for health services and manpower. Need increased for nurses with broader and more scientifically based education because of technological developments. Recommended continuation of training support and inclusion of construction grants for schools of nursing and new support for planning, recruitment and research.
Progress Report on Nursing Training, 1970. US/DHEW, August 1970	Reported on significant increase in number of nursing students and nursing personnel. January 1970 700 000 RNs employed, 20 000 higher than Surgeon General's Consultant Group's projection but well below optimal goal. Implied improvement due to federal financial support.
Evaluation of Nurse Training Act, September 1974 (unpub)	Since passage of the NTA 1964 graduates from nursing schools preparing as RNs increased by 50%. Provided detailed analysis of relationship between federal financial support to nursing schools and student enrollments.
Report to the Congress, Nurse Training, 1974. DHEW Pub. no. (HRA)75–41, 1975	Nursing moving into community and assuming expanded roles. Correction of uneven distribution of nursing ranks and expertise a top priority. Provided detailed financial data on operation of NTA.
First Report to the Congress, February 1977, Nurse Training Act of 1975. DHEW Pub. no. (HRA)78–38, February 1978	Presented detailed data on various approaches to projecting nursing supply, distribution and requirements. State-by-state analyses revealed wide variation in ratios of RNs to population. Pointed out increased demand had absorbed increased supply.
Second Report to the Congress, March 15th, 1979 (Revised) Nurse Training Act of 1975. DHEW Pub. no. (HRA)79–45	Highlighted uneven geographical distribution of nursing personnel. Contained detailed description of various modelling approaches to determining supply and requirements. Projected that aggregate supply and demand would be in balance by 1985.

Year and title	Major findings
Third Report to the Congress, February 1982, Nurse Training Act 1975. DHHS Pub. no. (HRA)82–7	Provided updated projections from the various methodologies, particularly criteria-based model developed by the Western Interstate Commission on Higher Education for which new criteria determined by panel of experts (November 1980). Projections for 1990, using the new criteria, indicated that requirements for RNs substantially exceeded supply, particularly for nurses with advanced education.
Report to the President and Congress on the Status of Health Personnel in the US, May 1984. DHHS Pub. no. HRS–P–OD–84–4	Agreed with findings of the 1983 nursing study by Institute of Medicine, National Academy of Sciences. Recommended limiting federal support to areas amenable only to federal intervention or to areas where support could serve as a catalyst to private, state and local sectors. These included support to nurse administrators, educators, clinical specialists and nurse practitioners.
Fifth Report to the President and Congress on the Status of Health Personnel in the US, March 1986, Report on Nursing. NTIS Accession no. HRP 0906804	Contains projections of criteria-based requirements model using criteria developed in 1984 for WICHE. Notes increase in intensity of nursing care in hospitals. Discusses possible impact of change in financing of care – trend towards prospective reimbursement.
Sixth Report to the President and Congress on the Status of Health Personnel in the United States, June 1988, Nursing. DHHS Pub. no. HRS–P–OD–88–1	Reported that despite drop in number of those applying to enroll in schools of nursing, supply of nurses had continued to increase. Support of federal government to nursing education had contributed to this increase. Despite increase there were signs that nursing shortage had reappeared. Hospitals were also reporting problems of recruitment and retention. A Secretary's Commission was appointed to address these problems.
Seventh Report to the President and Congress on the Status of Health Personnel in the US, October 1989. DHHS Pub. no. HRS–P–OD–90–1	Includes a special section on the 'Nursing Shortage' that discusses recent evidence on the increase in shortage of nurses in various employment settings, particularly acute care. Presents findings and conclusions from the Secretary's Commission on Nursing (1988). Contains updated projections of nursing supply and requirements including projections based on the historical trend model and on criteria developed in 1988. Includes data from the March 1988 National Sample Survey of Registered Nurses.

their major findings and conclusions. Detailed study of these reports, which average over 150 pages in length, reveals the development of the methodology for projecting nursing supply and requirements from the rather simplistic approach of the Surgeon General's Consultant Group on Nursing to the sophisticated modelling approaches developed in the 1970s. While not strictly a planning study the Secretary of the US Department of Health and Human Services appointed a Commission on Nursing in 1987 to examine the reputed shortage of RNs. The Commission issued its final report in 1988, declaring that a nursing shortage did indeed exist but that it was primarily a result of increase in demand for nurses and not of a contraction in supply.

NURSING PLANNING STUDIES BY NON-FEDERAL ORGANIZATIONS

While the federal government has played a major role in conducting planning studies there have been several non-federal studies that have evaluated nursing supply and requirements and have also made recommendations for the future. The 1923 Goldmark Report has already been mentioned. A 1948 report by Esther Lucille Brown, 'Nursing for the Future', criticized the quality of nursing education and recommended that basic nursing education be moved into the mainstream of higher education. One result of the Brown report was the establishment of an accreditation programme for schools of nursing. A 1975 study by the National League for Nursing, 'Nurses for a Growing Nation', made projections of nursing needs for 1970 based on the ratio in the 75 percentile of the state ratios of nurses to population.

In 1967, partially as a follow-up to the Surgeon General's Consultant Group on Nursing report, the National League for Nursing and the American Nurses' Association established a National Commission for the Study of Nursing Education. Its final report, published in 1970, 'An Abstract for Action', did not make statistical projections for the future but recommended the organization of state planning committees for nursing education to promote preparation for expanded practice. It also encouraged creation of a National Joint Practice Commission with state counterparts to facilitate communication between nurses and physicians.

In 1983 the Congressionally-ordained Institute of Medicine of the National Academy of Sciences (an independent advisory body to the government) completed a two-year study of nursing. The report, 'Nursing and Nursing Education: Public Policies and Private Actions', essentially concerned with advising Congress on the future of federal financial support for nursing education, emphasized the need for advanced preparation of nurses in view of the growing complexity of nursing as well as research. Federal support for basic nursing education, to increase the overall supply, was not viewed as necessary since aggregate supply and demand was expected to be in balance for the remainder of this decade. Also, in 1983, the report of the National Commission on Nursing, 'Summary Report and Recommendations', by the American Hospital Association, was issued, recommending improvements in nursing management and career incentives as a means of improving the quality of nursing care in hospitals.

This brief overview of nursing planning studies has shown that considerable effort has been expended to obtain an adequate base and develop useful methodologies for evaluating and planning nursing needs and resources. From one perspective this effort may be seen as 'overkill' since many studies seem to repeat findings and conclusions of other investigations. Considering the size of and complexities within the nursing profession the planning effort is really not overdone. Then, too, large sums of public monies have been expended on nursing and the attempt to enhance the cost-effectiveness of resources devoted to nursing is understandable. The value of this planning effort is probably high, considering the improvement in the balance of supply and demand, the significant increase in educational preparation of nurses, the creation of new categories of nurse to serve in expanded roles created by technological advances and some improvement in geographical distribution of nurses, although some areas unfortunately remain poorly supplied.

The central focus of nursing planning studies, whether orientated to a state, as in state surveys, or to the national level, as in the various Reports to Congress, is analysis of future nursing supply and demand (the attempt in planning is to achieve a balance between supply and demand). As viewed by one of the models developed by the Western Interstate Commission on Higher Education for the Division of Nursing (1978) the relationship between nursing supply and demand is complex and requires an expensive database and sophisticated modelling. In the final section of this chapter current methodology for analyzing future nursing supply and demand, as utilized by the federal government, will be briefly described. The term 'requirements' will be used to describe two contrasting approaches – one that essentially projects 'demand' in the economic definition of the term and one that projects 'need' according to professional judgement.

METHODOLOGY FOR PROJECTING NURSING SUPPLY REQUIREMENTS

The supply model provides three projections for each state and for the US as a whole:

1. Nurse population: nurses with current licences to practice;
2. Nurse supply: those practising nursing full or part time;

3. Full-time equivalent supply: those practising full time plus one-half the number of nurses practising part time.

Each projection is subdivided into highest educational level achieved: associate degree or diploma, baccalaureate, master's degree and doctorate. In addition the model accounts for age of the nurse in terms of ten age groupings.

The model for making these projections takes account of the following variables for which assumptions about future behaviour are made:

1. Inputs from the education system (new graduates, past RN baccalaureates and higher degree graduates);
2. The number of new licences;
3. Net losses or gains due to lapsed and reinstated licences;
4. The proportion of the nurse population employed in nursing (activity rate), according to age group of the nurse.

It is clear that assumptions made by the supply model for future projections are dependent on the availability of a substantial amount of data.

REQUIREMENTS PROJECTIONS

Two main approaches are utilized (Table 20.3 below). One, the historical trend-based model, projects future requirements in the utilization of services and resources, modified by expected changes in the health care system. Projections are provided for states and for the nation. Requirements are analyzed for major health care settings, community hospitals, other hospitals, nursing homes, physicians' offices, community health agencies, health maintenance organizations, nursing education and all other settings combined. Projections are based on trends in three main variables: population components, services provided *per capita* and num-

Table 20.3 Full-time equivalent RN supply and requirements: for the years 2000, 2010 and 2020 (in thousands)

	2000	2010	2020
Supply	1 624	1 621	1 403
Historical-trend-based requirements	1 967	2 142	2 278
Criteria-based requirements*	2 102	–	–

* Based on 'lower-bound' projections, using more constrained criteria than 'upper-bound' projections. Projections for 2010 and 2020 are not available.

Source: US Department of Health and Human Services (1990) *Seventh Report to the President and Congress on the Status of Health Personnel in the United States.* Washington D.C.: GPO.

bers of full-time equivalent RNs and LPNs per unit of service provided. Among the various data sources needed for these projections the sample surveys of RNs play an important role.

The other approach to projecting requirements is the criteria-based model. The focus here is on the number of nursing personnel according to educational level needed to meet particular nursing service goals. Essentially this model is an elaboration of the methodology employed in the state surveys of needs and resources and used on a partial basis to make national estimates by the Surgeon General's Consultant Group on Nursing and more completely in the project by the Western Interstate Commission on Highest Education, WICHE project in the 1970s. Also called a 'professional judgement' model, the criteria-based approach requires a panel of experts to determine the projection criteria, namely nursing service goals and levels of educational preparation goals. Three sets of goals have been produced for applying the criteria-based model on the national level, the first by a panel of experts convened in 1977 as part of the WICHE project, the second in 1980 and the latest in 1984, which has made projections for the years 1990 and 2000. Although the national panels of experts prepared projections for the states a number of states have used their own panels of experts to arrive at state-specific criteria-based projections. The recently completed study by the Mid-Atlantic Regional Nurses Association is an example.

COMPARISON OF PROJECTIONS

Table 20.3 summarizes national projections for supply and requirements, comparing for the latter the historical trend-based and the criteria-based projections. For both 1990 and 2000 the criteria-based projections indicate a shortage of RNs and a surplus of LPNs. The historical trend-based projections show a surplus of both categories. An important difference between the two requirements' projection is the higher number of nurses for nursing homes and community health according to the criteria-based model. This model also projected higher numbers of nurses in hospitals. Considering the striking changes taking place in the health care industry the criteria-based model, which looks to the future, may indeed be more realistic than the trend-based model, which gives considerable attention to the past.

Part Five

Conclusions

21
Conclusions

The purpose of this book was to present the salient features of the nursing systems of the UK, Canada and the US. A concise overview was presented of the history of nursing – the evolution of education, practice, research and planning – in the three countries. Since these countries have significantly different health systems the book's authors attempted to reveal differences, if any, in the way nursing has evolved and how it is practised, which may be related to the nature of the health systems.

There is a timeliness to the discussion of comparative health systems. In many countries throughout the world there is considerable concern about such fundamental issues as the escalating costs of health care and the efficacy and effectiveness of this care. In the US for example, health care costs have risen to 12% of the gross national product, the highest percentage in the world. Yet the efficacy and the equity of this expenditure are questionable. A high proportion of Americans are dissatisfied with their health care because of fragmented services and questionable outcomes from highly technological and expensive care. Moreover at least 30 million people in the US have no health insurance and face formidable barriers to access to health care. And the number of people in this plight is growing. In the past year much attention has been given in the US to examination of other health systems, especially Canada's system of national health insurance, as possible directions in which the US should go.

While physicians and politicians play major decision making roles in shaping, directing and changing a nation's health system, it is the profession of nursing that is the dominant group of health care providers in the three countries studied in this book, as well as in most countries throughout the world. It has been said, for example, that hospitals exist primarily to provide nursing care to the sick. Thus study of the role of nursing within the context of a health care system is important to an understanding of the system and assessing its advantages and disadvantages, especially as it might be applied from one country to another.

In an orderly and logical way this book presents a survey of the essential characteristics of nursing in the three countries. It was the original intention to present in the closing pages of the book an in-depth analysis of these differences and similarities in the health systems, which range from one heterogeneous, largely private system (US) to a homogeneous, nationalized health service (UK). The analysis has been limited, however, by the unavailability of timely and comparable data on such important topics as job satisfaction, career development and cost-effectiveness of nursing services. These are important topics for further research. The information presented in this book can serve as a valuable backdrop to such research.

From the data presented in this book it is possible to draw some conclusions about the similarities and dissimilarities among the three systems and to make a few generalizations about which aspects might be usefully applied from one country to another. However it is clear that there are more similarities than differences, notwithstanding major differences in the health systems of the three countries. The nursing systems of the UK, Canada and the US are similar in the way nurses are educated, the way in which nursing is organized and practised and the direction in which the profession is moving. Moreover the socio-demographic characteristics of nurses in the three countries, for example the predominance of middle class women, are similar. In the broadest outlines it is difficult to see the impact of the varying health systems on nursing, although obviously differences do exist.

This chapter will present the major similarities in the characteristics of nursing in the three countries, the major differences, and an assessment of characteristics that might be beneficially transferred from one country to another, and will conclude with recommendations for future studies.

SIMILARITIES IN NURSING

The three countries, in addition to having a common language (French is also an official language in Canada), a democratic system of government, an educated population and reasonably high standards of living for most citizens, have evolved nursing systems strongly influenced by the teachings of Florence Nightingale. To a greater or lesser extent all three countries are moving away, some say liberating themselves, from strict adherence to Miss Nightingale's influences.

While the UK still largely prepares nurses in the system proposed by Nightingale, in which students serve as apprentices and much of the education is provided in hospitals, there are indications that the future will see a change towards moving nursing education into academic institutions, as is happening in Canada and the US. In the US 35% of all employed registered nurses (RNs) hold at least a bachelor's degree from a college or university. In Canada the figure is 12%, and in the UK only 5% of registered nurses hold college or university degrees. The UKCC's Project 2000 report (United Kingdom Central Council for Nursing, Midwifery and Health Visiting, 1986) would significantly reduce the service contribution of students as well as advancing the academic validity of nursing education. Reports by the Royal College of Nursing (RCN) and English National Board (ENB) recommend transferring nursing education into the mainstream of higher education, as is occurring in Canada and the US. Entry into practice for professional nurses in the future will likely be a baccalaureate degree in all three countries, although this will be likely to occur later in the UK than in the others.

Nursing roles in the three countries are expanding, although the largest share of nurses, 65–80%, are still employed in acute care settings in hospitals, many in staff nurse positions. Advanced nursing and specialized roles such as nurse practitioners, nurse clinicians and clinical nurse specialists are proliferating, particularly in Canada and the US. An increasing proportion of these nurses are employed in ambulatory care settings. Moreover nurses are assuming a greater number of administrative and managerial positions.

The impact of technology on nursing is substantial in all three countries. Although especially notable in the US, critical care units have increased in number, requiring a high intensity of nursing care and knowledge of complex equipment.

Public health and community health nursing, with emphasis on health promotion and disease prevention, are receiving more attention, although less than 10% of the total nursing workforce in the three countries is employed in these important specialties.

Shortages of nurses are, to a greater or lesser extent, prevalent in all three countries. Demographics have played a role in this situation. Declining birthrates, beginning in the late 1960s, have reduced the pool of applicants to nursing schools. Also employment opportunities for women have expanded in many fields, making recruitment into nursing more difficult. Demand for nursing is also increasing at a time when growth in supply has slowed down. The ageing of the population in all three countries is an important factor in increased demand; technological advance is another.

Concern with rising costs of health care, especially in the US, has stimulated cost-containment efforts. In the US the concept of 'managed care' and the growth of health maintenance organizations have changed, although in a limited way, the free-wheeling nature of the health care delivery system. Also controls in the US over hospital charges and physicians' fees, which are being implemented for older patients insured by the federal government, brings the health system a little closer to the Canadian system.

Nursing research in the three countries has expanded from very modest beginnings and has moved from preoccupation with 'management improvement' type studies that focused on issues of nursing organization, workload and staffing to clinically-orientated studies based on nursing theories and models that are attempting to lay down the scientific basis of nursing.

Concern with professional issues is high in the three countries. These include the aforementioned 'entry into practice' debate and moving nursing education into the mainstream of higher education. Another concern is the quality of nursing care – how to measure it and how to improve it. The standards of nursing service and nursing education have undoubtedly been raised by the emphasis on quality in these areas.

DISSIMILARITIES IN NURSING

The many obvious dissimilarities among the nursing systems of the three countries are largely superficial and are due to the different stages of development. For example in the UK the nursing service to patients that students provide is an integral part of their educational experience. In the US and Canada the apprenticeship model was eliminated after the Second World War and very few hospital-based schools of nursing remain. Project 2000 will bring the UK closer to the US and Canada, although this will create serious funding and manpower problems as replacements for student services will be required. The greater rapidity with which both Canada and the US were able to change from apprenticeship to educational models might well be due to less involvement of government in the area of direct services to patients, the greater availability of and 'easier' entry to institutions of advanced education, the less entrenched notions of the Nightingale model of nursing and consequent agressiveness of nurses to share in the direction of their 'destinies', and the greater availability of funding for nursing education. Also the apparent greater resistance to change found in the UK might be explained by its structure of society, as opposed to those in Canada and the US.

Another difference is the greater number of nurse-midwives in the UK compared to Canada and the US. In recent years midwifery has been growing in the latter countries due, in part, to the recognition that nurse-midwives are a valuable resource for care in underserved areas. Another difference that will become less striking in the future is the larger proportion of nurses with formal postgraduate education in the US compared to the UK and Canada. Over 6% of employed US nurses have postgraduate degrees, including nearly 5000 with doctorates (there are 46 doctoral programmes). Postgraduate education for nurses in Canada is expanding: 2000 nurses have earned master's degrees and the first doctoral programme in nursing was recently established. In the US the greater number of postgraduate courses is probably due, oddly enough,

Dissimilarities in nursing

to the direct intervention and funding of the government. Politically US nurses have pushed hard for increased funding resources in this area. Although postgraduate education for nurses in the UK lags behind, efforts by the RCN and ENB, as well as the impact Project 2000, should help to close the gap. Canada and the UK also differ from the US in the funding of nursing education. Their nursing schools are publicly funded whereas in the US one third of all nursing education programmes are privately funded.

Even when differences in the supply of nurses are examined, what first appear to be differences become less so when the situation is more thoroughly investigated. Because of differences in the way data are collected, including varying definitions of the registered nurse as well as the timing of data collection, it is difficult to make precise comparisons of the nursing supply in the three countries. The best estimate of the number of employed registered nurses (full-time equivalents) per 100 000 population in the three countries is:

UK	263*
Canada	570**
US	546**

* Includes registered nurses and health visitors.
** Includes only registered nurses.

These data reveal that the US and Canada employ twice as many RNs *per capita* as the UK. One explanation for this seeming difference is the shorter length of stay of patients in acute care hospitals in Canada and the US than in the UK. Thus, on a given day, a patient doubtless has more intense need for nursing care in these countries than in the UK. Another explanation is the need to consider the mix of nursing personnel who provide nursing services. If enrolled nurses are added to the registered nurse population in the UK and their equivalents in Canada (nursing assistants) and the US (licensed practical nurses), the following numbers of nursing personnel (full-time equivalents) per 100 000 population become:

UK	399
Canada	887
US	686

This makes the quantitative nursing manpower picture more dissimilar among the three countries. To bring it a little closer it is necessary to account for all personnel who provide nursing services, including students, pupils and unqualified personnel in the UK, orderlies in Canada and nursing aides and orderlies in the US. The numbers of total nursing personnel per 100 000 population are estimated as follows:

UK	690
Canada	1001
US	847

Another view of the difference in nursing manpower is to estimate numbers of nurses in community health work – district nursing in the UK. This comparison reveals the varying emphases on services provided in non-institutionalized settings. Although the largest share of nursing manpower in each country is found in hospitals, including acute and long-term care settings, there is a growing proportion who work in the community setting. As the following figures show Canada has the highest per 100 000 population number of community-orientated nurses, and the UK the least, by a considerable margin:

UK	17
Canada	52
US	38

To characterize the three nursing systems is to say first that there are many similarities between Canada and the US. These include the trend over the past 30 years towards the movement of nursing education into higher education and the credentialling of an increasing number of nurses with academic degrees. Canada and the US are similar in the volume of nursing resources that are available relative to their populations as well as in levels of pay and benefits, which have increased in recent years.

Although the impact of the different health systems on nursing cannot be precisely described by currently available data, a few generalizations are possible:

1. There is greater homogeneity in training, registering, staffing, management and distribution of nurses in the UK under the National Health Service, practically the sole employer of nurses, than in the US and Canada. Some diversity does exist among the four countries comprising the UK, but they are alike in many fundamental ways.
2. Change in the system of nursing is probably slower to occur in the UK because unified control of the health system may not permit as much experimentation with alternative ways of delivering service as in the more widely diverse US environment.
3. There is very likely to be a closer relationship between nursing service and nursing education in the UK and Canada than in the US, although an effort has been made in the US in recent years to foster coordination of service and education through interchanges of staff and other programmes.
4. Although health care expenditure *per capita* varies considerably all

countries are concerned with rising health care costs. Shortages of nursing personnel exist under the different health systems. With increasing demands for health care in the future nursing shortages will continue.
5. Awareness has increased of the importance of programmes of health promotion and disease prevention in improving health status and reducing needs for health care. Nurses can play a significant role in these programmes even though the major emphasis continues to be on acute care.

This book has presented a survey of nursing in three countries, not an in-depth analysis. Only original research can address the numerous, important and provocative issues and questions suggested by this survey. The book, therefore, concludes with a list of topics that could profitably serve as the basis for further research:

1. Differences in the socioeconomic backgrounds of students recruited into schools of nursing;
2. Differences in job stability and job satisfaction;
3. The political activity of nurses;
4. The productivity of nurses;
5. Variations in the quality of nursing care;
6. The trend towards specialization in nursing and its impact on primary care;
7. The use of innovative nursing models;
8. Relationships between nurses and doctors and other health care providers;
9. The impact of longer lengths of stay in acute care hospitals in the UK and Canada;
10. The relationship between costs and benefits of nursing care;
11. The impact of public funding on nursing education and research.

References

Abdellah, F.G. and Levine, E. (1965) *Better Patient Care Through Nursing Research*. New York: Macmillan.

Able Smith, B. (1960) *A History of the Nursing Profession*. London: Heinemann.

Able Smith, B. (1978) *NHS The First Thirty Years*.

Advisory Committee on Nursing Manpower (1980) *Report on Nursing Manpower*. Ontario: Ministry of Health.

Advisory Committee on Nursing Workforce (1988) *Report of the Advisory Committee on Nursing Workforce* (2 vols.). St. John's: Newfoundland Minister of Health and Newfoundland Hospital and Nursing Home Association.

Agnew, G.H. (1974) *Canadian Hospitals 1920 to 1970*. Toronto: University of Toronto Press.

Alberta Association of Registered Nurses (AARN) and Alberta Hospital Association (AHA) Joint Committee on Nursing Manpower Issues (1985) *Position Paper on Quality of Working Life*. AARN and AHA, Edmonton, Alberta.

Alberta Association of Registered Nurses (1991) PhD in Nursing Approved, *AARN Newsletter*, **47** (1): 5.

Alexander, M.F. (1980) *Nurse Education. An Experimentation in the Integration of Theory and Practice in Nursing*. PhD thesis, University of Edinburgh.

Allemang, M. (1986) The development in ideas of nursing education in Canada. In: J. Allen and M.F. Thibaudeau (eds.), *Proceedings of the Colloquium on Nursing Research*, Pt. 1, McGill University, Montreal, pp. 5–22.

Allemang, M. and Cahoon, M.C. (1974) Nursing education research in Canada. In: J.J. Fitzpatrick and R.L. Taunton (eds.), *Annual Review of Nursing Research*, vol. 4, Springer Publishing Company, New York, pp. 261–78.

Allen, M. (1982a) Design to evaluate a model of nursing across primary care settings: a comparative systems approach. In: J.O. Godden and M.C. Cahoon (eds.), *Decision-Making in Nursing Research. Proceedings of the Third National Conference on Research in Nursing*, University of Toronto, Toronto, pp. 27–47.

Allen, M. (1982b) A model for nursing: a plan for research development.

In: *Research – A Base for the Future: Proceedings of the 1981 International Conference*, Edinburgh, Scotland, September 1981, University of Edinburgh, Edinburgh, pp. 315–30.

Allen, M. (1986a) The relationships between graduate teaching and research in nursing. In: S.M. Stinson and J.C. Kerr (eds.), *International Issues in Nursing Research*, Croom Helm, London, pp. 151–67.

Allen, M. (1986b) The contribution of nursing to science in Canada. In: K. King, E. Prodrick and B. Bauer (eds.), *Nursing Research: Science for Quality Care, Proceedings of the 10th National Research Conference*, April 9–11, University of Toronto, Toronto, pp. 5–14.

Allen, M. and Reidy, M. (1971) *Learning: The First Five Years of the Ryerson Nursing Program*, Toronto. Registered Nurses Association of Ontario.

Allen, M. and Thibaudeau, M.F. (eds.) (1973) *Actes du colloque sur la recherche infirmière, 1973*. Montreal: Université de McGill. (Also available in English by the same authors.)

Allessandro, E.J. (1988) Comparable worth and nursing. *Nursing Management*, December 19(12): 72I–72J, 72L, 72N–72P.

American Hospital Association, *Summary Report and Recommendations*, AHA Chicago, USA.

American Nurses' Association (1965) *Position Paper on Education for Nursing*. New York: American Nurses' Association.

American Nurses' Association (1985) *Facts About Nursing 84–85*. Kansas City: American Nurses' Association.

Anderson, O.W. (1984) Health services in the US. In: T.J. Litman and L.S. Robins, *Health Politics and Policy*, John Wiley, New York, pp. 67–80.

Arnett, R.H., Cowell, C.S., Doridoff, L.M. and Freeland, M.S. (1985) Health spending in the 1980s: adjusting to financial incentives, *Health Care Financing Review*, **6**, 1–26.

Armer Committee (1955) Working party on the training of District Nurses. Report from the Ministry of Health, Scotland.

Athlone Committee Report (1939) Inter departmental Committee on Nursing Services, HMSO, London.

Attridge, C. and Callahan, M. (1987) *Women in Women's Work: Nurses' Perspectives on Quality Work Environments* (Research Report #1). University of Victoria, Faculty of Human and Social Development, Victoria.

Award, D., Griener, G., Langstaff, J. (1985) Hospital ethics Committees: survey reveals characteristics. *Dimensions*, **62**.

Baly, M. (1977a) *Nursing Past into Present*. London: Bostford.
Baly, M. (1977b) *Nursing and Social Change*, London: Heinemann.
Baly, M. (1980) *Nursing and Social Change* (2nd edn.) Heinemann, London.
Barnard, K. (1984) Nursing research related to infants and young chil-

dren. In: H.H. Werley and J.J. Fitzpatrick (eds.), *Annual Review of Nursing Research*, vol. 1, Springer Publishing Company, New York, pp. 3–25.
Baumgart, A.J. (1988) The nursing workforce in Canada. In: A.J. Baumgart and Larsen (eds.), *Canadian Nursing Faces the Future; Development and Change*, Moseby, Toronto, pp. 39–62.
Bendall, E.R.D. (1975) *So You Passed Nurse. An Exploration of Some of the Assumptions on Which Written Examinations Are Based.* London: Royal College of Nursing.
Bendall, E.R.D. and Raybould, E.A. (1969) *A History of the GNC for England and Wales.* London: H.K. Lewis.
Besel, L. (1985) CNA Connection. *The Canadian Nurse*, **81** (6): 7.
Bethune, P. (1991) Personal communication, Ontario Ministry of Health.
Bisson, A. (1991) Personal communication, Canadian Nurses Foundation.
Bonds (1984) Provision of nursing care to elderly people in nursing homes, Newcastle upon Tyne Polytechnic, UK.
Brown, E.L. (1948) *Nursing for the Future*, Russel Sage Foundation, New York.
Brimmer P. (1986) The American Nurses' Association: its role in research. In: S.M. Stinson and J.C. Kerr (eds.), *International Issues in Nursing*, Croom Helm, London, pp. 289–312.
Buchan, W. (1771) *Domestic Medicine or the Family Physician*, 2nd edn. Thomas Dobson, Philadelphia.
Burdett, H.C. (1901) *Burdett's Annual*. London:
Burdett, H.C. (1905) *Selection Committee on Registration*, London.
Burgess, M.A. (1928) *Nurses, Patients and Pocketbooks, Committee on the Grading of Nursing Schools.* National League for Nursing Education, New York.

Cahoon, M.M. (1986) Research developments in clinical settings: a Canadian perspective. In: S.M. Stinson and J.C. Kerr (eds.), *International Issues in Nursing Research*, Croom Helm, London, pp. 182–204.
Canada Health Act (1984) Ottawa: Health and Welfare Canada. Canada (1972–73). *The Community Health Centre in Canada*, vols. 1–3 (Hastings Report). Ottawa: Information Canada.
Canada 1981 Major Causes of Death (1986) Health and Welfare Canada, Ottawa.
Canada Health Manpower Inventory (1984) Ottawa: Health and Welfare, National Health and Welfare Canada.
Canadian Council on Hospital Accreditation (1983) *Aims and Objectives*. Ottawa: Canadian Council on Hospital Accreditation.

Canadian Council on Hospital Accreditation (1984) *Standards for Accreditation of Canadian Health Care Facilities*. Ottawa: Canadian Council on Hospital Accreditation.

Canadian Hospital Directory (1988) Ottawa: Canadian Hospital Association.

The Canadian Nurse (1986) CNA's Ginette Rodger appointed to MRC. *The Canadian Nurse*, **82**: 12.

Canadian Nurses Association (1978) *Position Statement on the Clinical Nurse Specialist*. Ottawa: Canadian Nurses Association.

Canadian Nurses Association (1979) *National Seminar on Doctoral Preparation for Canadian Nurses*. Ottawa: Canadian Nurses Association.

Canadian Nurses Association (1980) *A Definition of Nursing Practice and Standards for Nursing Practice*. Ottawa: Canadian Nurses Association.

Canadian Nurses Association (1982a) *Entry to Practice of Nursing: A Background Paper*. Ottawa: Canadian Nurses Association.

Canadian Nurses Association (1982b) *Nursing in Canada*. Ottawa: Canadian Nurses Association.

Canadian Nurses Association (1982c) *Role of the RNA – A Response to the Task Force*. Ottawa: Canadian Nurses Association.

Canadian Nurses Association (1982d) *Statement on Physician Assistants*. Ottawa: Canadian Nurses Association.

Canadian Nurses Association (1983a) *Ethical Guidelines for Nursing Research Involving Human Subjects*. Ottawa: Canadian Nurses Association.

Canadian Nurses Association (1983b) *Position Paper on the Role of the Nurse Administrator and Standards for Nursing Administration*. Ottawa: Canadian Nurses Association.

Canadian Nurses Association (1984a) *Biennial Meeting Folio of Reports*. Ottawa: Canadian Nurses Association.

Canadian Nurses Association (1984b) *Brief to the House of Commons Standing Committee on Health, Welfare and Social Affairs in Response to the Proposed Canada Health Act 1984*. Ottawa: Canadian Nurses Association.

Canadian Nurses Association (1984c) *Entry to Practice Newsletter*, **1** (1): 1–5.

Canadian Nurses Association (1984d) *Entry to Practice Newsletter*, **1** (3): 1–2.

Canadian Nurses Association (1984e) *Entry to Practice Newsletter*, **1** (5).

Canadian Nurses Association (1984f) *Entry to Practice Newsletter*, **1** (14).

Canadian Nurses Association (1984g) *Entry to Practice Newsletter*, **1** (15).

Canadian Nurses Association (1984h) *Exploring the Future of Hospitals in Canada: A Definition Study*. Ottawa: Canadian Nurses Association.

Canadian Nurses Association (1984i) *A Five-Year Plan for the Development of Nursing Research in Canada*. Ottawa: Canadian Nurses Association.

Canadian Nurses Association (1984j) *Position Paper on Specialist Roles in Maternal – Infant Nursing*. Ottawa: Canadian Nurses Association.

Canadian Nurses Association (1984k) *Research Imperative for Nursing in Canada: A Five-Year Plan Towards the Year 2000*. Ottawa: Canadian Nurses Association.

Canadian Nurses Association (1985a) *Approximate Union Membership and Membership Dues*. Ottawa: Canadian Nurses Association.

Canadian Nurses Association (1985b) *Canadian Hospital Inventory*. Ottawa: Canadian Nurses Association.

Canadian Nurses Association (1985c) *Code of Ethics for Nursing*. Ottawa: Canadian Nurses Association.

Canadian Nurses Association (1985d) *Compilation of Information on Nursing Research Committees*. Unpublished report.

Canadian Nurses Association (1985e) *A National Plan for Nursing Administration in Canada*. Ottawa: Canadian Nurses Association.

Canadian Nurses Association (1985f) *Nursing Programs and Entrance Requirements at Canadian Universities*. Ottawa: Canadian Nurses Association.

Canadian Nurses Association (1985g) *Sources of Funds for Nursing Education, Nursing and Health-Related Research Projects*. Ottawa: Canadian Nurses Association.

Canadian Nurses Association (1986a) *Biennial Meeting Folio of Reports*. Ottawa: Canadian Nurses Association.

Canadian Nurses Association (1986, 1987) *Index of Canadian Nursing Research/Index de Recherche Infirmière au Canada*. Ottawa: Canadian Nurses Association.

Canadian Nurses Association (1987) *Entry to Practice Newsletter*, **1** (7).

Canadian Nurses Association (1988a) *Biennial Meeting Folio of Reports*. Ottawa: Canadian Nurses Association.

Canadian Nurses Association (1988b) *Nursing in Canada*. Ottawa: Canadian Nurses Association.

Canadian Nurses Association (1988c) *Position Paper on the Role of the Nurse Administrator and Standards for Nursing Administration*. Ottawa: Canadian Nurses Association.

Canadian Nurses Association (1989) *Objectives and Activities for Entry to Practice for 1989*. Ottawa: Canadian Nurses Association.

Canadian Nurses Association (1990) *Canadian Nurses Association: Research Imperative for Nursing in Canada. The Next Five Years 1990–1995*. Ottawa: Canadian Nurses Association.

CAPNA Special Committee (1984) *The Present and Future of the Practical Nurse/Nursing Assistant in the Canadian Health Care System*. CAPNA, Ottawa.

Central Policy Unit, The Citizen's Charter (1991) HMSO, London.

Carson, R., McGuire, B. and Lamb, C. (1987) *Descriptive Study of Demographic Characteristics and Job Satisfaction of British Columbia Registered Nurses with Three Educational Backgrounds.* Vancouver: Registered Nurses Association of British Columbia.

Chadwick, E. (1842) *The Sanitary Conditions of the Labouring Population of Great Britain.*

Clark, K. (1986) *Midwifery: A CNO Policy Background Paper.* Toronto: Toronto College of Nurses.

Clark, W. (1985) New computers at Toronto General could replace doctor's hospital charts. *Globe and Mail*, November 27, p. A10.

Cole, D. and Postgate, R. (1961) *The Common People.* London: Methuen & Co.

College of Nurses (1985) *The Standards and Levels of Nursing Practice Including the Assumptive Base: A Discussion Paper.* Toronto: College of Nurses.

Collinge, J. (1988) *Report on Nursing Manpower, Retention and Turnover in Hospitals of the M.J.H.I. with Recommendations.* Montreal: Task Force on Nursing Manpower, Montreal Joint Hospital Institute.

Committee on the Grading of Nursing Schools (1934) *Nursing Schools – Today and Tomorrow.* New York: Committee on the Grading of Nursing Schools.

Committee for the Study of Nursing Education (1923) *Nursing and Nursing Education in the United States.* New York: Macmillan.

Conroy, D.M. and Hibberd, J.M. (1983) Areas of Cooperation and conflict between nursing associations and negotiating bodies. In: International Council of Nurses, *Cooperation and Conflict*, International Council of Nurses, Geneva.

Council for Nursing Assistants (1987) *Task Force Report on the Present and Future Role of the Nursing Assistant.* St. John's, Newfoundland: Council for Nursing Assistants.

Crichton, A. (1981) *Health Policy Making. Fundamental Issues in the United States, Canada, Great Britain, Australia.* Ann Arbor, MI: Health Administration Press.

Department of Health and Social Security, (1981) *Handbook of Policies and Priorities for the Health and Personal Social Services in England.* London: HMSO.

Department of Health and Social Security (1949) *Report of the Working Party on Midwives.* London: HMSO.

Department of Health and Social Security (1969) *Report of the Halsbury Committee.* London: HMSO.

Department of Health and Social Secuirty (1972) *Report of the Committee on Nursing* (Briggs Report). London: HMSO.

Department of Health and Social Security (1977a) *Extending Role of the*

Clinical Nurse – Legal Implications and Training Requirements, HC (77) 22. London: HMSO.

Department of Health and Social Security (1977b) *Nursing in Primary Health Care*. CNO(77)8. DHSS Chief Nursing Officer's Letter, London HMSO.

Department of Health and Social Security (1978) *NHS The First Thirty Years*. London: HMSO.

Department of Health and Social Security (1980) *Report of the Standing Commission on pay comparability. Report No. 3, Nurses and Midwives (Chairman: H.A. Clegg)*. London: HMSO.

Department of Health and Social Security (1983) Nurse Manpower Planning: Planning Approaches and Techniques, HMSO, London.

Department of Health and Social Security (1981) *Care in Action*. London: HMSO.

Department of Health and Social Security (1984) *Health and Personal Social Services Statistics*. London: HMSO.

Department of Health and Social Security (1984, 1985) *Performance Indicators*. London: HMSO.

Department of Health and Social Security (1986) *Neighbourhood Nursing. A Focus on Care* (Cumberlege Report). London: HMSO.

Department of Health – England (1991) The Health of the Nation, HMSO, London.

Department of Health – England (1989) Working for Patients, HMSO, London.

Department of Health, Working for Patients, Education and Training (1989).

Department of Health, The Patient's Charter (1991) HMSO, London.

Strategy for Nursing. Nursing Division Department of Health, 1989, London.

Department of Health and Social Services (1983) *Nurse Manpower Planning: Planning, Approaches and Techniques*. London: HMSO.

Department of Health and Social Services – Northern Ireland (1984) *Health and Personal Social Services Statistics*.

Department of Health and Social Services – *Nursing in the Eighties*. Chief Nursing Officer's Report.

Department of Health (1991) Using Information in Managing Nursing Resources, Nursing Division. London: HMSO.

Department of Health and Human Services (1972) *Planning for Nurses, Needs and Resources*, Washington DC: GPO.

Dick, D., Harris, B., Lehman, A. and Savage, R. (1985) *Getting into the Act: The Canadian Nurses' Experience*. Paper presented at the 18th Quadrennial Congress of the International Council of Nurses, Tel Aviv, Israel, June 15–21.

Donnison, J. (1977) *Midwives and Medical Men*. London: Heinemann.
The DPA Group Inc. (1987) *The Future of Nursing Assistants in New Brunswick*. Fredericton, Association of New Brunswick Registered Nursing Assistants.
Dunnell and Dobbs *Nursing Working in the Community*. London HMSO.

English National Board (1985) *Professional Education/Training Course, Consultation Paper*. London: ENB.
Etzone, A. (ed.) (1969) *The Semi-Profession and Their Organisations*. New York: Macmillan and Free Press.

Faux, S. (in press) *Nurse Researchers in Clinical Settings in Canada*. London, Ontario: University of Western Ontario.
Federal Security Agency (1948) *The Nations Health*, Washington DC: GPO.
Field, P.A. and Morse J.M. (1985) *Nursing Research: The Application of Qualitative Approaches*. London: Croom Helm.
Field, P.A. and Stinson, S.M. (1986) *A Beginning Survey of Selected Characteristics of Canadian Nursing Masters' Programs*. Unpublished thesis, Edmonton. School of Nursing, *University of Alberta*.
Flaherty, J. (1985) The future. In: *Introduction to Nursing Management: A Canadian Perspective*, Canadian Hospital Association, Ottawa, pp. 211–32.
Flaherty, M.J. (1979) *Employment for Registered Nurses in Canada: Current Status*. Ottawa: Canadian Hospital Association.
Flexner, A. (1910) *Medical Education in the United States and Canada*. Carnegie Foundation for the Advancement of Teaching, Bulletin no. 4, Washington, DC.
Flint, C. (1986) *Sensitive Midwives*, London: Heinemann.
Fortin, F., Taggart, M.E., and Kerouac, S. (1983) *Une Experience Assistée par Ordinateur D'Auto-apprentissage du Cours D'Introduction a la Recherche*. Montreal: Université de Montreal.
Fortin, F., Taggart, M.E., Gervais, N. and Kerouac, S. (1984a) *Introduction à la Recherche ERPO – SOI 3385. Module 1 – Le Problème*. Montreal: Université de Montreal.
Fortin, F., Taggart, M.E., Gervais, M. and Dalpe, M. (1984b) *Introduction à la Recherche ERPO – SOI 3386. Module 2 – La Recension des Ecrits*. Montreal: Université de Montreal.
Foucault, M. (1967) *Madness and Civilisation*.
Framework of Audit for Nursing Services, Nursing Division, Dept of Health 1991.
Frazer, D. (1973) *The Evolution of the British Welfare*. London: Macmillan.
Frazer, J.G. (1890) *The Golden Bough*, London: Macmillan. Reprinted 1981 by Avenel Books, New York.

Frazer, W.P. (1947) *Duncan of Liverpool*. London: Macmillan.
Fretwell, J.E. (1985) *Freedom to Change. The Creation of a Ward Environment*. Royal College of Nursing Research Series. London: Royal College of Nursing.

Gagnon, M. (1973) *Catalogue de L'expostion Commemorative du Tricentenaire de la Mort de Jeanne Mance, Fondatrice de L'Hotel Dieu de Montreal 1673–1973*. Montreal: McGill Press.
General Nursing Council Minutes (1949) London: General Nursing Council.
Gibbon, J.M. and Mathewson, M.S. (1947) *Three Centuries of Canadian Nursing*. Toronto: Macmillan.
Giovannetti, P. (1973) Measurement of patients' requirements for nursing services. In: E. Levine (ed.), *Research on Nurse Staffing in Hospitals*, Government Printing Office, Washington, DC, pp. 41–56.
Giovannetti, P. (1991) Nurse researchers (Letters/Courrier). *The Canadian Nurse*, **87** (2): 10.
Glass, H. (1985) *The Future of Health Care in Canada and Nursing's Role Within It: A Background Paper*. Ottawa: Canadian Nurses Association.
Gooden, J.O. and Cahoon, M.C. (eds.) (1974) *Decision-making in Nursing Research, Proceedings of the Third National Conference on Research in Nursing*. Toronto: University of Toronto, Faculty of Nursing.
Gornick, M., Greenberg, J.N., Eggers, P.W. and Dobson, A. (1986) Twenty years of Medicare and Medicaid. *Health Care Financing Review 1985 Annual Supplement*. Washington DC: GPO.
Gosselin, R. (1984) Decentralization/reorganization in health care: the Quebec experience. *Health Care Management Review*, Winter.
Grantham, M.A. and Allan P. (1986) *The Clinical Promotion Project Between the Nursing Divisions of the Victoria General Hospital and the University of Alberta Hospital, Edmonton*. Paper presented at the Second National Joint Conference for Nurses in Education, Administration and Continuing Education, Ottawa, January 29–31.
Gray, C. (1985) Doctors and health insurance: the British experience. *Canadian Med Assoc J*, **132**: 442–4, 447–8.
Griffin, G.J. and Griffin, J.K. (1969) *Jensen's History and Trends of Professional Nursing*, 6th edn. Saint Louis, MO: C.V. Mosby Co.

Hacker, C. (1974) *The Indomitable Doctors*. Toronto: Clarke Irwin.
Hamrin, E. (ed.) (1983) Research: a challenge for nursing practice. In: *Proceedings of the Fifth Workgroup of European Nurse Researchers Meetings, Uppsala, Sweden, August 11–14, 1982*. Uppsala: Swedish Nurses' Association.

Hansard, R. (1985) *Chief Officer Career Profile*, Institute of Manpower Studies Report III. Brighton: University of Sussex.
Hartley, K. and Goodwin, L. (1985) The Exchequer Cost of Nurse Training, University of York.
Hastings, J. et al. (1981) Canadian health administrators study. *Canadian Journal of Public Health*, **71** suppl. 1.
Hastings, J.E.F. (1985) Canada's health care system. In: *Introduction to Nursing Management: A Canadian Perspective*, Canadian Hospital Association, Ottawa, pp. 1–38.
Hastings, J.E.F. and Mosley, W. (1966) *Organized Community Health Services (A Special Study for the Royal Commission on Health Services*. Queen's Printer, Toronto, Canada.
Hastings, J.E.F. and Vayda, E. (1984) Health service organization and delivery: promise and reality. In: *Proceedings of Health Policy Conference on the Canadian Health Care System*, Banff Centre of School of Management, Banff, Alberta, August.
Hayward, J. (1975) Information – a prescription against pain. Royal College of Nursing, London.
Health and Personal Social Services Statistics (1986).
Henderson, V. (1984) Personnal communication.
Hodgson, M. and Ormerod, C. (1985) Case mix management – management tool of the future? *The Canadian Nurse*, **81**: 10.
House of Commons Select Committee on the Registration of Nurses. Report, proceedings and minutes of evidence 1904–1905.
House of Commons (1986) *Debate on the National Health Service (Management)* Official Report no. 14, March, 1986, London: HMSO.
Hutt, R. (1985) *Chief Officer Career Profile*, Institute of Manpower Studies Report III. Brighton: University of Sussex.

Imai, R. (1981) *Today's Realities: Who Requires Care – Who Provides Care? Background paper for the Taskforce on the Role of the RN*. Toronto: College of Nurses of Ontario.
Institute of Medicine (1983) *Nursing and Nursing Education: Public patients and private actions*, National Academy of Sciences, Washington DC.
International Labour Organisation (1981) *Nursing Personnel Recommendation*. Geneva: International Labour Organisation.

Jacobsen, A., of Mercer/Hickling Johnston (1986) *Final Report: Utilization of Registered Nursing Assistants in Alberta*. Edmonton: Alberta Association of Registered Nursing Assistants.
Johns, E. and Pfefferkorn, B. (1934) *An Activity Analysis of Nursing*. New York: Committee on the Grading of Nursing Schools.

Jones, K. (1953) *Lunacy Law and Conscience*. London: Routledge and Kegan Paul.

Kahn, J. and Westley, W.A. (1984) *The Working Environment in Canadian Hospitals: Constraints and Opportunities*. Government of Canada, Ministry of Labour, Ottawa, Canada.

Kalish, P.A. and Kalish, B.J. (1978) *The Advance of American Nursing*. Boston: Little, Brown.

Kalish, P.A. and Kalish, B.J. (1982) *Politics of Nursing*. Philadelphia: Lippincott.

Keddy, W. and Wolnik, S. (1985) Monitoring and evaluating organizational effectiveness. In: *Introduction to Nursing Management: A Canadian Perspective*, Canadian Hospital Association, Ottawa, pp. 125–47.

Kerr, J.C. (1986) Structure and funding of nursing research in Canada. In: S.M. Stinson and J.C. Kerr (eds.), *International Issues in Nursing Research*, Croom Helm, London, pp. 97–112.

Kerr, J.C. (1978) *Financing University Nursing Education in Canada*. Unpublished PhD thesis, University of Michigan, Ann Arbor, MI.

Kikuchi, J.F. and Simmons, H. (1986) A science in jeopardy. In: K. King, E. Prodick and B. Bauer (eds.), *Nursing Research: Science for Quality Care*, University of Toronto, Faculty of Nursing, Toronto, pp. 28–31.

King, F. (ed. (1971) *First National Conference on Research in Nursing Practice: Proceedings of the [First] National Nursing Research Conference, Ottawa, February 16–18, 1971*. Vancouver: School of Nursing, University of British Columbia.

King, K., Prodrick, E. and Bauer, B. (eds.) (1986) *Nursing Research: Science for Quality Care. Proceedings of the Tenth National Nursing Research Conference, Toronto, April 9–11, 1985*. Toronto: Faculty of Nursing, University of Toronto.

Klein, R. (1985) Why Britain's Conservatives support a socialist health care system. *Health Affairs*, **4**: 44.

Kogan, M. and Henkel, N. (1983) *Government and Research: The Rothschild Experiment in a Government Department*. London: Heinemann.

Kratz C.R. (1978) *Care of the Long-Term Sick in the Community, Particularly Patients with Stroke*. Edinburgh: Churchill Livingstone.

Kravitz, M. and Laurin, J. (eds.) (1984) *La Recherche Infirmière au Service de la Pratique. Actes du 9e Colloque· National, 12, 13, et 14 Octobre, 1983*. Montreal: McGill University School of Nursing.

Lalonde, M. (1974) *A New Perspective on the Health of Canadians*. Ottawa: Information Canada.

Lamb, A.M. (1977) Baillier and Tindall, Primary Health Nursing, a

description of the work of HV.DN domestic midwives and school nurses.
Lamb, M. (1981) *Nursing Education in Canada and the Canadian Nurses Association: An Historical Abstract.* Ottawa: Canadian Nurses Association.
Lamb, M. and Stinson, S.M. (1991) *Canadian Nursing Doctoral Statistics: 1989 Update.* Toronto: Canadian Nurses Association.
Larsen, J. and Stinson, S.M. (1979) *Canadian Nursing Doctoral Statistics, 1979.* A Report to the Policy Committee of the Kellogg National Seminar on Doctoral Preparation for Canadian Nurses.
Larsen, J. and Stinson, S.M. (1980) *Canadian Nursing Doctoral Statistics, 1980.* Toronto: Canadian Nurses Association.
Leatt, P. (1981) *Education for Nursing Administration in Canada: A Discussion Paper.* Ottawa: Canadian Nurses Association.
Leatt, P. (1982) Educational Preparation for nursing administration in Canada. *Health Management Forum.*
Leatt, P. (1985a) Management education for nurses in Canada. *Journal of Health Administration Education*, **3**: 3.
Leatt, P. (1985b) Management functions and roles. In: *Introduction to Nursing Management: A Canadian Perspective*, Canadian Hospital Association, Ottawa, pp. 53–790.
Leatt, P. **(1987)** *Medical Staff Organization in Canadian Hospitals* (1987) Toronto: University of Toronto.
Leatt, P. (1986) *Multi-institutional Arrangements in Ontario Hospitals.* Paper presented at the 8th Jean-Yves Rivard Colloqium, University of Montreal, October.
Lemieux-Charles, L. (1980) *A Blueprint for Nursing: A Report to the Council of the Colleges of Nurses.* Toronto: College of Nurses of Ontario.
Lemieux-Charles L. (1981) *Turnover Survey*, Toronto General Hospital, Toronto.
Lemieux-Charles, L. (1983) Nursing Staff Survey. Toronto: Toronto General Hospital.
Lemieux-Charles, L and Lamb, M. (1986) 'Addressing the Educational Needs of Nurse Administrators', *Dimensions in Health Service*, **63**, 13–15.
LeTouze, D. (1984) Hospital bed planning in Canada: a survey analysis. *International Journal of Health Services*, **14**: 105–26.
Levesque, L. (1981) Rehabilitation of the chronically-ill elderly: a method of operationalizing a conceptual model for nursing. In: R.C. MacKay and G. Zilm (eds.), *Research in Practice: Proceedings of the National Nursing Research Conference, October 22–24, 1980*, School of Nursing, Dalhousie University, Halifax, pp. 22–34.
Levine, E. and Wright, S. (1957) New ways to measure personnel turnover, **31**, 38–42.

Levine, E (1983a) Nursing in the UK and the USA. *Nursing Times*.
Levine, E. (1983b) *The Registered Nurse Supply and Nurse Shortage*. Background Paper to Institute of Medicine, National Academy of Sciences. Washington DC: National Academy Press.
Levine, E. (1985) Some issues in nursing productivity. In: F.A. Shaffer (ed.), *Costing Out Nursing: Pricing Our Product*, National League for Nursing, New York, pp. 237–53.
Levine, E and Abdellah, F.G. (1984) DRGs: a recent refinement to an old method. *Inquiry*, **21**: 105–12.
Levine, E. (ed.) (1973) *Research on Nurse Staffing in Hospitals*. Washington, DC: GPO.
Levit, K.R. Lazenby, H., Waldo, D.R. and Daridoff, L.M. (1985) National health expenditures, 1984. *Health Care Financing Review*, **7**: 1–35.
Levitt, R. and Wall, A. (1984) *The Reorganised National Health Service*, 3rd edn. London: Croom Helm.
Lomba (1977) *Primary Health Nursing*. London: Baillière Tindall.
Lovell, V. (1981) *I Care that VGH Nurses Care! A Case Study and Sociological Analysis of Nursing's Influence on the Health Care System*. Vancouver: In Touch Publications Ltd.
Lowry, B. (1983) Project overview and framework. *Dimensions*, **60**.

McGuire, J. (1977) *The Expanded Role of the Nurse*. Unpublished Paper Prepared for the Royal Commission on the National Health Service.
MacKay, R.C. and Zilm, G. (eds.) *Research in Practice: Proceedings of the National Nursing Research Conference, October 22–24, 1989*. Halifax: Dalhousie University, School of Nursing.
McKeown, T. (1976) *The Modum Rise of Population*. London: Arnold.
McKervill, H.W. (1985) Equal pay for work of equal value. *The Canadian Nurse*, **81** (7): 24–6.
MacPhail, J. (in press). International nursing research. *Journal of Professional Nursing*.
Manitoba Association of Licensed Practical Nurses (1989) *Future Practical Nursing Education*. Winnipeg: Manitoba Association of Licensed Practical Nurses.
Marshall, E.D. and Moses, E.B. (1965) *The Nation's Nurses Inventory of Professional Registered Nurses*. New York: American Nurses' Association.
Medical Research Council (1985) *Report of the MRC Working Group in Nursing Research*. Ottawa: Medical Research Council.
Medical Research Council (1986) *MRC Grants and Awards Guide: 1986–87*. Ottawa: Medical Research Council.
Medical Research Council (1990) *Report of the President, 1989–1990*. Ottawa: Medical Research Council.

Memorandum (1971)

Meltz, N. and Marzetti, J. (1988) *The Shortage of Registered Nurses: An Analysis in a Labour Market Context*. Toronto: Registered Nurses Association of Ontario.

Miller, L. (1951) Medical and hospital care in Newfoundland. *Canadian Medical Association Journal*, **64**: 52–5.

Ministère de la Santé et des Services Sociaux du Quebec (MSSSQ) (1987) *La main d'oeuvres en soins infirmiers. Rapport du comité d'etude*. Quebec: Ministère de la Santé et des Services Sociaux du Quebec.

Ministry of Health (1947) *Report of the Working Party on the Recruitment and Training of Nurses*. London: HMSO.

Ministry of Health (1953) Annual Report, London: HMSO.

Ministry of Health (1955) Working Party on the Training of District Nurses (Armer Committee) Report, Ministry of Health and Department of Health, Scotland.

Ministry of Health (1966) *Senior Nursing Staff*, Ministry of Health, London: HMSO.

Ministry of Health (1969) *Management Structure*, London: HMSO.

Ministry of Health (1969) *Management Structure in the Local Health Authority Nursing Service*. London: HMSO.

Ministry of Health of British Columbia (1983) *Diploma-Nurse – Baccalaureate Nurse: Is There a Difference? Report on a Descriptive Study of College R.N. Programs and the Generic B.S.N. Program*. Victoria: Ministry of Education.

Ministry of Health & Scottish Home and Health Department (1966) *Report of the Committee on Senior Nursing Staff* (The Salmon Report). London: HMSO.

Ministry of Labour (1990) *Policy Directions Amending the Pay Equity Act*. Ministry of Labour, Government of Ontario, Toronto.

Ministry of National Health and Welfare (1983) *Preserving Universal Medicine*. Ottawa: Ministry of National Health and Welfare.

Morgan, M., Colman, M. and Manning, N. (1985) *Sociological Approaches to Health and Medicine*. London: Croom Helm.

Mussallem, H.K. (1965) *Nursing Education in Canada*, Royal Commission on Health Services. Ottawa: Queen's Printer.

Mussallem, H.K. (1968) *The Lamp and the Leaf* Canadian Nurses Association, Ottawa.

Nasan, C. (1986) *Ontario Council on Community Health Accreditation*. Personal communication.

National Academy of Sciences, Institute of Medicine (1983) *Nursing and Nursing Education: Public Policies and Private Actions*. National Academy Press, Washington, D.C.

National Audit Office (1985) *Control of Nursing Manpower Report*. London: HMSO.
National Board of Prices and Incomes (1968) *Report, 1968* (Cmnd 3585).
National Commission for the Study of Nursing and Nursing Education (1970) An abstract for action, McGraw-Hill, New York.
National League for Nursing (1975) *Nurses for a Growing Nation*, National League for Nursing, New York.
National League for Nursing (1986) *Nursing Data Review 1986*. National League for Nursing, New York.
National League for Nursing (1990a) *Nursing Data Source*. New York: National League for Nursing.
National League for Nursing (1990b) *Nurses Student Census 1989*. National League for Nursing, New York.
National League for Nursing Education (1937) *A Study of the Nursing Service in Fifty Selected Hospitals*. The United Hospital Fund of New York, New York.
National League for Nursing Education (1948) *A Study of Nursing Service on One Children's and Twenty-One General Hospitals*. New York: National League for Nursing Education.
National Organization & Professional Health Workers and National Hospital Institute (1979) *Proceedings of the First Conference of European Nurse Researchers: Collaborative Research and its implementation in Nursing*. Utrecht: National Hospital Institutes of the Netherlands.
NGA Research Associates (1986) *Utilization of Certified Nursing Assistants in Saskatchewan*. Regina: Saskatchewan Nursing Assistant Association.
Norton, D. (1962) *An Investigation of Geriatric Nursing Problems in Hospitals*. National Corporation for the Care of Old People.
Norton, D. (1970) By accident or design? A study of equipment development in relation to basic nursing problems. ELS Livingstone, Edinburgh.
Nuffield Provincial Hospitals Trust (1953) *The Work of the Nurse in Hospital Wards*. Nuffield Provincial Hospitals Trust, London.
Nurses Association of New Brunswick (1988) *Presentation on Concerns of Nurses in New Brunswick to the Nursing Human Resources Advisory Committee*. Fredericton: Nurses Associations of New Brunswick.
Nurses and Midwives Whitley Council (1955) *Staff Side Minutes* (NMC43).
Nursing Studies Research Unit, University of Edinburgh (1982) *Research – A Base for the Future: Proceedings of the 1981 International Conference, Edinburgh, Scotland, September 1981*. Edinburgh: University of Edinburgh, Nursing Studies Research Unit.

Office of Population and Census Survey (1981) *Statistics Household Survey*

10% Sample. London: Office of Population and Census Survey (HMSO).

Office of Population and Census Survey (1984) *Household Survey 1% Sample*. London: Office of Population and Census Survey (HMSO).

Ontario Association of Registered Nursing Assistants (1985/6) *RNA Utilization*. Ottawa: Canadian Nurses Association, H.K. Mussallem Library.

Ontario Hospital Association (1985) *Nursing Manpower Survey 1985*. Ontario Hospital Association, Toronto.

Ontario Nurses Association (1982a) *The Role of the RNA – A Response to the Taskforce*. Toronto: Ontario Nurses Association.

Ontario Nurses Association (1982b) *Presentation to the Commission of Inquiry into Part-Time Work*. Toronto: Ontario Nurses Association.

Ontario Nurses Association (1982c) *Presentation to the Commission of Inquiry into Part-time Work*, ONA, Toronto.

O'Toole, J. (1981) *Making America Work: Productivity and Responsibility*. Continuum Publishing Co., New York.

Oulton, J. (1991) Personal communication, University of Toronto, Toronto.

Paech, G. (1986) *Bitter Memories and Legal Lessons*. An Address Given to the 1986 Graduating Class of Baccalaureate Nursing Students, University of Western Ontario, London, Ontario, Canada, March 7.

Parry-Jones, W.L. (1972) *The Trade in Lunacy*.

Pater, J. (1985) *The Making of the NHS*. London: Kings Fund.

Pay Equity Commission (1989) *Pay Equity in Ontario: Some Facts*. Ontario: Pay Equity Commission.

Payne, L. (1986) The meaning of health: a phenomenological perspective. In: K. King, E. Prodrick and B. Bauer (eds.), *Nursing Research: Science for Quality Care*, Faculty of Nursing, University of Toronto, Toronto, pp. 32–9.

Pembury, S.E.M. (1980) *The Ward Sister – Key to Nursing. A Study of the Organisation of Individualised Nursing*. RCN Research Series, London: Royal College of Nursing.

Performance Indicators (1984).

Pfefferkorn, B. and Rovetta, C. (1940) *Administrative Cost Analysis for Nursing Service and Nursing Education*. New York: National League for Nursing Education.

Poulton, K. (1981) *Perception of Wants and Needs by Nurses and Their Patients*. Unpublished PhD thesis, Surrey University.

Powell, E. (1976) *Medicine and Politics: 1975 and after*. Kent: Pitman Medical.

Prince, J.E. (1982) *Florence Nightingale's Reform of Nursing 1860–1887*, Unpublished PhD thesis, University of London.

Pringle, D. (1991) Personal communication, University of Toronto.
Public Service Alliance of Canada (1982) Technological change. *The Review*, **59** (2): 11.

RCN (1979) Extended Role of the Clinical Nurse, RCN, London.
Redfern (1991) *Nursing Elderly People*. Edinburgh: Churchill Livingston.
Registered Nurses Association of British Columbia (1987) *Registered Nurse Manpower Planning Guide*. Vancouver: Registered Nurses Association of British Columbia.
Registered Nurses Association of Ontario (1982a) *Background Paper on Baccalaureate Nursing Preparation: Entry Level to Practice as a Registered Nurse*. Toronto: Registered Nurses Association of Ontario.
Registered Nurses Association of Ontario (1982b) *Submission to the Commission of Inquiry into Part-Time Work*. Toronto: Registered Nurses Association of Ontario.
Registered Nurses Association of Ontario (1985) *Education for Excellence. Volume II – Background Papers Concerning the Entry to Practice Position*. Toronto: Registered Nurses Association of Ontario.
Registered Nurses Association of Ontario (1988a) *Gender Discrimination in Female Dominated Establishments With No Male Comparison Groups*. Toronto: Registered Nurses Association of Ontario.
Registered Nurses Association of Ontario (1988b) *Sorry No Care Available Due to Nursing Shortage: A Prescription for Reforming Human Resources Planning in Health Care*. Toronto: Registered Nurses Association of Ontario.
Registered Nurses Association of Ontario (1990) *Pay Equity: What It Means to You*. Toronto: Registered Nurses Association of Ontario.
Roberts, M.M. (1954) *American Nursing, History and Interpretation*. New York: Macmillan.
Robinson, S. (1980) *Midwifery Manpower*. London: University of London, Nursing Education Research Unit.
Rodwin, V.C. (1984) *The Health Planning Predicament*. Berkeley: University of California Press.
Roemer, M.I. (1985) *National Strategies for Health Care Organization, A World Overview*. Ann Arbor, MI: Health Administration.
Roswell, G. (1982) Changing trends in labour relations: effects on collective bargaining for nurses. *International Nursing Review*, **29** (5):
Royal College of Nursing (1984) *What the RCN Stands For*. London: Royal College of Nursing.
Royal College of Nursing (1985) *The Education of Nurses: A New Dispensation*, Commission on Nursing Education. London: Royal College of Nursing.

Royal College of Nursing (1979) *Extended role of the Clinical Nurse*. London: RCN.
Royal Commission on the Costs of Health Services, (1965). Ottawa: Queen's Printer.
Royal Commission on the Cost of Health Services, (1982). Ottawa: Queen's Printer.
Royal Commission on Health Services, Volumes I, II (1965) Ottawa: Queen's Printer.
Royal Commission on the National Health Service (1979) Chairman: A. Merrison. London: HMSO. 1979.
Rubin, S. (1981) the expanded role nurse. Part I – Role theory concepts. *Canadian Journal of Nursing Administration*, **1** (2): 23–7.
Schaffer, A. (1985) Nurses' new role: patient's advocate. Globe and Mail, April 19, p. 7.
Schieber, G.J. and Poullier, J.P. (1989) International health care expenditure trends, 1987. *Health Affairs*, **8** (3): 169–77.
Schurr, M.C. and Turner J. (1982) *Nursing – Image on Reality*. London: Hodder and Stoughton.
Scottish Home and Health Department (1980) *Health Priorities in the Eighties*. Edinburgh: Scottish Home and Health Department.
Scottish Home and Health Department (1986) *Scottish Health Statistics 1984*. Edinburgh: Scottish Home and Health Department.
SFN (1989) Nursing Division, Department of Health.
Sethi A.S., Dimmock, S.J. and Roswell, G. assisted by Birkwook, P., Chenier, H., Graydon, W., *et al.* (1985) *Comparative Collective Bargaining Strategies Among Nurses in Canada. Part 1 – Canada*. Unpublished manuscript, Masters in Health Administration Programme, University of Ottawa, Ottawa, Canada.
Sikorski, J. (1986) What's in a title? *College Communique*, **11** (2): P. 2.
Simly, M.B. (1951) *Charitable Effort in Liverpool in the 19th Century*. London:
Simpson H.M. (1981) If I could alter one thing: the first Winifred Raphael memorial lecture, London: RCN.
Smith, F.B. (1982) *Florence Nightingale, Reputation and Power*. London: Croom Helm.
Soderstrom, L. (1978) *The Canadian Health System*. London: Croom Helm.
Stapleton, M.F. (1986) Ward sisters – another perspective: their ongoing educational needs. London: RCN.
Starr, P. (1982) *The Social Transformation of American Medicine*. New York: Basic Books.
Statistics Canada (1990a) *Registered Nurses Management, 1989*. Ottawa: Statistics Canada.

Statistics Canada (1990b) *The Research Imperative for Nursing in Canada: A 5-Year Plan Towards the Year 2000*. Ottawa: Canadian Nurses Association.

Stinson, S.M. (1977) Central issues in Canadian nursing research. In: B. LaSor, M.R. Elliot (eds.), *Issues in Canadian Nursing*. Prentice-Hall of Canada, Scarborough, Ontario, pp. 3–42.

Stinson, S.M. (1975) Some notes on selected issues and alternatives regarding nursing research organizations in Canada. In: G. Zilm, S. Stinson, M. Steed, P. Overton, (eds.), *Development and Use of Indicators in Nursing Research: Proceedings of the 1975 National Nursing Research Conference*. Edmonton: University of Alberta, School of Nursing.

Stinson, S.M. (1978) Alternative health administration/nursing collaborative models: the University of Alberta. In: C.H. Slater (ed.) *The Education and Roles of Nursing Service Administrators*. W.K. Kellogg Foundation, Battle Creek, MI, pp. 51–64.

Stinson, S.M., Lamb, M. and Thibaudeau, M.F. (1990) Nursing research: the Canadian scene. *International Journal of Nursing Studies*, **27** (2): 105–22.

Stinson, S.M., Larsen, J. and MacPhail, J. (1984) *Canadian Nursing Doctoral Statistics: 1982 Update*. Ottawa: Canadian Nurses Association.

Stinson, S.M., MacPhail, J. and Larsen, J. (1988) *Canadian Nursing Doctoral Statistics: 1986 Update*. Ottawa: Canadian Nurses Association.

Stinson, S.M., Kerr, J.C., Giovannetti, P., Field, P.A. and MacPhail, J. (eds.) (1986) *New Frontiers in Nursing Research: Proceedings of the International Nursing Research Conference, Edmonton, Alberta, Canada, May 7 and 9*. Edmonton: University of Alberta, Faculty of Nursing.

Storch, J., Hazlett, C.B. and Stinson, S.M. (1977) *A Canadian Survey for Nurses Engaged in Research in 1976*. Edmonton: Division of Health Services Administration, University of Alberta.

Task Force Reports on the Cost of Health Services in Canada, vols. I–III (1969). Ottawa: Queen's Printer.

Taylor, M. (1978) *Health Insurance and Canadian Public Policy: The Seven Decisions that created the Canadian Health Insurance System*. McGill-Queen's University Press, Montreal.

Thibaudeau, M.F. and Marchak. N. (eds.) (1973) *L'Enseignement au Malade*. Les Presses de l'Université de Montreal, Montreal.

Thibaudeau, M.F., Kerouac, S. and Fortin, F. (1980) *La Recherche Infirmière au Quebec. Rapport du Colloque Tenu à la Faculté des Sciences Infirmières, Université de Montreal, 24–25 Avril, 1980*. Université de Montreal, Montreal.

Thompson, C., and LeTouze, D. (1984) Hospital capital shows signs of old age, part 2. *Dimensions*, **61** (2): 19–22.

Thurston, N. and Tenove, S. (1987) *Nursing Research in Canadian Teaching Hospitals*. Paper presented at the International Nursing Research Conference, Washington, DC. October 13–16.

Thurston, N., Tenove, S. and Church, J. (1987) *Nursing Research in Canadian Teaching Hospitals*. Calgary: Foothills Hospital.

Tibbitts, H.J. and Levine, E. (1953) *Health Manpower Sourcebook. 2. Nursing Personnel*. Washington, DC: GPO.

Tocqueville, A.C.H. de (1835, 1840) *De la democratie en Amerique*, parts 1 and 2. Published in English by Phillips Bradley, New York, 1945.

Tooley, S.A. (1906) *The History of Nursing in the British Empire*. Bousfield & Co. London.

United Kingdom Central Council for Nursing, Midwifery and Health Visiting 1986) *Project 2000. A New Preparation for Practice*. London: United Kingdom Central Council for Nursing, Midwifery and Health Visiting.

United States Department of Health, Education and Welfare (1956) *Design for State-Wide Nursing Surveys*, Washington, DC: GPO.

United States Department of Health, Education and Welfare (1959) *Professional Nurse Traineeship, Part I*. Washington, DC: GPO.

United States Department of Health, Education and Welfare (1964) *Nurses for Leadership*. Washington, DC: GPO.

US Department of Health and Human Services (1964) *Smoking*. Washington, DC: GPO.

US Department of Health and Human Services (1981) *Prevention*. Washington, DC: GPO.

US Department of Health and Human Services (1983) *Report to the President and Congress on the Status of Health Personnel in the United States*, vols. I and II. Washington, DC: GPO.

The United States Department of Health and Human Services (1986) *The National Institutional Conference on Nursing Productivity*, GPO Washington, DC, p. 60.

US Department of Health and Human Services (1988) *The Registered Nurse Population, An Overview*. Washington, DC: GPO. (See also previous sample survey reports – 1977, 1980, 1984.)

United States Department of Health and Human Services, Bureau of Health Professions Manpower (1989) *Seventh Report to the President and Congress on the Status of Health Personnel in the United States*. Washington, DC: GPO.

United States Department of Health and Human Services, Division of Nursing (1986) *Preliminary Data from the National Sample Survey of Registered Nurses*. November 1984. Unpublished.

US Department of Health and Human Services, Secretary's Commission

on Nursing (1980) Support Studies and Background Information, vol. III. Washington, DC: GPO.
US Department of Health and Human Services, Secretary's Commission on Nursing (1988) *Final Report*, vol. I. Washington, DC: GPO.
United States President's Commission on the Health Needs of the Nation (1952) *Building America's Health. A Report*. Washington DC: GPO.
US Department of Health and Human Services, National Center for Health Statistics (1991). Health United State, 1990. Washington DC: GPO.
US Department of Health and Human Services (1990) the Registered Nurse Population, Washington, DC: GPO, p. 60.
US Public Health Service, Division of Nursing (1969) *Health Manpower Sourcebook. 2. Nursing Personnel*. Washington, DC: GPO.
US Public Health Service (1979) *Healthy People. The Surgeon's Report on Health Promotion and Disease Prevention*. Washington, DC: GPO.
United States Surgeon General's Consultant Group on Nursing (1963) *Towards Quality in Nursing: Needs and Goals*. Washington, DC: GPO.

Van Loon, R.J. (1978) From shared cost to block fundings and beyond: the politics of health insurance in Canada. *Journal of Health, Politics, Policy and Law*, **2**: 454.

Wallace, J. (1983) *Commission of Inquiry into Part-Time Work*. Government of Canada, Ministry of Labour, Ottowa.
Washington Post (1986). March 13.
Watkin, B. (1978) *The National Health Service, The First Phase*. London: George Allen and Unwin.
Webb, S. and Webb, B. (1911) *English Poor Law History*. London: Cass.
Weir, G.M. (1932) *Survey of Nursing Education in Canada*. Toronto: University of Toronto Press.
Welsh Office (1985) *Health and Personal Social Services Statistics for Wales 1984.*: Welsh Office, Cardiff.
Western Interstate Commission on Higher Education (1978) *Nursing Resources and Requirements: A guide to state-level planning*, Denver, Co. WICHE.
White, R. (1985) *The Effects of the NHS on the Nursing Profession, 1948–1961*. London: Kings Fund.
Wilensky, H.L. (1964) The Professionalization of everyone? *American Journal of Sociology*, **70**: 137–58.
Willman, M. (1991) Personal communication, University of British Columbia, Vancouver.
Wilmot, V. (1986) Health science policy, health research and nursing

research funding. In: S.M. Stinson and J.C. Kerr (eds.), *International Issues in Nursing Research*, Croom Helm, London, pp. 76–96.

Woodham Smith, C. (1950) *Florence Nightingale 1820–1910*. London: Constable & Co. Ltd.

Woodward, J. (1974) *To do the sick no harm: A study of voluntary hospital systems*. Routledge and Kegan Paul, London.

Wood, R. (1947) Ministry of Health land offers, Working Party on recruitment and Training – Report. London: HMSO.

Woods, G. (1986) *RNA Utilization in Ontario*. Toronto: Ontario Association of Registered Nursing Assistants.

World Almanac 1991 (1990) New York: Pharos Books.

World Almanac 1992 (1991) New York: Pharos Books.

World Health Organisation (1976) *Declaration of Alma Ata. Health for All by the Year 2000*. 1976 Health Assembly. Geneva: World Health Organisation.

World Health Organisation (1983) *Manpower Statistics*. Geneva: World Health Organisation.

Youell, L. (1986) A question of balance. *The Canadian Nurse*, **82**: 3.

Zilm, G.N., Larose, O. and Stinson, S.M. (eds.) (1979) *Ph.D. Nursing. Proceedings of the Kellogg National Seminar on Doctoral Preparation for Canadian Nurses*. Ottawa: Canadian Nurses Association.

Index

Abel Smith, B. 34
Abdellah, F. 261, 265
Aberdeen, Lady 120
Acute care 238–9
Agency for Health Care Policy and Research (US) 265
Alberta Association of Registered Nurses (AARN) 185
Alberta Foundation for Nursing Research 188
Alcott, L. M. 208
American Association of Colleges of Nursing 259, 277
American Association of Critical Care Nurses 259
American Hospital Association (AHA) 277
  Association of Nurse Executives 259
American Medical Association (AMA) 212, 215
  Council on Medical Education 210
American Nurses' Association (ANA) 185, 202, 209, 255–6, 276–7
  American Academy of Nursing 258
  American Nurses Foundation 258
  Cabinet on Nursing Research 264
  Inventory of Registered Nurses 275
  Nurses Coalition for Action in Politics 258
  position paper 217
American Public Health Association (APHA) 209
Arnstein, M. 264
Association of British Nurses 48
Association of Supervisors of Midwives 96
Association of Universities of Colleges of Canada 139

Athlone, Lord 50

Battle, W. 45
Beveridge, William 50
von Bismark, O. 18
Blue Cross/Blue Shield 19, 212
Boer War 121
Boston Training School for Nursing 209
Briggs Report (UK) 56, 99, 105
British Hospital Association (BHA) 44
British North American Act 119–20
British Medical Association (BMA) 31
Brown, E. L. 282
Buchan, W. 208
Burgess, M. 211–12

Canada
  Bond Program 126
  demographics 9, 11, 125–6
  nursing settings 146
  nursing assistants 148–9
  nursing workforce 121, 128
  trends in organization of health services 127–8
  type of government 125
Canada Health Act, 1984 23, 125, 164, 171–2
Canadian Association of Practical and Nursing Assistants (CAPNA) 149
Canadian Association of University Schools of Nursing (CAUSN) 134, 156, 178–9, 183, 186–7, 201
Canadian College of Health Service Executives (CCHSE) 156, 201
Canadian Conference on Nursing, 1957 130

Canadian Council on Hospital
　　Accreditation (CCHA) 154–5
Canadian Foundation for
　　Advancement of Teaching 210
Canadian Health Administration
　　Study 156
Candian Hospital Association (CHA)
　　139, 153–4, 156, 175, 201
Canadian International Classification
　　of Diseases (CICD) 153
Canadian International Development
　　Agency 175
Canadian Long Term Care
　　Association (CLTA) 155
Canadian Medical Association (CMA)
　　122, 129, 154–6, 175
Canadian Military Sisters 121
Canadian National Association of
　　Trained Nurses 122
Canadian Nurses Association (CNA)
　　122 129–32, 139, 141, 150–3,
　　158–9, 162, 164, 178
　　code of ethics 152–3
　　entry to practice 141–4, 202–3
　　forerunner (CNATN) 122
　　politics 171–5
　　standards for practice 150–1
　　The Canadian Nurse 122
　　unions 163
　　Weir Report 122, 129
Canadian Nurses Foundation (CNF)
　　178–9, 186
Canadian Nursing Research Group
　　(CNRG) 186
Canadian Public Health Association
　　(CPHA) 151, 156, 201
Canadian Red Cross Society 130
Cartier, J. 117
Carnegie Foundation for
　　Advancement of Teaching 210
Case-mix groupings (CMGs) 153
Central Midwives Board 49, 52
　　Nursing Development Units, NHS
　　88–9
Chadwick, E. 42
Citizens' Charter (UK) 72
　　Patients' Charter 72, 87

Civil Nursing Reserve (UK) 50
Civil War (US) 208
Clegg Report 1980 (UK) 96
Clinical grading 88
Clinical ladders 170
College of Nursing (UK) 49
College of Nurses of Ontario 198–9
Commission on Graduates of Foreign
　　Nursing Schools 257–8
Commission of the Sanitary
　　Conditions of the British Army 99
Committee for Study of Nursing
　　Education (Goldmark Report) 211
Committee of Nursing Services 1938
　　50
Committee on the Grading of Nursing
　　Schools 211–13
Community health care (home health
　　care) 218
Comprehensive Health Planning Act
　　1966 273
Conference of University Principals
　　182
Connecticut Training School for
　　Nursing 209
Consumerism 33–4
Costs
　　escalation 218–22
Council of District Nursing 45
Council of Training of Health Visitors
　　43, 52
County Asylum Act, 1808 (UK) 40, 46

Dalhousie University 121
Davis, C. 261
Department of Defense (US) 222
Department of Health (formerly and
　　Social Security) (UK) 61, 90, 101,
　　110–14
Department of Labor (US) 222
Department of National Health and
　　Welfare (NHW) (Canada) 122
Department of Veterans Affairs (US)
　　213, 222
DeTocqueville, A. 5

Diagnosis Related Groups (DRGs)
(US) 14, 30–1, 153, 221, 242, 245, 248
Dimock, S. 209
Dix, D. 208

Economics, national 7–8
Edinburgh University
  first international nursing research conference 185
Education of nurses
  advanced study 61, 129, 137–8, 231–2
  baccalaureate programs 134–5
  collaboration between education and service 235–6
  costs 61–2
  degrees 68
  diploma programs 132–4, 136
  faculty 231–2
  funding 59–62, 143–4, 232–3
  graduate and higher education 61
  health pick-up 69
  model baccalaureate program 141
  nursing assistant programs 139–42
  nursing management 139
  role of government 236
  see also Nursing education
Education Act, 1944 40
Education Advisory Groups (EAG) 60–1
Emergency Nursing Committee (UK) 50
English National Board 56–9, 291
  Entry to Practice 202, 234–5
Environmental protection 30
Environmental Protection Agency (US) 222
Epidemics
  early immigrants, Canada 117–9
  US South 210
  Great Britain 41
Etzioni, A. 92

Federal Hospital Insurance and Diagnostic Services Act, 1957 123
Federal Medical Care Act, 1968 123–4

Fenwick, B. 43
Fleming, A. 213
Flexner, A. 210
  Flexner Report 210–11
Fidler, N. D. 129–30
Formation des checheurs aide à la recherche (FCAR) 188
Future of nursing research 188–9

General and Marine Hospital (Canada) 120
General Nursing Council (UK) 46–7, 50, 52, 94, 105
General Nursing Register 105
Gilbert Act, 1782 40
Girard, A. M. 130
Goldmark, J. 225
  Report 211, 263, 282
Government
  and health care 212–13
  public policy 261–2
Grew, Nehemiah 40
Grey Nuns (*Soeurs Grisse*) 118–19, 120
Gross National Product 7
Guertin, C. 118
Guy's Hospital 43

Halsbury Committee Report 1974 (UK) 96
Health authorities 52, 59–60, 103
Health care
  costs 13–15, 124–5
  cost-containment 126
  facilities 29
  providers 27–8
  public (or consumer) 33–4
  quality 15
  technology 12–13, 28–9
Health care systems
  characteritistics 21, 22, 34–5
  evolution 18–20
  financing 24–5
  government involvement 22–23, 123–8
  licensing 30
Health indicators 223–4

Health insurance
　origins 13, 122–5, 212
Health of the nation 1991 (UK) 87, 109
Health maintenance organization,
　(HMO) 25, 212, 220–1
Health promotion,
　and disease prevention 15–16
Health personnel 11–12
Health services
　cost-containment 245
　organization 25–7
Health Science Resource Center 184
Health Visitors Association 93
Helen K. Mussallem Library 184
Henderson, Virginia 264
Hierarchy
　of nurses 242–4
Higher education
　financing 59–62
　Polytechnics and Colleges Funding Council (PCFC) (UK) 61
Hill-Burton construction program (US) 215, 273
Hospital for Sick Children, Canada 173–5
Hospital Insurance and Diagnostic Services Act, 1957, Canada 19
Hospital Medical Records Institute 153
Hospital Corporation of America 23
Hospital Survey and Construction Act of 1947 (Hill-Burton) 215, 273
Hotel Dieu of Quebec 117
Hotel Dieu of Montreal 118
Hubou, M. 117
Humana 23

Indian Health Service, PHS 9
Institute of Nursing (Bishopsgate) 43
Interagency Conference on Nurses Statistics (US) 277–8
International Classification of Diseases (ICD) 24
　common taxonomy 8
International Council of Nurses (ICN) 48, 173, 185

Inventory of Registered Nurses (US) 275
International Nursing Research Conferences 184

Johns, E. 121
Johns Hopkins University 210
Johnson, L. B. 218
Joint Board of Clinical Nursing Studies (UK) 105
Joint Commission for Accreditation of Hospitals (JCAH) (US) 31

Kaiserwerth 43, 48
Kellogg, W. K., Foundation 266
King's College 48
King's Fund Centre 90
Koch, R. 209

LeLonde, M. 15–16, 127
Levine, Eugene 256, 265
Licensed practical nurse supply 242
Licensure 257–8
Locke, J. 6
Local Government Board Act, 1871 42
London Hospital 44
Lunacy Acts 1845, 1890, 1980 (UK) 46
　Amendment Act, 1861 40, 46
Machin, M. 120
Mack, T. 120
Manitoba Association of Licensed Practical Nurses (MALPN) 149
Marine Hospital Service 208
Matrons' Council of Great Britain and Ireland 48
McGill University 129, 137, 182–3
McMaster University 185, 188
Medical Care Act, 1966 (Canada) 19, 125
Medical Research Council (MRC) (Canada) 102, 107, 177–8, 187
Medicare/Medicaid 3, 14, 19, 30, 218–19, 240, 266
Medico-Psychological Association 46
Mental Deficiency Acts 1913, 1936 (UK) 40, 46
Mental Health Act, 1959 (UK) 47

Index

Mental Illness Act, 1946 (UK) 40
Mental health 40
  nursing 46-7
  hospitals 45-6
Massachusetts Board of Health 209
Metropolitan Poor Law Act, 1867 (UK) 40
Mid-Atlantic Regional Nurses Association (US) 278, 285
Midwifery 151-2
  training 68
Midwives Act 1902 (UK) 49
Ministry of Health (UK) 42, 45, 50
Ministry of Higher Education and Science (Canada) 182
Mitchell, C. 120
Modelling
  types of 284-5
  use in planning 283-5
Montreal General Hospital 118-19, 120

National Academy of Sciences, Institute of Medicine (NSA, IOM) (US) 221, 264-5
  Report 282-3
National Advisory Council on Nurse Training (US) 261
National Board of Prices and Incomes Report in 1968 (UK) 96
National Commission for the Study of Nursing Education (CSNE) (US) 282
National Commission on Nursing (NCN) (US)
  Summary Report and Recommendations 283
National Council Licensure Examination (US) 234
National Council of Nurses of the United Kingdom (NCNUK) 48
National Council of Vocational Qualifications (NCVQ (UK) 67-8
National Council of State Boards of Nursing (NCSBN) (US) 258-9, 277

National Federation of Licensed Practical Nurses (NFLPN) (US) 259
National Federation of Nurses Unions (NFNU) (Canada) 164
National Health Grant Program (NHGP) (Canada) 29
National Health Insurance Act 1911 (UK) (Development) 19
National Health Planning and Resources Development Act of 1974 (US) 274
National Health Research and Development Program (NHRDP) (Canada) 177-8, 185
National Health Service (UK) 19, 29, 33, 35, 44-5, 50-5, 63
  budget 53-4
  community services 86-7
  intakes to nurse training 64, 66
  National Audit Office 110, 114
  nursing education 46-7
  nursing workforce 63, 73-88, 91
  personnel 27, 52
  planning 109-12
  reform 1991 89
  settings 75-87
  qualifications for nurse training 57-8
National Health Service Act 1946 (NHS) (UK) 50
National Health Service and Community Care Act 1990 (UK) 54
National Health Service Corps (NHSC) (US) 30
National Health Service Reorganisation Act 1974 (UK) 51, 52
National Health Service Trusts (UK) 55
National Insurance Act 1948 (UK) 44
National League for Nursing (NLN) (formerly National League for Nursing Education) (US) 31, 209, 228, 259-66, 263-4
  Nursing Date Review 277

National Nursing Research
    Conference (NNCRs) (Canada)
    183-6
National plan for nursing
    administration in Canada,
    position paper 200-1
National Research Council (NRC)
    (Canada) 177
National Sample Surveys
    Registered Nurses 277
    Licensed Practical Nurses 277
National Science and Engineering
    Research Council (NSERC)
    (Canada) 178
National Student Nurses Association
    (NSNA) (US) 259
Newfoundland Council for Nursing
    Assistants (Canada) 149
New England Hospital for Women
    and Children (US) 209
Nightingale, F.
    influence on nursing 5, 48, 99,
    199-200, 208-9, 225
Northern Ireland National Board
    (UK) 56-9
Nuffield Provincial Hospitals Trust
    (UK) 100
Nurse Training Act 1943, 1964 (US)
    214, 217-18, 279-80
Nurse education
    continuing education 69
    post-registration 68-9
    historical evolution 225-6
    Northern Ireland 70-1
    Scotland 70-1
    statutory framework (UK) 56-7
    Wales 70-1
    see also Education of Nurses
Nurse educators 144-5
Nurse researchers
    numbers 180
Nurses
    administrators 155-6
    characteristics 251-3
        demographics 158-9
    clinical nurse specialist 244, 250

Nurses—*cont.*
    distribution of workforce 237-9
    education 161, 251-2
    expanding role 87-8, 245
    Federal government 244-6
    hierarchy 242-6
    in politics 97-8, 259-60
    job satisfaction 256-7
    nurse practitioner 243-4, 250
    licensed practical nurse 242, 248
    registrations 48-50, 132
    roles 248-51
    salary issues 166-9, 253-6
    shortages 50, 246
    specialties 77-87
    unemployed 253
    unions 93, 96, 163-4
Nurses Act 1949, 1957 (UK) 51
Nurses, Midwives and Health Visitors
    Act 1979 (UK) 45, 52, 56, 104
Nurses Registration Act 1919 (UK) 40,
    46, 49
Nurses Salary Committee (UK) 50
Nursing
    collaboration with other groups 175
    comparisons 289-95
    education
        post-graduate 293
    licensure 162
    part-time 283-5
    planning 217, 283-5
    politics 97-8, 171-5
    professional specialities 77-8
    salaries 44, 96-7, 164-5
    settings 83-7, 247-8
    status 175-6
    supply and demand models and
        methodology 283-5
    workload 32
Nursing and Midwifery Negotiating
    Council (UK) 95-6
*Nursing and Nursing Education: Public
    Policies and Private Actions* (US)
    282-3
Nursing Research (US) 264, 269
Nursing research
    research awards 267

Nursing research—*cont.*
  clinical research centers 103–4
  development 100–1, 177–8, 263–5
  educational programs 104–5, 180, 183, 214, 251–2
  funding 101–2, 186–8, 263–5
  information dissemination 106–7, 269–70
  libraries 184–8
  literature 183–4
  organizations 101–4, 178–9, 263–7
  priorities 108, 199–203, 270–2
  role of CNA 182–8
  Steinberg Collection (UK) 107
  supply and demand models and methodology 283–5
  types of studies 267–9
  voluntary organizations 187
Nursing Research Grants Program, PHS (US) 216
Nursing Resources and Requirements: A Guide for State-Level Planning (US) 278
Nursing services
  demand 190–3
Nursing Theory Congress 1986 (Canada) 151

Ontario Association of Registered Nursing Assistants (Canada) 148–9
Ontario Association on Community Health Accreditation (Canada) 155
Ontario College of Nurses (Canada) 150
Ontario Department of Health (Canada) 130
Ontario Hospital Labor Disputes Arbitration Act (Canada) 165
Ontario Ministry of Health (Canada) 187
Ontario Nurses Association (Canada) 170
Ontario Pay Equity Act 1988 (Canada) 167
Order of Nurses of Quebec (ONQ) (Canada) 184–5

Pasteur, L. 2, 209
Pay Equity Commission (Canada) 167–8
Peer review groups (PROs) (US) 31
Petty, W. 40
Planning
  balancing supply and demand 193–8
  blueprint of nursing 198–9
  database 276–8
  early methodology 274–6
  history 273–8
  methodology for requirements and supply 283–5
  role of government 274–5
  role of nursing organizations 196–8
Planning For Nursing Needs and Resources (US) 278
Policy
  governmental 109–12
Poor Law Amendment Act 1834 (UK) 40
Poor Law Board Act 1847 (UK) 40, 42
Powell, E. (UK) 98
President's Commission on Health Needs of the Nation (US) 217
Preventive health care 237–8
Prince Edward Island Nurses' Act (Canada) 164
Professional associations 184–6, 258–9
Professional Institute of the Public Service of Canada 164
Professional standards review organizations (PRSOs) 30–1
Project 2000 (UK) 57, 62–5, 77, 83, 93, 98
  futures staffing 'mixes' 63–5
  impact of proposals 65
  proposed education standards 62–3
Public health
  first nurse 117
Public Health Act of 1848, 1872, 1875 (UK) 40, 42

Quaker Society 45

Quality
 of working life of nurses 168–9
Quebec Council of Universities (Canada) 182
Queen Victoria Jubilee Nursing Institute (UK) 43, 45

Rathbone, W. 43
Reed, W. 210
Red Cross 121
Regional Hospital Boards (UK) 51
 of British Columbia (Canada) 172–3
Registered Nurses Association of Ontario (Canada) 143, 166–7, 160–70, 174–5
Registration of Doctors Act 1858 (UK) 40
Registration of Nurses Act 1919 (UK) 46
Regulated Health Professions Act (Canada) 152
Report of the Committee on Nursing (UK) 104–5
Reports to Congress (health manpower) (US) 280–1
Review Body Reports (UK) 96–7
Right to strike (Canada) 165
Robert Wood Johnson Foundation (US) 266
Roentgen, W. 209
Rothschild, Lord 101
Royal British Nurses Assocation 49
Royal College of Midwives (UK) 93
Royal College of Nursing (UK) 31, 49, 93, 103, 291
 Report 1979 88
Royal College of Nursing Research Society (UK) 107
Royal Commission of 1871 (UK) 42
Royal Commission on Health Services (Canada) 130
 Nursing Reports 1964 131
Royal Commission on the NHS (UK) 52
Royal Sanitary Association [UK] 42–3
Ryerson, G. (UK) 121
Ryerson Polytechnical Institute (Canada) 137

Salmon Report (UK) 52, 94–5
Saskatchewan Registered Nurses Association (SRNA) (Canada) 163–4
Saskatchewan Hospital Services Plan (Canada) 123
Scottish Health Visitors Association 96
Scottish National Board 56–9
Secretary's Commission on Nursing (US) 15
Service Employees International Union (Canada) 163–164
Shephard, I. J. (Canada) 118
Sigma Theta Tau International Honor Society 185
Sisters of Providence (Canada) 120
Social Sciences and Humanities Research Council (SSHRC) (Canada) 178
Social Security Act 1935 (US) 215
Social Work and Nurse Visitor Training Act 1962 (UK) 43
Society of Health (formerly Royal Sanitary Association) (UK) 43
Spanish American War 210
Statistics Canada 190
St. Bartholomew's Hospital (UK) 40
St. Thomas's Hospital (UK) 43, 48
St John's House (UK) 48
Strategy for Nursing 1989 (UK) 72, 89
Surgeons General's Consultant Group on Nursing (US) 217, 279, 285

Toronto General Hospital (Canada) 120
 School of Nursing 122
Treatment Acts 1930, 1946 (UK) 40
Tuke, W. 45
Twining, L. 40

United Kingdom
 constitution 5
 demographics 55, 75
 legislation 40
 nursing settings, 75–87

United Kingdom—*cont.*
 population 9, 11, 55, 75–6
 parliamentary system 6
 unions 93, 96
United Kingdom Central Council for Nursing, Midwifery and Health Visiting (UKCC) 52, 56–60, 67, 73, 93, 111
United States
 Army Nurse Corps 210
 Cadet Nurse Corps 214
 demographics 224
 history of nursing 202–22
 Department of Health and Human Services (formerly Health, Education and Welfare) 222
 Public Health Service 213
  annual budget 223
  Division of Nursing Resources 214, 264, 274–6
  Division of Nursing Education 214
  Division of Nursing 216, 223, 265–79
  Health Care Financing Administration 261, 265–6
  legislation 219
  increased functions 215
  National Centre for Health Statistics 277
  National Center for Nursing Research 261, 265–9, 270–2
  National Institutes of Health 215, 265, 269–70
  Pure Food and Drug Act 213
 'mixed' health system 3
 Navy Nurse Corps 210
 population 9, 11
 Surgeon General 16
  Surgeon General's Consultant Group on Nursing 217, 279, 285
Universite de Montreàl (Canada) 137, 184
University of Alberta (Canada) 137, 139, 182, 184

University of British Columbia (Canada) 121, 129, 143, 182
University of Calgary (Canada) 185
University of Laval (Canada) 184–5
University of Leithbridge (Canada) 185
University of Manitoba (Canada) 122
University of Minnesota (US) 211
University of Saskatchewan (Canada) 139
University of Toronto (Canada) 182, 188
Universities Funding Council (UK) 61

Vancouver General Hospital (Canada) 121, 172–3
Victorian Order of Nurses (VON) (Canada) 120–1
Voluntary Aids Detachment (VAD) (UK) 49

War and nursing 121
Weir Report 122, 129
 recommendations 122
Welsh National Board 56–9
Western Interstate Commission on Higher Education (WICHE) 278–80, 283, 285
Whitley Council (UK) 50, 93, 95–6
Workgroup of European Nurse Researchers 185
Working Party on the Recruitment and Training of Nurses (UK) 97, 100
World Health Organization
 Alma Ata Declaration 108–9
World War I 121, 213
World War II 50, 121, 130, 139, 213, 225

Yale University (US) 211
York Retreat (UK) 45
York University (Canada) 139